Handbook of
Psychopharmacology

Volume 14

Affective Disorders:
Drug Actions in Animals and Man

Handbook of
Psychopharmacology

Volume 14

Affective Disorders:
Drug Actions in Animals and Man

Edited by

Leslie L. Iversen
Department of Pharmacology
University of Cambridge

Susan D. Iversen
Department of Psychology
University of Cambridge

and

Solomon H. Snyder
Departments of Pharmacology and Psychiatry
The Johns Hopkins University
School of Medicine

PLENUM PRESS • NEW YORK AND LONDON

Library of Congress Cataloging in Publication Data

Main entry under title:

Handbook of psychopharmacology.

   Includes bibliographies and indexes.
   CONTENTS: v. 1. Biochemical principles and techniques in neuropharmacology.
—v. 2. Principles of receptor research. — v. 3. Biochemistry of biogenic amines. —
v. 4. Amino acid neurotransmitters. — v. 5. Synaptic modulators. — v. 6. Biogenic
amine receptors. — v. 7. Principles of behavioral pharmacology. — v. 8. Drugs,
Neurotransmitters, and Behavior. — v. 10. Neuroleptics and Schizophrenia. — v.
11. Stimulants. — v. 12. Drugs of Abuse. — v. 13. Biology of Mood and Antianxiety
Drugs. — v. 14. Affective Disorders: Drug Actions in Animals and Man. 1. Psychopharmacology. I. Iversen, Leslie Lars. II. Iversen, Susan D., 1940-   III.
Snyder, Solomon H., 1938   [DNLM: 1. Psychopharmacology. QV77 H236]
RC483.1136   615'.78   75-6851
ISBN 0-306-38934-7 (v. 14)

© 1978 Plenum Press, New York
A Division of Plenum Publishing Corporation
227 West 17th Street, New York, N.Y. 10011

Printed in the United States of America

CONTRIBUTORS

THOMAS P. DETRE, *Department of Psychiatry, University of Pittsburgh School of Medicine, and Western Psychiatric Institute and Clinic, Pittsburgh, Pennsylvania*

R. R. FIEVE, *Lithium Clinic and Metabolic Research Unit, Columbia Presbyterian Medical Center; Milhausen Depression Center Program, Atchley Pavilion; Foundation for Depression and Manic Depression, New York, N.Y.*

SAMUEL GERSHON, *Neuropsychopharmacology Research Unit, New York University–Bellevue Hospital Center, New York, N.Y.*

NELSON HOWARD HENDLER, *Department of Neurological Surgery and Department of Psychiatry and the Behavioral Sciences, The Johns Hopkins University School of Medicine, and The Johns Hopkins Hospital, Baltimore, Maryland*

DAVID J. KUPFER, *Department of Psychiatry, University of Pittsburgh School of Medicine, and Western Psychiatric Institute and Clinic, Pittsburgh, Pennsylvania*

ROBERT A. MAXWELL, *Department of Pharmacology, Wellcome Research Laboratories, Burroughs Wellcome Co., Research Triangle Park, North Carolina*

H. L. MELTZER, *Lithium Clinic and Metabolic Research Unit Columbia Presbyterian Medical Center; Milhausen Depression Center Program, Atchley Pavilion; Foundation for Depression and Manic Depression, New York, N.Y.*

DENNIS L. MURPHY, *Clinical Neuropharmacology Branch, National Institute of Mental Health, Bethesda, Maryland*

BARON SHOPSIN, *Neuropsychopharmacology Research Unit, New York University–Bellevue Hospital Center, New York, N.Y.*

RICHARD F. SQUIRES, *Research Laboratories, A/S FERROSAN, Sydmarken 1-5, DK-2860 Soeborg, Denmark*

FRIDOLIN SULSER, *Vanderbilt University School of Medicine and Tennessee Neuropsychiatric Institute, Nashville, Tennessee*

HELEN L. WHITE, *Department of Pharmacology, Wellcome Research Laboratories, Burroughs Wellcome Co., Research Triangle Park, North Carolina*

PREFACE

Underlying the design of the *Handbook of Psychopharmacology* is a prejudice that the study of drug influences on the mind has advanced to a stage where basic research and clinical application truly mesh. These later volumes of the *Handbook* are structured according to this conception. In certain volumes, groups of drugs are treated as classes with chapters ranging from basic chemistry to clinical application. Other volumes are assembled around topic areas such as anxiety or affective disorders. Thus, besides chapters on individual drug classes, we have included essays addressing broad areas such as "The Limbic–Hypothalamic–Pituitary–Adrenal System and Human Behavior" and "Peptides and the Central Nervous System."

Surveying these diverse contributions, one comes away with a sentiment that, far from being an "applied" science borrowing from fundamental brain chemistry and physiology, psychopharmacology has instead provided basic researchers with the tools and conceptual approaches which now are advancing neurobiology to a central role in modern biology. Especially gratifying is the sense that, while contributing to an understanding of how the brain functions, psychopharmacology is a discipline whose fruits offer genuine help to the mentally ill with promises of escalating benefits in the future.

L.L.I.
S.D.I.
S.H.S.

CONTENTS

CHAPTER 2

Monoamine Oxidase, Monoamine-Oxidase-Inhibiting Drugs, and
Human Behavior

DENNIS L. MURPHY

CHAPTER 3

Tricyclic and Monoamine Oxidase Inhibitor Antidepressants:
Structure–Activity Relationships

ROBERT A. MAXWELL and HELEN L. WHITE

CHAPTER 4

Tricyclic Antidepressants: Animal Pharmacology (Biochemical and Metabolic Aspects)

FRIDOLIN SULSER

CHAPTER 5

Tricyclic and Monoamine-Oxidase-Inhibitor Antidepressants:
Clinical Use

DAVID J. KUPFER and THOMAS P. DETRE

CHAPTER 6

Lithium Pharmacology and Physiology

NELSON HOWARD HENDLER

CHAPTER 7

Lithium: Clinical Considerations

BARON SHOPSIN and SAMUEL GERSHON

CHAPTER 8

Lithium Prophylaxis and Experimental Rubidium Therapy in
Affective Disorders

R. R. FIEVE and H. L. MELTZER

1

MONOAMINE OXIDASE INHIBITORS: ANIMAL PHARMACOLOGY

Richard F. Squires

1. INTRODUCTION

The animal pharmacology of the monoamine oxidase inhibitors (MAOIs*) has been reviewed previously by Zirkle and Kaiser (1964), Biel *et al.* (1964), Pscheidt (1964), Horita (1967), and Jacob and Simon (1968).

1.1. Localization

In mammals, MAO activity is found in most organs including liver, brain, kidney, heart, intestine, lung, salivary gland, gonads, and various kinds

---

* Abbreviations used in this chapter. ACTH: adrenocorticotrophic hormone; AMPT: α-methyl-p-tyrosine (or its methyl ester, H 44/68); BOL: 2-bromlysergic acid diethylamide; DA: dopamine; DBH: dopamine-β-hydroxylase; DDC: diethyldithiocarbamate; DMPEA: β-(3,4-dimethoxyphenylethylamine); DMT: *N,N*-dimethyltryptamine; FRF: follicle-stimulating-hormone-releasing factor; FLA-63: bis(4-methyl-*l*-homopiperazinyl thio carbonyl) disulfide; FSH: follicle-stimulating hormone; GABA: γ-aminobutyric acid; HCG: serum gonadotropin; 5-HIAA: 5-hydroxyindoleacetic acid; 5-HT: 5-hydroxytryptamine, serotonin; 5-HTP: 5-hydroxytryptophan; L-dopa: dihydroxyphenylalanine; LH: luteinizing hormone; LRF: luteinizing-hormone-releasing factor; MAO: monoamine oxidase; MAOI: monoamine oxidase inhibitor; 5-MeODMT: 5-methoxy-*N,N*-dimethyltryptamine; MIF: melanocyte-inhibiting factor (L-prolyl-L-leucyl-glycinamide); NA: noradrenaline; PCPA: p-chlorophenylalanine (or its methyl ester, H 69/17); PEA: β-phenethylamine; PGO: pontogeniculooccipital; PS: paradoxical sleep; REM: rapid eye movement; SH: spontaneously hypertensive; TRH: thyrotropin-releasing hormone.

Richard F. Squires • Research Laboratories, A/S FERROSAN, Sydmarken 1-5, DK-2860 Soeborg, Denmark.

of smooth muscle (Zeller, 1951; Davison, 1958; Blaschko, 1952, 1963; Glenner et al., 1957; Koelle and Valk, 1954; Squires, 1972b) where it is mostly bound to mitochondria and localized in the mitochondrial outer membrane (Schnaitman and Greenawalt, 1968; Greenawalt, 1972). Histochemical studies have shown that MAO activity occurs in a large variety of cell types including smooth muscle fibers, mucosal epithelial cells, renal tubule cells, hepatic cells, various types of neurons, and glia (Koelle and Valk, 1954; Glenner et al. 1957; Consolo et al., 1968; Giacobini and Kerpel-Fronius, 1970; Robinson, 1967, 1968, 1972; Furness and Costa, 1971). In the brain MAO is found in some, but not all, types of neurons, and in glia. Very high MAO activity has been found by several investigators in the locus coeruleus (Robinson, 1968; Shimizu et al., 1959; Bouchaud and Jacque, 1971; Bloom et al., 1972), a region containing a high density of NA-containing perikarya (Dahlström and Fuxe, 1964).

There is additional evidence demonstrating the presence of MAO in certain types of neurons:

1. After depletion of amines by reserpine the concentrations of NA, DA, and 5-HT can be increased in neurons normally containing these transmitters, in vitro and in vivo, only after MAO has been inhibited (e.g., Dahlström and Fuxe, 1964; Hamberger et al., 1964; Sachs, 1970; Corrodi and Fuxe, 1967; Fuxe and Ungerstedt, 1967; Lichtensteiger et al., 1967; Fuxe et al., 1968). Formaldehyde-induced fluorescence in 5-HT neurons increases after administration of various MAOIs alone (Dahlström and Fuxe, 1964; Fuxe et al., 1968; Bartonicek, 1966, 1970).

2. Determined histochemically by the tetrazolium method of Glenner et al. (1957) as well as biochemically, MAO activity accumulates proximal to a ligature of rat sciatic nerve (Dahlström et al., 1969; Dahlström, 1972).

3. Considerable MAO activity is associated with synaptosomes (De Lores Arnaiz and De Robertis, 1962; Barondes, 1966; Neidle et al., 1969; Coyle and Snyder, 1969a; Baldessarini and Vogt, 1971; Tabakoff et al., 1974; Daly and Aprison, 1974; Jansen et al., 1974).

4. MAO activity decreases, to varying degrees, after denervation of various organs. After superior cervical ganglionectomy MAO activity is reduced in the pineal and salivary gland of the rat (Snyder et al., 1965; Goridis and Neff, 1971a; Neff et al., 1974; Neff and Goridis, 1972). In the pineal, ganglionectomy reduces MAO-A about 70% while leaving MAO-B essentially unchanged (Goridis and Neff, 1971a,b; Neff and Goridis, 1972; Neff et al., 1974). The superior cervical ganglion contains almost exclusively MAO-A (Goridis and Neff, 1971a,b), and immunosympathectomy of rats reduces MAO in this ganglion to 10% of control values while reducing MAO to a smaller extent in spleen, submaxillary glands, kidneys, and liver (Klingman, 1966). Immunosympathectomy did not reduce MAO in retina, pineal, or hypophysis using tryptamine as substrate. Surgical denervation also reduces MAO-A activity in the nictitating membrane of the cat (Jarrott and Langer, 1971), the submaxillary gland, iris, and vas deferens of the rabbit, as

well as the vasa deferentia of the rat and guinea pig (Jarrott, 1971). 6-Hydroxydopamine denervation of rat mesenteric artery leads to a selective decrease in MAO-A (Goridis and Neff, 1974).

There is now good agreement that MAO-A is the predominant form of MAO in sympathetic nerves.

1.2. Function

The two most important physiologic functions of MAO seem to be (1) inactivation of toxic amines, both endogenously formed and of exogenous origin, and (2) participation in regulating the intracellular concentrations of biogenic amines (Bhagvat *et al.*, 1939; Koelle and Valk, 1954; Arioka and Tanimukai, 1957; Davison, 1958; Zeller, 1951; Kopin, 1966; Bloom *et al.*, 1972; Squires, 1972*b*).

Because of its localization in the walls of blood vessels (Bloom *et al.*, 1972; Glenner *et al.*, 1957; Koelle and Valk, 1954; Arioka and Tanimukai, 1957; Owman and Rosengren, 1967; Dyer and Weber, 1971; Tarver *et al.*, 1971; Gillespie, J. S., 1973) MAO may also participate in maintaining the blood–brain barrier and, in general, helping to protect tissues from circulating amines.

1.3. Mechanisms

It now seems probable that increases in the concentration of the endogenous neurotransmitter 5-HT in brain play a preponderant role in many of the pharmacologic effects of the MAOIs. This is perhaps to be expected since after general MAO inhibition the concentration of 5-HT in the brains of all species investigated increases more than those of other known neurotransmitters such as NA and DA, which are also substrates for MAO (Pletscher, 1957; Spector *et al.*, 1958, 1960*a,b*; Brodie *et al.*, 1959; Wiegand and Perry, 1961; Gey and Pletscher, 1961; Dubnick *et al.*, 1962; Jori *et al.*, 1963; Spector, 1963; Uchida and O'Brien, 1964; Corrodi, 1966; Valzelli and Garattini, 1968; Javoy *et al.*, 1972, 1973; Yang and Neff, 1974). Increases in the concentrations of NA and DA also play important roles in some of the pharmacologic effects of the MAOIs. In some functional or behavioral systems (e.g., ovulation, male copulatory behavior) a catecholamine and 5-HT may play antagonistic roles, while in others (e.g., suppression of PGO waves; antagonism of electroshock-, Metrazol-, and sound-induced convulsions; centrally mediated reduction in blood pressure) a catecholamine and 5-HT may exert similar effects. This requires the use of selective inhibitors of catecholamine and 5-HT synthesis (e.g., AMPT and PCPA), respectively, or of precursors such as 5-HTP or L-dopa, which selectively increase the concentrations of 5-HT and DA, respectively, to elucidate the mechanisms by which an MAOI exerts its effect.

Other biogenic amines such as tryptamine (Hess *et al.*, 1959; Sjordsma *et al.*, 1959*a,b*; Tedeschi, D. H., *et al.*, 1959; Tedeschi, R. E., *et al.*, 1959; Green, H., and Sawyer, 1960; Eccleston *et al.*, 1966; Martin *et al.*, 1972, 1974, 1975; Saavedra and Axelrod, 1973, 1974*a*; Snodgrass and Horn, 1973; Marsden and Curzon, 1974; Snodgrass and Iversen, 1974; Philips *et al.*, 1974; Boulton and Baker, 1975; Sloan *et al.*, 1975), PEA (Saavedra, 1974; Boulton and Baker, 1975), and octopamine (Kakimoto and Armstrong, 1962; Molinoff and Axelrod, 1969, 1972; Molinoff *et al.*, 1969; Kopin *et al.*, 1964, 1965; Osumi and Fujiwara, 1969; Saavedra and Axelrod, 1974*b*; Saavedra *et al.*, 1974), which are normally present in tissues in very low concentrations, increase severalfold after inhibition of MAO, especially together with the administration of the corresponding amino acid precursor. Accumulation of one or more of these amines may also be involved in some of the pharmacologic effects of the MAOIs. For example, the accumulation of octopamine in sympathetic nerves may contribute to the hypotensive effects of certain MAOIs (e.g., Kopin *et al.*, 1964). Although they are substances of considerable interest, physiologic roles for endogenous tyramine, octapamine, PEA, phenethanolamine, and tryptamine remain to be established.

Thus the MAOIs may produce pharmacologic effects by:

1. Increasing the levels of catecholamines or 5-HT or both.
2. Increasing the levels of an endogenous microamine—such as tyramine, octopamine, PEA, phenethanolamine, tryptamine, or *N*-methylhistamine—which under normal conditions is deaminated by MAO.
3. Preventing the deamination of an exogenous amine which releases one (or more) of the endogenous amines from their natural stores.
4. Preventing the deamination of an exogenous amine which acts directly on a specific receptor.
5. A combination of the mechanisms described above.

After the discovery of two main types of mitochondrial MAO, MAO-A and MAO-B (Johnston, 1968; Knoll and Magyar; 1972; Squires, 1968, 1972*b*; Gorkin and Romanova, 1968; Hall *et al.*, 1969; Fuller *et al.*, 1970; Fuller and Roush, 1972; Fuller, 1968, 1972; Christmas *et al.*, 1972; Goridis and Neff, 1971*a,b*; Yang and Neff, 1973, 1974; Neff and Goridis, 1972; McCauly and Racker, 1973), it has become of obvious interest to investigate the pharmacology of the selective MAOIs. NA, DA, and 5-HT are all deaminated mainly by MAO-A, which is selectively inhibited by clorgyline, Lilly 51641, harmine, and harmaline. PEA and benzylamine, on the other hand, are deaminated mainly by MAO-B, which is selectively inhibited by deprenyl or low doses/concentrations of pargyline. Tryptamine, tyramine, and kynuramine, for example, seem to be deaminated about equally well by MAO-A and MAO-B.

Only those pharmacologic effects which appear likely to be dependent

on the inhibition of MAO will be considered in this review. Some criteria for
a pharmacologic effect to be related to MAO inhibition are: (1) the effect is
produced by at least two structurally different MAOIs; (2) the effect has a
time course paralleling MAO inhibition or another parameter, such as an
increased amine level, which is known to depend on MAO inhibition; and (3)
antagonism of long-term effects by the simultaneous administration of a
reversible, short-duration inhibitor (e.g., harmine) (see Biel *et al.*, 1964).

2. INHIBITION OF 5-HT AND CATECHOLAMINE SYNTHESIS

After inhibition of MAO brain levels of 5-HT, NA and DA increase to
new steady-state levels, the largest increase being for 5-HT (see above). That
the concentrations of these amines do not increase above a limiting value,
even after repeated daily doses of an MAOI (Spector *et al.*, 1958, 1960*a,b*;
Brodie *et al.*, 1959; Spector, 1963), suggests that biosynthesis of these amines
is regulated by negative feedback mechanisms, one of which may be
inhibition by an amine of the corresponding amino acid hydroxylase (e.g.,
Nagatsu *et al.*, 1964).

Pretreatment with MAOIs has been reported to inhibit the synthesis of
NA (Neff and Costa, 1966; Lin *et al.*, 1969), DA (Javoy *et al.*, 1972, 1973),
and 5-HT (Macon *et al.*, 1971) from their amino acid precursors in brain *in
vivo*, as well as 5-HT synthesis from L-tryptophan *in vitro* (Hamon *et al.*,
1972, 1973). This inhibition of catecholamine and 5-HT synthesis by MAOIs
seems to be due to inhibition of tyrosine hydroxylase and tryptophan
hydroxylase, respectively, by increased intraneuronal concentrations of un-
bound catecholamines and 5-HT. However, NA and especially DA synthesis
seem to be more tightly regulated by feedback inhibition than 5-HT
synthesis: both NA and DA synthesis are significantly inhibited when their
concentrations in brain reach about 150% of control values (Lin *et al.*, 1969;
Javoy *et al.*, 1972, 1973), while the synthesis of 5-HT does not appear to be
significantly inhibited before its concentration in brain approaches about
300% of control values (Macon *et al.*, 1971). Very little inhibition of 5-HT
synthesis *in vivo* is found with 5-HT concentrations near 200% of control
(Lin *et al.*, 1969; Millard *et al.*, 1972). That 5-HT synthesis from L-
tryptophan is inhibited by increasing 5-HT concentration intraneuronally is
strongly suggested by the finding (Hamon *et al.*, 1972, 1973) that synthesis
inhibition in striatal slices *in vitro* by 5-HT added to the incubation medium
could be significantly reversed by chlorimipramine, a potent inhibitor of 5-
HT uptake (Carlsson, 1970). Similarly, tyrosine hydroxylase in synaptosomes
from rat striatum is effectively inhibited by DA added to the incubation
medium and this inhibition is almost entirely reversed by benztropin

(Christiansen and Squires, unpublished), inhibitor of the neuronal DA pump (Coyle and Snyder, 1969*b*).

3. INHIBITION OF SPONTANEOUS FIRING OF 5-HT NEURONS

Aghajanian *et al.* (1970) reported that four MAOIs (pargyline, tranylcypromine, phenelzine, and iproniazid) administered intraperitoneally progressively inhibited the spontaneous firing rate of single raphe neurons in the rat. The time course of this inhibition parallels MAO inhibition since pargyline, tranylcypromine, and phenelzine, known to inhibit MAO rapidly, produced essentially complete inhibition of raphe activity within 30–40 min, while iproniazid, an MAOI with a slow onset of action, required between 1 and 2 hr to produce maximum inhibition of raphe activity. The inhibition of raphe activity, produced by all four MAOIs, was prevented by selective depletion of brain 5-HT with PCPA, indicating that the inhibitory effect of the MAOIs is dependent on increases in the concentration of 5-HT in the raphe neurons and subsequent leakage to the outside. Other drugs which increase the concentration of 5-HT inside or outside the 5-HT neuron such as L-tryptophan (Aghajanian, 1972), 5-HT reuptake blockers (such as amitriptyline, imipramine, and chlorimipramine) (Sheard *et al.*, 1972), and chlorpheniramine (Bramwell, 1974), as well as *p*-chloroamphetamine (Sheard, 1974) and *p*-chlormetamphetamine (Bramwell, 1974), both potent releasers of 5-HT from neurons, and 5-HTP (Jacobs *et al.*, 1975) also inhibit raphe firing, probably by activating inhibitory 5-HT autoreceptors located on the raphe neuronal membrane (Aghajanian *et al.*, 1972; Haigler and Aghajanian, 1974). The progressive inhibitory activity of pargyline on raphe firing, which alone requires 30–40 min to become maximum, is greatly accelerated by pretreating with L-tryptophan, complete inhibition then occurring within 2 min (Bramwell, 1974).

4. INHIBITORY EFFECTS ON PARADOXICAL SLEEP AND PONTOGENICULOOCCIPITAL WAVES

Several MAOIs (harmaline, tranylcypromine, iproniazid, nialamide, pargyline, and phenylisopropyl hydrazide) have been reported to dramatically suppress paradoxical sleep (PS) for long periods in the cat while increasing slow-wave sleep (Jouvet *et al.*, 1965; Jouvet, 1969, 1972; Jones, 1972). Nialamide was also found (Mouret *et al.*, 1968) to inhibit PS in the rat. Tranylcypromine and iproniazid inhibit PS in the monkey (Reite *et al.*, 1969).

In humans, chronic treatment with phenelzine has been reported to greatly reduce or totally abolish rapid-eye-movement (REM) sleep (Bowers and Kupfer, 1971; Wyatt et al., 1969, 1971a,b; Dunleavy, 1973; Dunleavy and Oswald, 1973).

Pontogeniculooccipital (PGO) waves, which are normally associated with PS (Jouvet and Michel, 1959), can be induced in the waking state by reserpine and related amine-depleting agents (e.g., Ro 4-1284) as well as by treatment with the specific 5-HT depletor PCPA (Jouvet, 1967, 1969; Delorme et al., 1965; Jalfre et al., 1974; Monachon et al., 1972; Ruch-Monachon et al., 1975a–e; Jacobs et al., 1972) or by raphe lesions (Pujol et al., 1971). The PGO waves associated with normal PS as well as those induced by reserpine are inhibited by nialamide, pargyline (Jouvet, 1972), tranylcypromine, and pheniprazine (Jones, 1972). On the other hand, Ruch-Monachon et al. (1975c) found that nialamide, but, surprisingly, not pheniprazine, suppressed both PCPA and Ro-4-1484-induced PGO spikes.

Several lines of evidence suggest that both PS and PGO waves are subjected to inhibitory control by 5-HT as well as catecholamine systems: A number of drugs known to inhibit neuronal reuptake of 5-HT (Oswald, 1969), including imipramine (Khazan and Brown, 1970; Khazan and Sawyer, 1964; Toyoda, 1964; Passouant et al., 1973), amitriptyline (Hartmann, 1968; Oswald, 1969), Lilly 110140 (Slater et al., 1974), and, especially, chlorimipramine (Passouant et al., 1973), effectively suppress PS. The 5-HT precursor 5-HTP (Matsumoto and Jouvet, 1964; Jouvet, 1969) as well as the 5-HT releaser fenfluramine (Johnson et al., 1971) have been reported to reduce PS in cats. Substances which activate central catecholamine receptors (by various mechanisms), such as amphetamine, phenmetrazine, diethylpropion, methylphenidate (Oswald, 1968), and desmethylimipramine (Khazan and Brown, 1970; Jones, 1972), also suppress PS. Administration of L-dopa reduces the duration of REM sleep in man (Wyatt et al., 1970) and rat (Hartmann et al., 1971; Altier et al., 1975), while AMPT increases it in the cat (King and Jewett, 1968; Stein et al., 1974).

Similarly, waking PGO waves induced in cats by pretreatment with PCPA or Ro 4-1284 can be suppressed by a variety of 5-HT reuptake inhibitors, chlorimipramine being among the most potent (Jalfre et al., 1974; Ruch-Monachon et al., 1975a). Other drugs thought to activate certain central 5-HT receptors, such as LSD and related indoleamine hallucinogens (DMT, psilocybin, bufotenin, and yohimbine) (Ruch-Monachon et al., 1975a), 5-HTP, and L-tryptophan, as well as 5-HT itself injected intracerebroventricularly (Ruch-Monachon et al., 1975b), also suppress waking PGO waves. A number of substances which probably activate central catecholamine receptors (directly or indirectly), such as extremely small doses of clonidine (10–100 μg/kg), amphetamine, or β-tetrahydronaphthylamine, as well as intraventricular injections of NA and DA, have recently been reported to suppress PGO waves, while the α-adrenergic blocker phenoxybenzamine as well as AMPT and two DBH inhibitors increase the density of PGO waves

(Ruch-Monachon *et al.*, 1975*c*). Acute bilateral lesions of the locus coeruleus increased the density of PCPA-induced PGO waves (Ruch-Monachon *et al.*, 1975*c*). The observations that nialamide (Ruch-Monachon *et al.*, 1975*c*) and pargyline (Henriksen *et al.*, 1970) can suppress PCPA-induced PGO waves in the cat provide additional evidence for an inhibitory role of catecholamines.

Taken together, the findings cited above strongly suggest that the MAOIs suppress both PS and PGO waves by increasing both 5-HT and β-hydroxylated catecholamines in the brain. Some indirect evidence suggests that epinephrine may be one of the catecholamines involved (Fuxe *et al.*, 1974; Ruch-Monachon *et al.*, 1975*c*). It is clear that other neurotransmitters (e.g., GABA and AC) are probably also involved in regulating PS and PGO waves (Jouvet, 1969; Jacobs *et al.*, 1972; Ruch-Monachon, 1975*d,e*).

5. EFFECTS ON GROWTH AND DEVELOPMENT

Zor *et al.* (1965*a*) reported that chronic administration of a number of MAOIs, including pivhydrazine, nialamide, isocarboxazid, mebanazine, phenelzine, pargyline, pheniprazine, and tranylcypromine, decreases cartilage growth in normal rats. Pargyline did not depress cartilage growth in adrenalectomized rats unless they received hydrocortisone. Growth hormone prevented the inhibitory effect of pargyline on cartilage growth (Zor *et al.*, 1965*a*). Chronic mebanazine reduces the growth of cartilage, and the normal increase in body weight and pituitary weight in growing male rats (Zor *et al.*, 1965*b*). These inhibitory effects of mebanazine are only partly overcome by growth hormone, and are strongly potentiated by hydrocortisone. Mebanazine, particularly when administered together with hydrocortisone, inhibits the growth of seminal vesicles, dorsolateral prostates, and ventral prostates of male rats in all stages of growth (Zor *et al.*, 1968). It was suggested that these inhibitory effects of chronic MAOI inhibition might be due to interference with LH production and effectiveness (Zor *et al.*, 1966) as well as inhibition of growth hormone synthesis and increase in ACTH release from the pituitary (Zor *et al.*, 1965*b*).

Chronic treatment of immature female mice with iproniazid (1.5–2.5 mg/kg per day for 35 days) caused a highly significant decrease in the weight of the ovaries (~30% decrease, P ~0.001) with smaller but still significant decreases in uterus and vagina weights (Robson and Botros, 1961). The weights of the adrenal glands and kidneys, as well as overall body weight, were not affected by chronic iproniazid treatment. The livers, and especially spleens, of the chronically treated female mice were much enlarged as compared with the untreated controls. When iproniazid was given chronically (2.5 mg/kg s.c. daily for 14 days) to mature female mice there was no significant effect on body weight, but estrus was slightly inhibited and the weights of ovaries and uteri significantly reduced. Immature female mice were treated chronically (19–45 days) with small doses of three other MAOIs (H.P. 1325, heptylhydrazine, and nialamide). Like iproniazid, these MAOIs were highly active in delaying the onset of sexual maturity (appearance of estrus and vaginal opening) and significantly reduced the weight of ovaries, uteri, and vaginae without affecting whole-body weight (Robson and Botros, 1961). Also like iproniazid, nialamide treatment greatly increased the size of the spleen. When given daily for 14 days to mature female mice H.P. 1325 and heptyl hydrazine also reduced the weight of ovaries, uteri, and vaginae. Chronic administration of nialamide to virgin female rats has been reported to interfere with the estrus cycle, produce an almost permanent keratinization of the vagina, reduce the weight of the ovary and uterus, increase the number of giant basophil cells in the anterior pituitary, and produce hypertrophy of the glomerular zone of the adrenal gland (Tuchmann-Duplessis and Mercier-Parot, 1962). In the male rat testicular size and function are usually normal after chronic nialamide, but there are very pronounced changes in the anterior pituitary with large increases in the size and number of basophils. As in the female there is a hypertrophy of the glomerular zone of the adrenal gland. The fertility of male rats is greatly reduced by chronic nialamide (Tuchmann-Duplessis and Mercier-Parot, 1962). Chronic daily or twice-daily administration of 5-HT to immature or mature female mice produced effects very similar to those produced by the MAOIs (delay of vaginal opening and estrus, decrease in weights of ovaries, uteri, and vaginae, but only small reduction of total body weight) (Robson and Botros, 1961). It has also been found that chronic administration of 5-HT (25 mg/kg daily for 42–53 days) to weanling female rats delayed the time of vaginal opening and decreased ovarian weight ($P < 0.001$, in both cases) (O'Steen, 1965). Chronic daily administration of 5-HT (200–1000 μg/kg s.c. daily for 24 days) or iproniazid (1.5–2.5 mg/kg daily for 24 days) to immature male mice had no significant effect on growth and only slightly reduced the weight of the testes. In mice chronic iproniazid, but not chronic 5-HT, significantly reduced the weight of the seminal vesicles. Chronic iproniazid significantly increased the weights of the adrenals and, especially, the spleen, while chronic 5-HT increased the weight of the adrenals but decreased that of the spleen (Robson and Botros, 1961). It is interesting that chronic iproniazid treatment delays sexual maturity much less in male than in female mice.

A number of MAOIs have been reported to prevent nidation and interrupt pregnancy in the mouse (Poulson and Robson, 1963, 1964). Chronic administration of a phenelzine derivative (o-chloro-β-phenylethylhydrazine, WL 27) was found to interrupt the normal estrus cycle, delay the onset of estrus in immature female mice, and depress the weights of sex organs in immature and adult female mice as well as immature male mice. Chronic administration of WL 27 (15 mg/kg daily for 28 days) to adult male mice caused a slight but not significant decrease in the weights of the sex organs and adrenals and a highly significant increase in the weight of the spleen. It was suggested that the MAOIs depressed pituitary gonadotrophic activity (Poulson and Robson, 1964). Chronic systemic administration of 5-HT has also been reported to interrupt pregnancy in mice (Lindsay *et al.*, 1963). Jaitly *et al.* (1968*a,b*) suggested that the MAOIs may inhibit or interrupt pregnancy by a variety of actions: (1) ovulation and implantation may be blocked either by inhibition of LH release from the pituitary or by antagonizing the action of LH on the ovary; (2) pregnancy in the mouse may be interrupted on days 7–10 by a peripheral antiprogesterone action on the uterus, where there is a significant correlation between inhibition of MAO and the antifertility effect. The ability of phenelzine and some of its derivatives to interrupt pregnancy after implantation on days 7–10 can also be reversed by, in addition to progesterone, LH, or by estradiol (Jaitly *et al.*, 1968*a,b*), which may act by releasing LH.

Chronic administration of several MAOIs, including iproniazid, in large doses to male rats leads to testicular atrophy, reduction in weight of prostate and seminal vesicles, impairment of spermatogenesis, degeneration of germinal epithelium, and formation of giant cells (Zbinden and Studer, 1959).

Chronic treatment of male rats with pargyline (15 mg/kg daily for 10 days) did not alter whole-body, testicular, seminal vesicle, adrenal, prostate, pituitary, or pineal gland weights, but decreased MAO activity (5-HT substrate) in all organs (especially hypothalamus and pituitary) and caused tubular degeneration with suppression of mature spermatocyte formation in the testis (Urry and Dougherty, 1975). Administration of tranylcypromine (1.25 or 5 mg/kg daily for 6 days) to 12-day-old cockerels significantly reduced the weight of testes. LH, FSH, or corticosterone increased testes weight and all these substances seemed to antagonize the inhibitory effect of tranylcypromine (Forbes, 1970). The inhibitory effect of tranylcypromine on testis development in the cockerel is presumably due to inhibition of gonadotropin release as well as a blockade of the peripheral effects of LH.

6. INHIBITION OF OVULATION

Golden Syrian hamsters, exposed daily from birth to 12 hr light (06 :00–18 :00), display a remarkably regular 4-day estrus cycle, with ovulation occurring every fourth day between 13 :00 and 15 :00. A critical period was found, between 14 :00 and 16 :00, on the day before ovulation, before which hypophysectomy or administration of MAOIs blocked ovulation, and after which both procedures were ineffective (Alleva and Umberger, 1966; Alleva *et al.*, 1966). Phenylisopropylhydrazine, 50 mg/kg; tranylcypromine, 75 mg/kg; iproniazid, 400 mg/kg; and pargyline, 200 mg/kg, were all effective inhibitors of ovulation, and also produced marked behavioral excitement. Inhibition of ovulation seemed to be correlated with increases in the brain levels of 5-HT (Alleva *et al.*, 1966). Given during the critical period, AMPT, a selective inhibitor of catecholamine synthesis, also blocks ovulation in the hamster (Lippmann, 1968) and increases the length of diestrus from 2 to 3 days. Pargyline at a dose of 200 mg/kg i.p., but not 75 mg/kg, inhibits ovulation when given during the critical period. Neither dose interfered with the inhibitory effect of AMPT. It was concluded that a sufficiently low NA/5-HT ratio was required for inhibition of ovulation (Lippmann, 1968). Pargyline (50 mg/kg), administered before the critical period, has been reported to inhibit spontaneous ovulation in the rat (Meyerson and Sawyer, 1967, 1968). Mebanazine has also been reported to inhibit ovulation in the rat, an effect which is potentiated by 5-HTP, but not by L-dopa (Labhsetwar, 1972). A single injection of AMPT also blocks ovulation 100% in the rat.

Immature female rats (25 days old) can be induced to superovulate by treatment with serum gonadotropin (HCG). Nialamide, administered up to 1 hr before HCG, inhibits this superovulation (Kordon *et al.*, 1968; Kordon and Vassent, 1968; Kordon, 1969). Pretreatment with PCPA, but not with AMPT, antagonized the inhibitory action of nialamide. Similarly, 5-HTP, but not L-dopa, inhibits HCG-induced ovulation (Kordon *et al.*, 1968). Microinjections of nialamide into the mediobasal tuberal part of the hypothalamus, but not into the pituitary, inhibit ovulation and luteinization (Kordon, 1969). Also, the inhibitory effects of microinjected nialamide are prevented by pretreatment with PCPA, but not with AMPT. Thus it appears probable that inhibition of ovulation in HCG-treated immature female rats by MAOIs is due to increased levels of 5-HT in specific neuronal pathways in the brain.

Ovulation induced in immature female rats primed with pregnant mare's serum gonadotropin followed by progesterone can be blocked with intraventricular microinjections of 5-HT and this blocking can be prevented by simultaneous injection of LSD or DA (Zolovick and Labhsetwar, 1973). Acute systemic administration of 5-HT (50 mg/kg s.c.), but not of 5-HTP, to spontaneously ovulating sexually mature female rats, on the day preceding proestrus, inhibited ovulation, and this inhibitory effect could be prevented by administration of methysergide (Labhsetwar, 1971*a,b*). Systemic administration of 5-HT (25 mg/kg s.c.) also inhibits ovulation in immature female rats primed with pregnant mare's serum gonadotropin (O'Steen, 1964, 1965; Endersby *et al.*, 1970), an effect which is probably due to suppression of LH release from the hypophysis.

Thus available evidence suggests that a central 5-HT system participates in the inhibition of ovulation (O'Steen, 1964, 1965; Alleva *et al.*, 1966; Kordon and Vassent, 1968; Kordon *et al.*, 1968; Endersby *et al.*, 1970; Lippmann, 1968; Kordon, 1969; Labhsetwar, 1971*a,b*, 1972; Kalnins and Ruf, 1971; Kordon and Glowinski, 1972; Zolovick and Labhsetwar, 1973) at a critical period in the estrus cycle, while a central catecholamine, probably DA, system participates in triggering ovulation at the critical period. The mechanism seems to be an inhibitory effect of 5-HT on the release of the gonadotropin-releasing factors (FRF and LRF), which counteracts stimulation of release by catecholamines (McCann, 1970; Wilson, 1974; Ganong, 1974; McCann and Moss, 1975; Kamberi and Vellis, 1975).

7. EFFECTS ON LORDOSIS

In ovariectomized rats, estrus behavior (lordosis), in response to a mounting male, can be consistently produced by administration of estrogen followed about 48 hr later by progesterone (Boling and Blandau, 1939; Beach, 1942).

Meyerson (1964a) discovered that progesterone, but not estrogen, can be replaced by reserpine or tetrabenazine treatment, suggesting that one or more of the amines depleted by these substances exerts an inhibitory effect on the lordosis response. Pheniprazine, pargyline, and nialamide, as well as imipramine, were found to block this induced estrus behavior (Meyerson, 1964b, 1966; Lindström, 1970). Imipramine acted synergistically with nialamide or pargyline. Since 5-HTP, but not L-dopa, also inhibits estrus behavior (Meyerson, 1964b) it was concluded that the inhibitory effect of the MAOIs, as well as that of imipramine, was due to facilitation of central 5-HT neuronal transmission (Meyerson et al., 1973, 1974). This conclusion was further supported by the finding that selective inhibition of 5-HT synthesis by PCPA can replace progesterone treatment in the activation of estrus behavior in ovariectomized rats (Zemlan et al., 1973; Meyerson et al., 1973) and that this activation can be prevented by pretreatment of the rats with pargyline (Meyerson and Lewander, 1970). Lordosis behavior induced in castrated male rats by treatment with estrogen and tetrabenazine could also be blocked by nialamide (Larsson and Södersten, 1971).

There is some evidence that a catecholamine system may also be involved in suppressing female copulatory behavior: D,L-amphetamine (2.0 mg/kg s.c.) inhibited the estrogen/progesterone- as well as the estrogen/reserpine-activated lordosis response. A subeffective dose of amphetamine (1.0 mg/kg) acted synergistically with subeffective doses of pargyline or imipramine in inhibiting lordosis (Meyerson, 1968). These results suggest that the MAOIs may inhibit female copulatory behavior by increasing the levels of a catecholamine, as well as 5-HT, in the brain.

8. EFFECTS ON MALE COPULATORY BEHAVIOR

The MAOIs may have opposite effects on the copulatory behavior of male rats, depending on, among other factors, the relative concentrations of catecholamines and 5-HT in the brain (Gessa and Tagliamonte, 1973, 1974;

Malmnäs and Meyerson, 1971; Malmnäs, 1973, 1974). In otherwise un-treated intact or testosterone-treated castrated male rats, pargyline (Taglia-monte *et al.*, 1971c; Malmnäs and Meyerson, 1970, 1971), iproniazid, and nialamide (Dewsbury *et al.*, 1972) inhibited copulatory behavior, an effect which appears to depend on increased central 5-HT transmission since selective depletion of brain 5-HT by PCPA pretreatment increases homosex-ual mounting behavior in intact male rats (Sheard, 1969; Shillito, 1970; Gawienowski and Hodgen, 1971; Tagliamonte *et al.*, 1969), castrated rats (Bond *et al.*, 1972; Gessa *et al.*, 1970; Malmnäs and Meyerson, 1971), and intact cats (Ferguson *et al.*, 1970; Hoyland *et al.*, 1970). Depending on the experimental situation, administration of testosterone may increase mounting behavior in PCPA-pretreated animals (Malmnäs and Meyerson, 1971; Bond *et al.*, 1972; Gessa *et al.*, 1970; Del Fiacco *et al.*, 1974; Gawienowski and Hodgen, 1971). PCPA pretreatment can also increase heterosexual mounting (Malmnäs and Meyerson, 1971; Salis and Dewsbury, 1971; Del Fiacco *et al.*, 1974; Tagliamonte *et al.*, 1971c), but this increase seems to depend on the level of sexual performance before PCPA treatment (Whalen and Luttge, 1970). The stimulatory effect of PCPA or PCPA–pargyline on male copula-tory behavior should be most pronounced in situations where a stimulation is possible to detect, i.e., when the sexually vigorous male is presented with a normally inadequate sexual stimulus (Malmnäs and Meyerson, 1971; Whalen and Luttge, 1970), or a sexually sluggish male is presented with an adequate sexual stimulus (Malmnäs and Meyerson, 1971).

However, PCPA alone or in combination with pargyline shortens mount and ejaculation latencies in male rats and increases the number of intromis-sions per minute (Ahlenius *et al.*, 1971; Malmnäs, 1973) without changing other components of heterosexual behavior.

In castrated male rats PCPA synergizes with testosterone (Malmnäs and Meyerson, 1971) or estradiol (Luttge, 1975) in restoring heterosexual mount-ing behavior.

Administration of small doses of 5-HTP (1–25 mg/kg) abruptly stops compulsive homosexual mounting induced by PCPA pretreatment in rats (Tagliamonte *et al.*, 1969; Shillito, 1970; Gessa *et al.*, 1970; Malmnäs and Meyerson, 1971) and cats (Hoyland *et al.*, 1970; Shillito, 1970; Ferguson *et al.*, 1970). 5-HTP also suppresses the normal copulatory behavior of male rats with receptive females (Gessa and Tagliamonte, 1974) and potentiates the suppressive effect of pargyline on heterosexual mounting in the male (Malmnäs and Meyerson, 1971; Tagliamonte *et al.*, 1971c).

In male rats pretreated with PCPA the administration of a MAOI increases the frequency of compulsive homosexual mounting (Tagliamonte *et al.*, 1969, 1971c; Malmnäs and Meyerson, 1971), indicating that mounting behavior is facilitated by a catecholamine system and inhibited by a 5-HT system (Malmnäs and Meyerson, 1971; Malmnäs, 1973, 1974). Compulsive homosexual mounting behavior in male rats induced by PCPA and pargyline is also effectively stopped by 5-HTP (5 or 25 mg/kg) (Tagliamonte *et al.*,

1969; Malmnäs and Meyerson, 1971). Further evidence that copulatory behavior in the male is promoted by a catecholamine (probably DA) system is provided by the findings that apomorphine (0.5 mg/kg) and L-dopa (100 mg/kg combined with a peripherally acting decarboxylase inhibitor, Ro 4-4602) stimulate the copulatory activity of sexually sluggish male rats with receptive females (Gessa and Tagliamonte, 1974; Da Prada *et al.*, 1973; Malmnäs and Meyerson, 1972; Malmnäs, 1973, 1974).

9. 5-HT-DEPENDENT BEHAVIORAL SYNDROMES

A number of characteristic, 5-HT-dependent, behavioral syndromes which differ somewhat with species, and the treatment used to elicit them, now all appear to depend on the presence of a critical concentration of free 5-HT in the CNS. The 5-HT-dependent indoleamine syndromes closely resemble the behavioral syndromes produced by indoleamine hallucinogens such as LSD, DMT, 5-methoxy-*N,N*-dimethyl tryptamine (5-MeODMT), and bufotenin. It therefore seems reasonable to assume that all these behavioral states depend on the activation of the same receptors in the CNS. The indoleamine syndromes have been reviewed by Mantegazzini (1966).

The 5-HT-dependent behavioral syndromes can be produced by (1) a large dose of a nonselective MAOI alone, e.g., nialamide (Corrodi, 1966); (2) 5-HTP, usually in combination with an MAOI; (3) L-tryptophan together with an MAOI; (4) reserpine or tetrabenazine in animals pretreated with an MAOI; or (5) the combination of an MAOI and a 5-HT pump blocker.

9.1. MAOI Plus Reserpine or Tetrabenazine

In the pioneering investigations on the interactions between the MAOIs and reserpine it was discovered that administration of reserpine to mice, rats, guinea pigs, and rabbits (but not cats and dogs) pretreated with a variety of MAOIs resulted in a characteristic behavioral excitation instead of the sedation normally seen after the administration of reserpine alone (Brodie *et al.*, 1956; Chessin *et al.*, 1957; Shore and Brodie, 1957; Spector *et al.*, 1958, 1960a,b; Tedeschi, D. H., *et al.*, 1959; Tedeschi, R. E., *et al.*, 1959; Eltherington and Horita, 1960; Green, H., and Erickson, 1962; Plummer and Furness, 1963; Gylys *et al.*, 1963). In a classic study (Brodie *et al.*, 1956; Shore and Brodie, 1957), it was shown that when rabbits are given reserpine after pretreatment with iproniazid they become excited, hyperactive, have dilated pupils, and exhibit other signs similar to those seen after administration of LSD or large doses of 5-HTP. It was concluded that this behavioral syndrome in rabbits is associated with a high concentration of free 5-HT in the brain. Similar conclusions were reached by Chessin *et al.* (1957) and by

H. Green and Erickson (1962) using several other animal species. Scheel-Krüger and Jonas (1973) have described excitation of long duration in rats pretreated with nialamide followed by tetrabenazine. Continuous locomotion and absence of rearing and biting on the cage wires were noted. The role of 5-HT in this nialamide–tetrabenazine syndrome was not investigated, but it was found that spiramide (0.2 mg/kg) produced complete inhibition of all locomotor and stereotype activities, while aceperone and phenoxybenzamine attenuated locomotion, and scopolamine strongly potentiated both locomotion and stereotype activities. Recently, it has been shown (Squires, unpublished) that inhibition of both MAO-A and MAO-B, before administration of reserpine, is required for the production of the indoleamine syndrome in rats, while selective inhibition of MAO-A alone is sufficient to completely block the usual behavioral and amine-depleting effects of reserpine (see also Fuentes and Neff, 1975). The MAOI–reserpine syndrome is completely blocked by PCPA pretreatment and is potentiated by loading with L-tryptophan (Squires, unpublished), 2 hr after reserpine.

9.2. MAOI Plus L-Tryptophan

In pioneering studies, the administration of L-tryptophan to humans (Sjoerdsma et al., 1959a–c) and experimental animals (Hess et al., 1959; Hodge et al., 1964) pretreated with MAOI was found to cause behavioral excitation. The behavioral syndrome produced in rats pretreated with iproniazid, 1-phenyl-2-hydrazinopropane (JB 516), or nialamide after loading with large doses of tryptophan (800 mg/kg) was described in detail by Hess and Doepfner (1961). This syndrome includes continuous side-to-side head movements interrupted by occasional head twitches, tremor, and aimless locomotion. The hindpart is held relatively fixed, and circling, jerky movements are performed by continuous stamping or treading ("piano playing") with the forelimbs. The males usually exhibit penile erection and there is a tendency for the hindlimbs to abduct. Grooming, rearing, normal exploration, and social interaction are disrupted (Squires and Buus Lassen, 1975). Similar behavioral effects of tryptophan in rats pretreated with pargyline (Horita and Carino, 1970; Jacobs, 1974a,b; Jacobs et al., 1974; Weber, 1966), iproniazid (Weber, 1966; Ernst, 1972), tranylcypromine (Weber, 1966; Grahame-Smith, 1971a,b), β-phenylisopropylhydrazine (Weber, 1966), and nialamide (Squires and Buus Lassen, 1975) have been repeatedly observed. Related syndromes have been observed in mice (Corrodi, 1966; Modigh and Svensson, 1972), guinea pigs (Hodge et al., 1964), dogs (Himwich et al., 1972), and rabbits (Carlsson et al., 1969a,b). In humans, MAOIs plus tryptophan can cause neurologic, behavioral, and subjective mental changes (Lauer et al., 1958; Oats and Sjoerdsma, 1960; Sprince et al., 1963; Glassman and Platman, 1969).

Although there seems to be little correlation between the intensity of the

MAOI–tryptophan syndrome and the total concentration of 5-HT in brain (Hess and Doepfner, 1961; Weber, 1966; Horita and Carino, 1970; Grahame-Smith, 1971*a*), the syndrome can be completely blocked by pretreatment with PCPA or a decarboxylase inhibitor, Ro 4-4602 (Hodge *et al.*, 1964), indicating that its development is dependent on 5-HT formation (Horita and Carino, 1970; Grahame-Smith, 1971*a*, 1972; Modigh and Svensson, 1972; Jacobs, 1974*b*; Squires and Buus Lassen, 1975). Simultaneous inhibition of MAO-A and MAO-B, before administration of L-tryptophan, is required for the full expression of the indoleamine syndrome (Squires and Buus Lassen, 1975). Selective inhibition of MAO-A by clorgyline administration reduces the concentration of 5-HIAA in rat brain after L-tryptophan loading to only about 70% of control values. Selective inhibition of MAO-B by deprenyl alone had no effect on the deamination of 5-HT (e.g., 5-HIAA formation) in rat brain, but, in combination with clorgyline, reduced 5-HIAA to 20–30% of control values.

Since 5-HT seems to be deaminated almost entirely by MAO-A *in vitro* (Johnston, 1968; Hall *et al.*, 1969; Fuller *et al.*, 1970; Jarrott, 1971; Christmas *et al.*, 1972; Knoll and Magyar, 1972; Squires, 1972*b*), it has been suggested (Squires and Buus Lassen, 1975) that, *in vivo*, 5-HT may be converted, e.g., by *N*-methylation, to a derivative such as bufotenin which might be partly deaminated by MAO-B to 5-HIAA. According to this hypothesis the MAOI–tryptophan syndrome would be dependent on the formation of bufotenin or another *N*-alkylated 5-HT derivative. The formation of an *O*-methylated derivative of 5-HT does not seem to be involved in the indoleamine syndrome, since the small concentrations of apparent 5-methoxyindoleacetic acid in rat brain are essentially unaffected by clorgyline and deprenyl, singly or in combination (Squires, 1975). No direct evidence for the formation of larger amounts of *N*-alkylated derivatives of 5-HT in rat brain, after inhibition of MAO and L-tryptophan loading, seems to be available at present.

The role of the catecholamines in the expression of the indoleamine syndrome is unclear. In rats the hyperactivity and hyperpyrexia produced by MAOI plus L-tryptophan or by 5-MeODMT can be inhibited by chlorpromazine (Grahame-Smith, 1972). Although chlorpromazine is known to block central DA and NA receptors (Carlsson and Lindqvist, 1963; Andén *et al.*, 1972; Hyttel, 1974; Nybäck *et al.*, 1967, 1968), pimozide, which is thought to more selectively block DA receptors (Nybäck *et al.*, 1970), fails to block the indoleamine syndrome, while spiroperidol, another known DA-receptor blocker, effectively blocks it (Jacobs, 1974*a*; Jacobs *et al.*, 1974), suggesting that chlorpromazine and spiroperidol may inhibit various aspects of the indoleamine syndrome by blocking receptor types other than DA receptors. Spiroperidol is an extremely potent displacer of specific [³H]LSD binding to rat brain membranes *in vitro*, a property it shares with six classical 5-HT antagonists (Squires, unpublished). Administration of AMPT has been reported to partially antagonize hypermotility in mice induced by L-trypto-

phan and nialamide (Modigh and Svensson, 1972), but has no effect on the
syndrome produced in rats by pargyline plus L-tryptophan (Jacobs, 1974*b*).
Pretreatment of rats with high doses of AMPT or FLA 63 (an inhibitor of
DA-β-hydroxylase) before MAOI and L-tryptophan decreases body temperature and motor activity as measured by a motimeter, but tremor and some
movements of the head, forelimbs, and whole body still persist (Buus Lassen,
unpublished).

In rats pretreated with reserpine, an intense syndrome is produced by
subsequent inhibition of both MAO-A and MAO-B followed by L-tryptophan
loading (Squires, unpublished). Under these conditions NA and DA concentrations in rat brain are less than 20% of control values, while the concentration of apparent 5-HT is significantly higher than in untreated controls.
Taken together, the observations described above indicate that the catecholamines play only a minor role in the expression of the indoleamine syndrome.

Pretreatment with diphenylhydantoin (75 mg/kg) enhances and acceler-
ates the onset of the syndrome produced by tranylcypromine and L-
tryptophan, but not that produced by 5-MeODMT (Green, A. R., and
Grahame-Smith, 1975). Since diphenylhydantoin alone does not decrease the
turnover of 5-HT in brain, as does chlorimipramine, it appears that
diphenylhydantoin may act by promoting the release of 5-HT through an as
yet unknown mechanism.

Certain MAOIs administered alone can produce a 5-HT-dependent
indoleamine syndrome. A large dose (500 mg/kg) of nialamide produces a
characteristic indoleamine syndrome in mice (Carlsson and Corrodi, 1964;
Corrodi, 1966) which develops slowly and can be prevented by selective
inhibition of 5-HT, but not of catecholamine, synthesis. Similarly, a large
dose of pargyline (300–400 mg/kg i.p.) produced a severe syndrome,
provided the rats were kept at an environmental temperature of 29°C
(Carlsson *et al.*, 1965). PCPA pretreatment has been reported to protect mice
from the late, but not the early, toxic effects of tranylcypromine (Gessner
and Soble, 1972). Several MAOIs administered alone to rats produce typical
indoleamine syndromes the first signs of which appear several hours after
administration (Buus Lassen, unpublished). The slow appearance of the
syndrome after the administration of a MAOI alone seems to parallel the
slow accumulation of 5-HT in brain (Pletscher, 1957; Spector *et al.*, 1958,
1960*a*,*b*; Brodie *et al.*, 1959; Macon *et al.*, 1971). After inhibition of MAO the
rate of 5-HT accumulation is accelerated by L-tryptophan loading (Grahame-
Smith, 1971*a*), a maximum accumulation rate being reached with about 100
mg L-tryptophan/kg corresponding to a minimum delay before onset of the
syndrome of about 20 min. Even doses of L-tryptophan as low as 2.5 mg/kg
in tranylcypromine-pretreated rats produced marked hyperactivity which
began about 110 min after L-tryptophan administration. It is well known that
under normal conditions, the concentration of L-tryptophan in brain is rate-
limiting for 5-HT synthesis (Eccleston *et al.*, 1965; Squires, 1974): L-
tryptophan loading will increase the concentration of 5-HIAA in rat brain

two- to threefold and that of 5-HT somewhat less, indicating that tryptophan hydroxylase in brain is not saturated with substrate under physiologic conditions. It is also of interest that tryptophan hydroxylase is not saturated by the normal oxygen concentration in the brain (Davis *et al.*, 1973), and *in vitro* an atmosphere of pure oxygen stimulates tryptophan hydroxylase fivefold compared to activity in air (Green, H., and Sawyer, 1966). In contrast, tyrosine hydroxylase in brain is normally saturated with both oxygen and L-tyrosine (Fisher and Kaufman, 1972).

A number of drugs and treatments increase the concentration of L-tryptophan and, subsequently, of 5-HT and 5-HIAA in brain (Tagliamonte *et al.*, 1971a,b). One of these treatments, chronic lithium (Tagliamonte *et al.*, 1971a,b; Perez-Cruet *et al.*, 1971; Sheard and Aghajanian, 1970; Schubert, 1973; Iwata *et al.*, 1974; Poitou *et al.*, 1974), promotes the development of the indoleamine syndrome after inhibition of MAO with tranylcypromine or pargyline (Grahame-Smith and Green, 1974; Jenner *et al.*, 1975; Judd *et al.*, 1975) without L-tryptophan loading, an effect which may be due to the ability of lithium ion to increase the concentration of L-tryptophan in brain, stimulate its uptake into neurons (Knapp and Mandell, 1973), increase the rate of 5-HT synthesis by other mechanisms, or facilitate its release (Sheard and Aghajanian, 1970).

After MAO inhibition the initial (first 60 min) rate of 5-HT accumulation in the brains of lithium-pretreated rats was greater than in untreated controls (Grahame-Smith and Green, 1974; Jenner *et al.*, 1975; Judd *et al.*, 1975). Rubidium ion also produces the indoleamine syndrome, and increases the initial rate of 5-HT accumulation after inhibition of MAO in rats. In both respects rubidium ion is more potent than lithium ion (Judd *et al.*, 1975). Lithium–MAOI-induced hyperactivity is blocked by prior administration of PCPA (Grahame-Smith and Green, 1974) or AMPT (Judd *et al.*, 1975). The syndrome produced by 5-MeODMT is not potentiated by lithium pretreatment (Grahame-Smith and Green, 1974). Taken together, these results suggest that both lithium and rubidium ions act by stimulating 5-HT syntheses or release or both. Acute or chronic lithium administration does not seem to have any effect on 5-HT turnover (i.e., 5-HIAA concentration) in L-tryptophan-loaded rats or mice, or to affect the development of the indoleamine syndrome in L-tryptophan-loaded animals given graded doses of nialamide (Buus Lassen and Squires, unpublished), or in nialamide-pretreated mice given graded doses of L-tryptophan. These observations suggest that lithium ion may speed up the onset of the indoleamine syndrome by increasing the concentration of L-tryptophan in the brain. The mechanisms by which chronic lithium and rubidium induce long-lasting increases in the concentration of L-tryptophan in blood and brain are not yet understood. However, inhibition of tryptophan pyrrolase does not seem to be involved (Schubert, 1973).

Thyrotropin-releasing hormone (TRH, L-pyroglutamyl-L-histidyl-L-prolinamide) in doses of 1–2 mg/kg i.p. has also been reported to potentiate the

MAOI–tryptophan syndrome, as well as the characteristic hyperactive behavioral syndromes produced by MAOI plus l-dopa, 5-MeODMT, 4-methoxyamphetamine, and pentylenetetrazole (Green, A. R., and Grahame-Smith, 1974). Thus TRH, as well as another tripeptide, MIF, seem to produce rather nonspecific excitatory effects. It is puzzling that 1 or 2, but not 10, mg TRH/kg potentiates the MAOI–tryptophan syndrome.

9.3. MAOI Plus 5-HTP

The behavioral excitation produced in experimental animals by 5-HTP, which resembles the behavioral effects of LSD, is also dependent on the formation of 5-HT: pretreatment with an MAOI increases the concentration of 5-HT in brain after administration of 5-HTP and simultaneously potentiates its behavioral effects (Udenfriend et al., 1957a,b; Bogdanski et al., 1958; Horita and Gogerty, 1958; Horita, 1958; Randall and Bagdon, 1959; Corne et al., 1963; Weber, 1966; Henning and Rubenson, 1971; Mannisto et al., 1971; Ernst, 1972). The behavioral effects of 5-HTP administered alone can also be potentiated by blockers of neuronal 5-HT uptake such as chlorpheniramine (Carlsson and Lindqvist, 1969), chlorimipramine (Carlsson et al., 1969b; Modigh, 1973), and imipramine (Loew and Taeschler, 1965; Sanghvi and Gershon, 1970; Westheimer and Klawans, 1974). Buus Lassen (1972a) confirmed the potentiation of 5-HTP-induced behavioral excitation in mice by imipramine, chlorimipramine, chlorpheniramine, and nortryptyline and found that it was blocked by the 5-HTP-decarboxylase inhibitor NSD 1015, further demonstrating the dependence of 5-HTP-induced behavioral effects on 5-HT formation.

When rats or mice were pretreated with selective inhibitors of MAO-A and MAO-B (clorgyline and deprenyl, respectively), it was found that simultaneous inhibition of MAO-A and MAO-B was required for maximum potentiation of low doses of 5-HTP, while inhibition of MAO-A alone was sufficient to potentiate maximally the behavioral effects of high doses of 5-HTP. Selective inhibition of MAO-B by deprenyl did not potentiate even the highest doses of 5-HTP tested (Squires, unpublished).

Several lines of evidence suggest that the catecholamines play only a minor role in 5-HTP-induced behavioral excitation. In dogs, two DA antagonists, haloperidol and pimozide, are without effect on 5-HTP-induced excitation (Dunkley et al., 1972). In mice, the depletion of NA and DA from brain with α-methyl-m-tyrosine (Modigh, 1972) or with AMPT (Buus Lassen, 1972a) did not prevent 5-HTP-induced excitation. Protriptyline, a potent blocker of neuronal NA uptake with only a weak inhibitory effect on 5-HT uptake, failed to potentiate the behavioral effects of 5-HTP in mice, while chlorimipramine, a potent inhibitor of 5-HT uptake, was an active 5-HTP potentiator (Modigh, 1973). However, 5-HTP-induced behavioral excitation in mice is attenuated by chlorpromazine (Bogdanski et al., 1958), perphenazine, and spiramide (Buus Lassen, 1972a), but not by the 5-HT antagonists methysergide, cyproheptadine, and methergoline (Buus Lassen, 1972a).

The pyrogenic effects of 5-HTP and LSD in the rabbit are greatly attenuated by pretreatment with BOL (Horita and Gogerty, 1958). In the dog, the behavioral and cardiovascular effects of 5-HTP and yohimbine, which are potentiated by imipramine, are not reduced or prevented by methysergide, BOL, or cyproheptadine (Sanghvi and Gershon, 1970). Thus the receptors involved in the expression of 5-HTP-induced behavioral excitation are not well characterized.

9.4. MAOI Plus 5-HT-Uptake Inhibitor

Toxic interactions between MAOIs and thymoleptic drugs in humans are well documented (e.g., Davies, 1960; Singh, 1960; Luby and Domino, 1961; Lee, 1961; Brachfeld et al., 1963). Similar toxic reactions can occur in humans treated with a combination of an MAOI and pethidine (Mitchell, 1955; Papp and Benaim, 1958; Palmer, 1960; Shee, 1960; Clement and Benazon, 1962; Craig, 1962; Taylor, 1962; Denton et al., 1962).

In mice pretreated with various MAOIs, including pargyline, phenelzine, iproniazid, tranylcypromine, and nialamide, toxic reactions occur after administration of pethidine (Gessner and Soble, 1973; Brownlee and Williams, 1963; Mustala and Jounela, 1966; Jounela, 1970; Rogers, 1971; Rogers and Thornton, 1969), chlorpheniramine, recipavrin, diphenhydramine, tripelennamine (Carlsson and Lindqvist, 1969), and chlorimipramine (Carlsson et al., 1969b). The symptoms produced by these combinations in the mouse include restlessness, convulsions, central excitation, hyperpyrexia (Jounela, 1970), extension and abduction of the hindlimbs, tremors, and side-to-side head movements (Carlsson and Lindqvist, 1969).

It was noted by Rogers and Thornton (1969) that pethidine toxicity in tranylcypromine-pretreated mice was related to the increase in the concentration of 5-HT in brain, and not to that of NA or DA. It was proposed that pethidine, and certain other potent analgesics, exert their toxic effects in MAOI-pretreated animals by releasing 5-HT. Jounela (1970) found that selective depletion of 5-HT from mouse brain by PCPA could prevent phenelzine–pethidine toxicity. The protective effect of PCPA pretreatment on MAOI–pethidine toxicity in mice was confirmed by Rogers (1971) and by Gessner and Soble (1973). Chlorpromazine has been reported to antagonize tranylcypromine–pethidine toxicity in mice (Gessner, 1973).

Similar toxic interactions between MAOIs and 5-HT pump blockers have been well described in rabbits. The MAOIs used include β-p-chlorophenylmercaptoethyl hydrazine (S 231) (Nymark and Møller Nielsen, 1963), tranylcypromine, nialamide (Carlsson et al., 1969b), phenelzine (Loveless and Maxwell, 1965; Sinclair, 1972a–c, 1973; Matilla and Jounela, 1973; Sinha et al., 1969; Dixit et al., 1970), and pargyline (Penn and Rogers, 1971; Fahim et *al.*, 1972; Gong and Rogers, 1973). The 5-HT-uptake inhibitors used in the rabbit studies included amitriptyline, pethidine (Nymark and Møller Nielsen, 1963), imipramine (Loveless and Maxwell, 1965; Sinha *et al.*, 1969; Dixit *et al.*, 1970; Sinclair, 1973), chlorpheniramine, bropheniramine, pheniramine, mepyramine, tripelennamine (Sinclair, 1972*c*; Carlsson and Lindqvist, 1969), chlorimipramine (Carlsson *et al.*, 1969*b*), and dextromethorphan (Sinclair, 1973).

In the rabbit the symptoms produced by the combination of an MAOI with a 5-HT pump blocker include hypermotility, excitation, erect ears, dilated pupils, exophthalmos, forced superficial respiration, clonic convulsions, hyperpyrexia, and tremors. Most of these symptoms are similar to those seen in rabbits after LSD or 5-HTP.

As mentioned in Section 9.3, the behavioral effects of 5-HTP in rabbits, including fatal hyperpyrexia, are also potentiated by 5-HT-uptake inhibitors (Sinclair, 1972*a,c*, 1973; Carlsson *et al.*, 1969*a,b*).

The 5-HT-uptake inhibitors which produce toxic reactions with MAOIs have been found active in several other tests for 5-HT uptake inhibition, including:

1. Inhibition of 5-HT uptake into identified 5-HT neurons *in vivo* after intraventricular injection (Carlsson *et al.,* 1968; Fuxe and Ungerstedt, 1968).
2. Inhibition of 5-HT uptake into brain slices (Blackburn *et al.*, 1967; Carlsson, 1970; Shaskan and Snyder, 1970; Ross *et al.*, 1972; Van Der Zee and Hespe, 1973), synaptosomes (Tissari and Suurhasko, 1971; Lidbrink *et al.*, 1971; Kannengiesser *et al.*, 1973; Korduba *et al.*, 1973; Ciofalo, 1974; Horn and Trace, 1974; Squires, 1974; Ross and Renyi, 1975), or blood platelets (Yates *et al.*, 1964; Todrick and Tait, 1969; Ahtee and Saarnivaara, 1971, 1973; Oxenkrug, 1973; Buczko *et al.*, 1974; Tuomisto, 1974; Ahtee, 1975).
3. Antagonism of 5-HT depletion from brain induced by *p*-chloromethamphetamine (Meek *et al.*, 1971), *p*-chloroamphetamine (Squires, 1972*a*; Fuller *et al.*, 1974*a,b*; Buus Lassen *et al.*, 1975), fenfluramine (Ghezzi *et al.*, 1973), 1-*p*-acetyldeoxyephedrine (Dubnick *et al.*, 1973), or 4-methyl-α-ethyl-*m*-tyramine (H 75/12) (Carlsson *et al.*, 1969*a*).
4. Reduction in the concentration of 5-HIAA, the main metabolite of 5-HT, in brain (Squires, 1971; Alpers and Himwich, 1972; Halaris *et al.*, 1973; Fuller *et al.*, 1974*a,b*; Ahtee, 1975; Buus Lassen *et al.*, 1975).

In the early studies with rabbits it was suggested that the toxic symptoms produced by MAOIs together with certain other drugs might be due to enhanced central 5-HT function (Loveless and Maxwell, 1965; Penn and Rogers, 1971). This suggestion was supported by the finding that PCPA pretreatment protected rabbits from the fatal hyperpyrexia usually produced by the administration of an MAOI followed by the administration of pethidine (Fahim *et al.*, 1972), chlorpheniramine (Sinclair, 1972*c*), *d*-methorphan (Sinclair, 1973), or imipramine (Gong and Rogers, 1973; Mattila and Jounela, 1973). Although PCPA pretreatment completely protects rabbits from the toxic phenelzine–pethidine interaction, subsequent administration of 5-HTP does not restore toxicity, as it does in the mouse (Jounela, 1970), despite high levels of 5-HT in brain (Mattila and Jounela, 1973).

The syndrome in rabbits has been reported to be blocked or attenuated by chlorpromazine (Dixit *et al.*, 1970; Sinclair, 1973), chlorisondamine, reserpine, and dibenzyline (Dixit *et al.*, 1970). The fatal hyperpyrexia induced in rabbits by phenelzine combined with chlorpheniramine (Sinclair, 1972*c*) or *d*-methorphan (Sinclair, 1973) can be blocked by PCPA pretreatment but not by pretreatment with AMPT. In contrast to the finding of Dixit *et al.* (1970), reserpine was reported to protect against the fatal hyperpyrexia induced by the phenelzine–chlorpheniramine combination (Sinclair, 1972*c*). Thus the role of the catecholamines in the expression of the indoleamine syndrome in rabbits is not clear at present.

Inhibition of both MAO-A and MAO-B seems to be required for the full development of pethidine toxicity in rabbits (Jounela and Mattila, 1975). Selective inhibition of MAO-A with clorgyline (1, 5, or 20 mg/kg) increases 5-HT and NA levels in rabbit brain to about the same extent as phenelzine, but does not give rise to excitation and hyperpyrexia together with pethidine. Selective inhibition of MAO-B with deprenyl (1–20 mg/kg) has little or no effect on 5-HT or NA levels, or on behavior after pethidine. However, when rabbits are pretreated with a combination of clorgyline and deprenyl (1 or 5 mg/kg, each), pethidine now causes excitation and hyperpyrexia similar to that seen after phenelzine pretreatment. These results are analogous to the effects of clorgyline and deprenyl pretreatment of rats loaded with L-tryptophan (Squires and Buus Lassen, 1975).

In the spinalized cat the combination of a MAOI (pheniprazine or pargyline) with imipramine resulted in a 250% increase in the spike height of the monosynaptic reflex at L7 (Clineschmidt, 1972). The MAOIs increased the levels of 5-HT in the cat spinal cord but left that of NA unaffected, suggesting that 5-HT is the amine mainly involved in this MAOI–imipramine interaction.

10. POTENTIATION OF INDOLEAMINE HALLUCINOGENS

Several indolealkylamines, which produce LSD-like behavioral effects, are deaminated by MAO *in vivo*. These effects can therefore be intensified and prolonged by pretreatment with MAOIs. The amines include DMT (Szara, 1956; Marderosian *et al.*, 1968; Lu *et al.*, 1974; Moore *et al.*, 1975), *N,N*-diethyltryptamine (Szara *et al.*, 1966), psilocin (4-hydroxy-*N,N*-dimethyltryptamine) (Kalberer *et al.*, 1962), and 5-methoxy-*N*-methyltryptamine (Taborsky and McIsaac, 1964). Bufotenin (*N,N*-dimethylserotonin), although a rather poor substrate for MAO (Blaschko and Philpot, 1953; Govier *et al.*, 1953), is deaminated to 5-HIAA to some extent *in vivo* (Gessner *et al.*, 1960; Sanders and Bush, 1967). The behavioral effects of bufotenin (50 mg/kg i.p.), an indoleamine syndrome plus cyanosis, are potentiated by inhibition of either MAO-A and MAO-B by clorgyline and deprenyl, respectively (Squires, unpublished).

5-MeODMT, one of the more potent indolealkylamine hallucinogens (Gessner *et al.*, 1961), is a constituent of plants used by South American Indians as hallucinogens in mysticoreligious ceremonies (Pachter *et al.*, 1959), and of the Australian grass *Phalaris tuberosa* (Gallagher *et al.*, 1964). Sheep grazing on this grass sometimes suddenly collapse and die, or develop a more chronic syndrome, phalaris staggers, of motor incoordination, convulsive spasms, nodding of the head, and dilatation of the pupils (Gallagher *et al.*, 1964).

Sheep are particularly sensitive to 5-MeODMT, 0.1 mg/kg injected into the jugular vein producing an intense syndrome. Similar symptoms are also induced in sheep by somewhat larger doses of bufotenin and DMT, also major constituents of *Phalaris tuberosa* (Gallagher *et al.*, 1964). 5-MeODMT is also highly toxic to guinea pigs, rats, and mice.

Grahame-Smith (1971*b*) found that 5-MeODMT produced a syndrome in rats very similar to that seen after a MAOI and L-tryptophan. The behavioral effects of 5-MeODMT can be potentiated by pretreatment with a MAOI, but not blocked by pretreatment with PCPA, indicating that 5-MeODMT produces its effects by acting directly on a particular receptor, not by releasing 5-HT. In the rat, about 54% of a 5 mg/kg dose is converted to 5-methoxyindoleacetic acid (Agurell *et al.*, 1969; Ahlborg *et al.*, 1968). The formation of 5-methoxyindoleactic acid from 5-MeODMT can be completely blocked by selective inhibition of MAO-A with clorgyline. Deprenyl, a selective inhibitor of MAO-B, has no effect on the deamination of 5-MeODMT, either alone or in combination with clorgyline (Squires, 1975). Thus, *in vivo* in rats, 5-MeODMT appears to be a highly specific substrate for MAO-A. Pargyline was reported to potentiate the stimulating effect of 5-MeODMT on locomotor activity in mice (Vasko *et al.*, 1974). The stimulating effects of DMT and, to a lesser extent, tryptamine, 5-methoxytryptamine, and bufotenin were also potentiated by pretreatment with pargyline.

11. TRYPTAMINE POTENTIATION

MAOIs potentiate the pressor response to tryptamine (Goldberg and Sjoerdsma, 1959; Eble and Rudzik, 1966) in the dog.

In rats intravenous injection of tryptamine (10–40 mg/kg) produces body tremors, bilateral placing-type clonic movements of forepaws, hunching of the back, backward locomotion, straub tail, dyspnea, and severe asymmetrical clonic convulsions (Tedeschi, D. H., *et al.*, 1959). These effects of tryptamine were originally found to be strongly potentiated by iproniazid and pheniprazine (JB-516) (Tedeschi, D. H., *et al.*, 1959), and were subsequently found to be potentiated by many other MAOIs (Green, H., and Sawyer, 1960; Gylys *et al.*, 1963; Biel *et al.*, 1964; Maxwell, D. R., *et al.*, 1961; Tedeschi, R. E., *et al.*, 1959; Tedeschi, D. H., *et al.*, 1960; Zirkle *et al.*, 1962; Zirkle and Kaiser, 1964).

Delini-Stula and Maitre (1975) found that the behavioral pattern produced by tryptamine in pargyline-pretreated rats (backward movements, tremor, vocalization, pronounced irritability, and characteristic stereotyped agitation) could be selectively modified by different types of psychotropic drugs. Phenothiazine and butyrophenone neuroleptics selectively inhibit stereotyped agitation and produce general depression at higher doses. Clozapine, on the other hand, inhibited the stereotypies but increased locomotor activity. Backward movements and tremor were inhibited by 5-HT antagonists (methysergide, cyproheptadine). Vocalization and irritability were suppressed by sedative drugs such as benzoctamine and promazine, as well as by high doses of β-blockers. Antihistaminics and α-blockers were without effect.

The occurrence, duration, and relative intensity of clonic convulsions produced by the injection of tryptamine into rats pretreated with MAOIs was correlated with the concentration of the amine in brain (Green, H., and Sawyer, 1960). In mice and cats intravenous tryptamine also produces excitement (Vane *et al.*, 1961). In the cat the symptoms produced by tryptamine, which include unsheathing of claws, hissing, snarling, mydriasis, retraction of eyelids, and convulsions, could be prolonged by pretreatment with pheniprazine (Vane *et al.*, 1961). When tryptamine is infused intravenously in man, at a rate of about 0.2–0.4 mg/kg per min, it produces physical and mental changes similar to those produced by LSD, but with much more rapid onset and termination (Martin and Sloan, 1970). Coppen *et al.* (1965) reported that intravenous infusion of tryptamine at a rate of about 0.02 mg/kg per min in depressed patients pretreated with isocarboxazid did not produce pronounced mental or physical changes, probably because of the low infusion rate. Intravenous infusion of tryptamine in dogs has also been reported to produce LSD-like symptoms (Martin and Eades, 1970) which are potentiated by pretreatment with MAOIs. These observations suggest that tryptamine and LSD act on some common receptors (Martin and Eades, 1970; Martin and Sloan, 1970).

Rather high doses of various neuroleptics (e.g., chlorpromazine and perphenazine) (Tedeschi, D. H., *et al.*, 1959, 1961) can antagonize tryptamine convulsions. However, the combination of neuroleptics with tryptamine elicits another set of abnormal symptoms including sitting up on the hind legs for about 60 sec, tremor, and hyperemia. LSD and BOL also attenuate tryptamine convulsions but induce backward locomotion, side-to-side head movements, and occasional tremors (Tedeschi, D. H., *et al.*, 1959).

Although it is known that tryptamine is deaminated by both MAO-A and MAO-B (Johnston, 1968; Squires and Buus Lassen, 1968) *in vitro*, harmine, a selective inhibitor of MAO-A, is by far the most potent potentiator of the convulsant effects of tryptamine in rats (Tedeschi, D. H., *et al.*, 1960), indicating that, *in vivo*, tryptamine may be deaminated almost entirely by MAO-A.

12. POTENTIATION OF PHENETHYLAMINE HALLUCINOGENS

Large doses (50–100 mg/kg) of PEA produce a stereotyped behavioral syndrome similar to that produced by *d*-amphetamine (Gunn and Gurd, 1940; Randrup and Munkvad, 1966, 1970; Sabelli *et al.*, 1975). Since PEA is a specific substrate for MAO-B (Yang and Neff, 1973, 1974; Wu and Boulton, 1975; Sabelli *et al.*, 1975; Sabelli and Mosnaim, 1974), pretreatment with selective inhibitors of MAO-B (deprenyl or pargyline) or nonselective MAOIs will potentiate the behavioral effects of PEA (Sabelli *et al.*, 1975; Braestrup *et al.*, 1975). Deprenyl, but not clorgyline (a selective inhibitor of MAO-A), produced amphetamine-like stereotyped behavior with PEA (40 mg/kg) (Braestrup *et al.*, 1975).

β-(3,4-Dimethoxyphenylethylamine) (DMPEA) produces no appreciable effects in humans in doses up to 600 mg p.o. (Hollister and Friedhoff, 1966; Shulgin *et al.*, 1966), but is rapidly deaminated to 3,4-dimethoxyphenylacetic acid in man and in rats (Shulgin *et al.*, 1966; Charalampous and Tansey, 1967; Schweitzer and Friedhoff, 1968). Levels of DMPEA in several organs of the rat are increased after inhibition of MAO with iproniazid (Vogel, 1967, 1968; Vogel and Horwitt, 1967). In the rat DMPEA increases climbing time in the rope-climbing test of Winter and Flataker (1951), this effect being intensified by pretreatment with iproniazid, and the delay in rope-climbing time was directly related to brain levels of DMPEA (Vogel and Horwitt, 1967).

A large number of highly potent hallucinogenic amphetamine derivatives are known (Shulgin *et al.*, 1969; Symthies *et al.*, 1967; Snyder *et al.*, 1971; Ho *et al.*, 1970; Shulgin *et al.*, 1971) which are resistant to deamination by MAO because of the methyl group in the α position. The corresponding phenethylamine homologues of these amphetamine hallucinogens should be substrates for MAO, and their behavioral effects should therefore be potentiated by MAOIs. The interactions of only a few of these phenethylamine derivatives with MAOIs seem to have been investigated. 2,5-Dimethoxy-4-methylphenethylamine, the homologue of the potent hallucinogen DOM (STP), was found by Ho *et al.* (1970) to be almost as potent as DOM in

disrupting conditioned behavior in the rat. It would be of interest to determine whether the behavioral effects of this and related PEA derivatives can be potentiated by MAOIs.

13. HYPOTENSIVE EFFECTS

This subject has been reviewed by Schoepke and Swett (1967).

The hypotensive effects of the MAOIs were first discovered and extensively studied in man (Gillespie, L., *et al.*, 1959; Orvis *et al.*, 1959, 1963; Maronde and Haywood, 1963; Brunjes *et al.*, 1963; Maxwell, M. H., 1963; Brest *et al.*, 1963; Sjoerdsma *et al.*, 1959a; Pennes and Hoch, 1957; Arnow, 1959; Moser *et al.*, 1964; Lader *et al.*, 1970). However, it has proved difficult to consistently demonstrate hypotensive effects of the MAOIs in experimental animals. Acute administration of Modaline (W 3207A) caused only a transient, biphasic change in the blood pressure and heart rate of the dog (Gylys *et al.*, 1963). Acute and chronic administration of pargyline to rats, cats, and dogs produced only slight reductions in blood pressure (Schoepke and Wiegand, 1963; Schoepke and Swett, 1967). In the spinalized cat acute administration of pargyline produces hypertension, while in the decerebrate cat the same treatment results in slight hypotension and bradycardia (Lynes, 1966). Both pargyline and iproniazid antagonized the striking hypertensive response to electrical stimulation in the medulla at a site defined by Lynes (1966). In a preliminary communication Spencer *et al.* (1960) reported that tranylcypromine and some other MAOIs produced a slight to moderate hypotension of relatively long duration (24–72 hr) in dogs.

Toda *et al.* (1962) reported that repeated intravenous administration of tranylcypromine (0.5 mg/kg) to amobarbital-anesthetized dogs produced acute pressor responses followed by acute hypotensive responses of very short duration on the fifth injection. A similar pattern of pressor, followed by depressor, responses after repeated intravenous administrations was observed with methamphetamine. Kaul and Grewal (1972) reported that several 3-amino-2-oxazolidinone derivatives, which are potent MAOIs *in vivo*, showed powerful antihypertensive effects in renal hypertensive rats, but concluded that the correlation between the two effects was not very good. Glavas *et al.* (1965) reported that administration of small doses of tranylcypromine (1 mg/kg) to anaesthetized rats caused rapid, transient hypotension, while larger doses of tranylcypromine (10 mg/kg), pargyline (25 mg/kg), or pheniprazine (10 mg/kg) caused persistent hypotension. Chronic administration of pargyline, together with various combinations of L-dopa and a peripheral decarboxylase inhibitor, to spontaneously hypertensive (SH) rats, in the drinking water, reduced blood pressure and increased the levels of NA in the brainstem, with a good correlation between the two effects (Yamori *et al.*, 1972).

Several mechanisms have been proposed to account for the hypotensive effects of the MAOIs: (1) ganglionic blockade, (2) adrenergic blockade, (3) induced subsensitivity of adrenergic receptors, (4) inhibition of NA release from nerve terminals, (5) accumulation of false transmitter substances (e.g., octopamine) in sympathetic nerve terminals, (6) increased NA transmission in the nucleus tractus solitarii (De Jong, 1974). Mechanisms 1–5 have been discussed in detail by Schoepke and Swett (1967). Mechanisms 1–4 are at present considered unlikely. Mechanisms 5 and 6 will be considered in greater detail here.

13.1. The False-Transmitter Hypothesis

Davey *et al.* (1963) showed that chronic, but not acute, treatment with nialamide resulted in reduced release of NA in response to stimulation of the sympathetic nerves of the perfused cat spleen. Day and Rand (1963) reported that after treatment with nialamide, repeated tyramine administration resulted in reduced response to sympathetic nerve stimulation. This occurred to a lesser extent when MAO was not inhibited. It was suggested that amines might accumulate in tissues following MAO inhibition resulting in impaired release of NA from the sympathetic nerve terminals. Kakimoto and Armstrong (1962) found that octopamine levels increased greatly in the brain, heart, spleen, and kidney of rabbits treated with iproniazid, and suggested that the beneficial effects of MAOIs in the treatment of angina pain might result from the accumulation of octopamine in the heart. Kopin *et al.* (1964) demonstrated that after treatment with pheniprazine, octopamine accumulated in the heart, spleen, and salivary gland of the cat, as well as the salivary gland of the rat. In both cat and rat denervation prevented the accumulation of octopamine in salivary glands after pheniprazine treatment, indicating that this accumulation took place in sympathetic nerves. After nialamide administration to mice, labeled tyramine is rapidly taken up by the heart and converted to octopamine, which is retained long after the tyramine has disappeared (Carlsson and Waldeck, 1963). After similar infusion of tritium-labeled tyramine into the splenic artery of the cat, subsequent stimulation of the splenic nerve resulted in marked release of octopamine into the splenic perfusate (Kopin *et al.*, 1964, 1965).

On the basis of the experiments described above, Kopin *et al.* (1964, 1965) proposed that accumulation of octopamine in sympathetic nerves might play a role in the antihypertensive effects of the MAOIs. Octopamine is known to have only about 1% of the pressor activity of NA in the dog (Lands and Grant, 1952).

In the absence of MAO inhibition small concentrations of octopamine occur naturally in several peripheral organs, where it is highly localized in sympathetic nerves (Carlsson and Waldeck, 1963; Molinoff and Axelrod, 1969; Molinoff *et al.*, 1969). Endogenous octopamine is unevenly distributed in rat, guinea pig, and human brain (Saavedra, 1974). The octopamine/NA ratio seems to be lower in brain than in several sympathetically innervated organs (e.g., heart and spleen) of the rat, both before and after treatment with a MAOI (Molinoff and Axelrod, 1969; Kakimoto and Armstrong, 1962), suggesting that the replacement of NA by octopamine after inhibition of MAO may occur to a greater extent in peripheral sympathetic nerves than in NA neurons in the brain.

13.2. Centrally Mediated Reduction of Blood Pressure

This subject has been recently reviewed by Van Zwieten (1973), Laverty (1973), and Day and Roach (1974b). Several lines of recent evidence now suggest that blood pressure and heart rate may be reduced by stimulation of central α-noradrenergic receptors, perhaps located in the area of the nucleus tractus solitarii in the medulla, or in the hypothalamus.

1. Microinjections of NA into the nucleus tractus solitarii decrease arterial blood pressure and heart rate in anaesthetized rats, effects which can be prevented by preceding injection of the α-blocker, phentolamine, at the same site (De Jong, 1974; De Jong *et al.*, 1975; Struyker Boudier *et al.*, 1975).

2. L-dopa combined with a selective peripheral inhibitor of dopa-decarboxylase reduces blood pressure in conscious, normotensive rats, an effect which can be blocked by central inhibition of dopa-decarboxylase and dopamine-β-hydroxylase, as well as by α-blockers, but not by DA-receptor blockers (Henning and Rubenson, 1970). L-dopa plus peripheral decarboxylase inhibitor also reduces blood pressure in pentobarbitone-anaesthetized and decerebrated (by midcollicular transection), but not in spinalized (at C7–Th1), rats (Henning *et al.*, 1972).

3. Clonidine may also reduce blood pressure by stimulating central α-receptors (Van Zwieten, 1973; Katic *et al.*, 1972; Schmitt *et al.*, 1971; Haeusler, 1973; Day and Roach, 1974a).

4. Chronic administration of pargyline together with various concentrations of L-dopa and peripheral decarboxylase inhibitor in the drinking water resulted in a wide range of NA concentrations in the brainstem of SH rats which correlated well with reductions in blood pressure (Yamori *et al.*, 1972).

5. SH rats have significantly lower levels of NA and aromatic acid decarboxylase in brain than normotensive controls (Yamori *et al.*, 1970).

In addition to reduction of blood pressure mediated by stimulation of α-noradrenergic receptors in the nucleus tractus solitarii, NA may also be able to increase blood pressure by acting on other types of central receptors, perhaps located in the hypothalamus (Przuntek *et al.*, 1971; Day and Roach, 1974a). 5-HT may also participate in central mechanisms reducing blood pressure, since PCPA administered intracisternally or systemically (Ito and Schanberg, 1972; Yamori *et al.*, 1972) tends to increase blood pressure. Conversely, the 5-HT precursors 5-HTP and L-tryptophan reduce blood pressure in cats (Flórez and Armijo, 1974), effects which were enhanced by pretreatment with tranylcypromine, and prevented by a decarboxylase inhibitor (Ro 4-4502). In dogs pretreated with MAOIs, 5-HTP also produced hypotension which could be prevented by general, but not not selective extracerebral, decarboxylase inhibition. The hypotensive action of 5-HTP was attenuated by pretreatment with either yohimbine or methysergide, but was unaffected by haloperidol (Antonnaccio and Robson, 1975). It has also been proposed that the central hypotensive effect of L-dopa can be in part mediated by central 5-HT release (Antonaccio and Robson, 1974).

Recently, direct evidence has been obtained which indicates that central epinephrine neurons may be involved in regulating blood pressure. Epinephrine caused a decrease in arterial blood pressure and heart rate when injected into the anterior hypothalamic region of rats (Struyker Boudier and Bekers, 1975). Epinephrine is 10 times more potent than NA in inducing these effects. Epinephrine nerve terminals have been located in the rat hypothalamus (Hökfelt *et al.*, 1974; Koslow and Schlumpf, 1974; Saavedra *et al.*, 1974). It has been suggested that clonidine may reduce blood pressure by stimulating central epinephrine receptors (Bolme *et al.*, 1974, 1975).

Thus the MAOIs may reduce blood pressure by a combination of mechanisms, the most important being (1) accumulation of octopamine in sympathetic nerves, and (2) increasing the concentrations of epinephrine, NA, and 5-HT in brain. It is of interest that the selective inhibitors of MAO-A, harmine and harmaline (Gunn, 1935; Pennes and Hoch, 1957), given intravenously to humans produce marked hypotension and bradycardia, while clorgyline, another selective inhibitor of MAO-A, produces bradycardia in man after tyramine ingestion (Lader *et al.*, 1970).

14. TYRAMINE POTENTIATION

MAOIs can modify the cardiovascular effects of tyramine. Several MAOIs potentiate the pressor effect of tyramine in the dog (Goldberg and Sjoerdsma, 1959; Toda *et al.*, 1962; Eble and Rudzik, 1966; Gerold, 1968), rat (Vanov, 1962; Tedeschi, D. H., and Fellows, 1964; Palm and Magnus, 1967; Rand and Trinker, 1968; Halliday *et al.*, 1968; Clarke, 1970; Patane and Arrigo Reina, 1970; Olsson and Schrold, 1971; Renton and Eade, 1972; Obianwu, 1969), cat (Kayaalp *et al.*, 1968), rabbit (Airaksinen *et al.*, 1966), and man (Pettinger and Oates, 1968). However, the development of tachyphylaxis to the pressor response of tyramine is more rapid in the nialamide-pretreated cat, rabbit, guinea pig, and rat (Davey *et al.*, 1963; Day and Rand, 1963). Similarly, the NA-depleting action of tyramine in rat heart is potentiated by pretreatment with pargyline (Spano, 1966). The development of tachyphylaxis to tyramine in the isolated guinea pig heart is associated with a decrease in the myocardial concentration of NA (Davey *et al.*, 1963).

Chronic pretreatment with pargyline (75 mg/kg per day for 7 days) strongly potentiated the contractile response of isolated guinea pig left atrial strips to tyramine (Antonaccio and Smith, 1967), and similar potentiation was seen after acute pretreatment with iproniazid or pheniprazine (Furchgott and Garcia, 1968). Iproniazid and nialamide increased the sensitivity of rabbit ear artery to intraluminally applied tyramine (De la Lande *et al.*, 1970). Administration of iproniazid, isocarboxazid, or clorgyline (a selective inhibitor of MAO-A) to depressed human subjects potentiated the mydriasis induced by 2% tyramine solution instilled into the eye (Bevan-Jones and Lind, 1971). Chronic administration of clorgyline (10–20 mg/day) markedly potentiated the bradycardia-inducing action of tyramine given orally to human volunteers (Lader *et al.*, 1970).

Severe hypertension has been reported in patients treated with MAOIs after eating cheese, beans, or certain yeast extracts (Blackwell, 1963; Blackwell *et al.*, 1965), and the tyramine content of these foods is considered to be the principal pressor substance involved (Blackwell and Mabbitt, 1965; Horwitz *et al.*, 1964).

The potentiation of the pressor action of tyramine by MAOIs may be only partly due to inhibition of tyramine's deamination by MAO, since other pressor amines, such as amphetamine, mephentermine, and ephedrine (Rand and Trinker, 1968; Elis *et al.*, 1967; O'Dea and Rand, 1969), which are not substrate for MAO are nevertheless potentiated by MAOIs. This potentiation seems likely to be due to increases in the concentrations of endogenous intraneuronal catecholamine (NA), which is released from its stores by the pressor amines (Elis *et al.*, 1967).

15. INTERACTIONS OF THE MAOIs WITH RESERPINE AND TETRABENAZINE

The early literature on MAOI–reserpine interactions was reviewed in detail by Biel *et al.* (1964) and Zirkle and Kaiser (1964). MAOI–reserpine-induced behavioral excitation was reviewed in Section 9.1. Pretreatment with MAOIs can prevent or attenuate many of the behavioral and physiologic changes induced by reserpine or tetrabenazine, including (1) depletion of cerebral NA, DA, and 5-HT; (2) sedation; (3) ptosis; (4) hypothermia; (5) depression of food-reinforced operant behavior (McKearney, 1968); (6) depression of avoidance responding (Heise and Boff, 1960; Bocknik *et al.*, 1968); (7) inhibition of DBH (Roth and Stone, 1968; Jonason and Rutledge, 1969); (8) reduction in threshold for electroshock and Metrazol convulsions (Prockop *et al.*, 1959*a,b*; Gray and Rauh, 1967; Rudzik and Mennear, 1966).

Prior inhibition of MAO-A alone appears to provide maximum protection against the usual effects of reserpine, administered subsequently (Pletscher *et al.*, 1959; Bocknik *et al.*, 1968; Fuentes and Neff, 1975; Squires, unpublished). Pretreatment with deprenyl (E-250), a selective inhibitor of MAO-B, is entirely without reserpine-antagonistic effect (Fuentes and Neff, 1975; Squires, unpublished). Simultaneous inhibition of MAO-A and MAO-B before the administration of reserpine produces the well-known behavioral excitation which is prevented by pretreatment with PCPA, and potentiated by L-tryptophan loading (Squires, unpublished).

However, when an MAOI is administered 2 hr or more after reserpine, most of the reserpine symptoms remain unchanged at least for several hours. Rats pretreated with reserpine followed by simultaneous inhibition of MAO-A and MAO-B and subsequent L-tryptophan loading also exhibit the indoleamine syndrome as described above. Under these conditions both NA and DA are low, while 5-HT is elevated. Unless both MAO-A and MAO-B are simultaneously inhibited the syndrome is not produced and the rats exhibit only reserpine symptoms (Squires, unpublished).

16. ANTICONVULSANT ACTIONS OF MAOIs

16.1. Electroshock and Metrazol Convulsions

Prockop et al. (1959a,b) were the first to report antagonism of electro-shock and Metrazol seizures in rats by several MAOIs. This finding has been confirmed by some investigators (P'an et al., 1961; Anderson et al., 1962; Chow and Hendley, 1959; Yen et al., 1962; Schlesinger et al., 1968b), but not by others (Bonnycastle et al., 1957; Kobinger, 1958; Lessin and Parkes, 1959; Sansone and Dell'Omodarme, 1963; Spoerlein and Ellman, 1961; Squires and Buus Lassen, 1968; Buus Lassen, 1972b).

However, the well-known ability of reserpine, tetrabenazine, and related amine depletors to facilitate electroshock and Metrazol seizures (Chen et al., 1954, 1968; Chen and Bohner, 1957, 1961; Prockop et al., 1959b; Lessin and Parkes, 1959; Schlesinger et al., 1968b; Azzaro et al., 1972; Wenger et al., 1973; Jobe et al., 1974) and to antagonize the anticonvulsant effects of various drugs (Gray et al., 1958, 1963; Rudzik and Mennear, 1965, 1966; Gray and Rauh, 1967, 1968, 1971) can be reduced or prevented by pretreatment with various MAOIs (Prockop et al., 1959a,b; Lessin and Parkes, 1959; Chen and Bohner, 1961; Gray et al., 1963; Rudzik and Mennear, 1965, 1966; Gray and Rauh, 1967; Chen et al., 1968; Pfeifer and Galambos, 1967).

The antagonism of electroshock and Metrazol seizures by 5-HTP in rats and mice is greatly potentiated by pretreatment with MAOIs (Prockop et al., 1959b; Lessin and Parkes, 1959; Chen and Bohner, 1961; Buus Lassen, 1972b).

Both 5-HT and catecholamines (especially NA) appear to play roles in determining the seizure thresholds for electroshock and Metrazol: L-dopa, especially when combined with iproniazid, was effective in reversing reserpine-induced facilitation of Metrazol seizures in mice (Chen and Bohner, 1961), and in reversing reserpine-induced antagonism of the protective effect of methazolamide against electroshock seizures (Gray *et al.*, 1963; Gray and Rauh, 1968). Reserpine antagonism of the antielectroconvulsive effect of acteazolamide can be prevented by pretreatment with α-methyl-dopa, while the antielectroconvulsive effect of acetazolamide is also antagonized by both α- and β-adrenergic blockers (Rudzik and Mennear, 1966). Substances which potentiate or release NA, such as imipramine, desipramine, amitriptyline, cocaine, and desoxyephedrine, antagonize the facilitating effect of tetrabenazine on electroshock seizures (Chen *et al.*, 1968). 5-HTP, together with a peripheral decarboxylase inhibitor (Ro 4-4602), protects rats from Metrazol-induced seizures (De La Torre *et al.*, 1970; De La Torre and Mullan, 1970). PCPA pretreatment facilitates Metrazol (De La Torre and Mullan, 1970; Alexander and Kopeloff, 1970; Meyer and Frey, 1973) and electroshock (Koe and Weissman, 1968; Gray and Rauh, 1971) convulsions. AMPT, disulfiram, and PCPA pretreatment potentiate and prolong the facilitating effect of reserpine on electroshock seizures (Gray and Rauh, 1971; Azzaro *et al.*, 1972; Wenger *et al.*, 1973). The anticonvulsant effect of imipramine is potentiated by L-dopa and 5-HTP (Chen *et al.*, 1968). Similarly, the anticonvulsant effects of 5-HTP are potentiated by imipramine, chlorimipramine, and nortriptyline (Buus Lassen, 1972*b*).

16.2. Audiogenic Seizures

In 1963 Plotnikoff *et al.* (1963) reported that six MAOIs (iproniazid, tranylcypromine, pheniprazine, α-ethyltryptamine, phenelzine, and nialamide) could protect mice from audiogenic seizures. Schlesinger *et al.* (1968*a*) confirmed that iproniazid and pheniprazine can protect seizure-susceptible (DBA/2J) mice from audiogenic seizures. Lehmann (1967) found that isocarboxazide, nialamide, harmaline, and tranylcypromine protected mice from the clonic phase of audiogenic seizures and, together with pyrogallol, also against the tonic phase. Iproniazid, while ineffective when administered alone, together with 5-HTP effectively protected rats from audiogenic seizures (Jobe *et al.*, 1973*b*).

Similar to electroshock- and Metrazol-induced convulsions, catecholamines and 5-HT both seem to be involved in determining the susceptibility of mice and rats to audiogenic seizures: reserpine, tetrabenazine, AMPT, and PCPA all increase the susceptibility of mice to audiogenic seizures (Lehmann, 1967; Schlesinger *et al.*, 1968*a*). In rats, the benzoquinolizine amine depletor, Ro 4-1284, as well as reserpine and PCPA, intensified audiogenic seizures (Jobe *et al.*, 1973*a,b*). Pretreatment with AMPT or DDC alone seems to have little effect on the susceptibility of rats to audiogenic seizures. However, these substances markedly potentiate and prolong the facilitating effect of Ro 4-

1284 (Jobe *et al.*, 1973*a*). Other drugs which release or potentiate NA or 5-HT or both (e.g., amphetamine, *p*-chlorometamphetamine, imipramine) also inhibit audiogenic seizures in rats and mice (Lehmann, 1967; Jobe *et al.*, 1973*a*).

16.3. Other Types of Seizures

One MAOI, JB-807, which was reported to antagonize electroshock and Metrazol seizures in mice, did not prevent caffeine or strychnine convulsions (Prockop *et al.*, 1959*b*). Picrotoxin-induced convulsions appear to be potentiated by nialamide and tranylcypromine, as well as by several thymoleptics, AMPT, and 5-HTP (Cowan and Harry, 1974). Pretreatment with PCPA does not seem to influence picrotoxin convulsions. Iproniazid was reported to facilitate and prolong lidocaine-induced seizures in mice, an effect which is potentiated by 5-HTP (De Oliveira and Bretas, 1974). Pretreatment with PCPA slightly inhibited lidocaine seizures.

16.4. Conclusions

Both endogenous 5-HT and catecholamines seem to be involved in the inhibition of electroshock, Metrazol, and audiogenic seizures, whereas these amine systems do not influence, or promote, caffeine, strychnine, picrotoxin, or lidocaine seizures. Inhibition of MAO-A alone may be sufficient to antagonize electroshock (Prockop *et al.*, 1959*b*) and audiogenic (Lehmann, 1967) seizures, since harmaline has an inhibitory effect on both seizure forms.

17. REFERENCES

AGHAJANIAN, G. K., 1972, Influence of drugs on the firing of serotonin-containing neurons in brain, *Fed. Proc. Fed. Am. Soc. Exp. Biol.* **31**:91–96.
AGHAJANIAN, G. K., GRAHAM, A. W., and SHEARD, M. H., 1970, Serotonin-containing neurons in brain: Depression of firing by monoamine oxidase inhibitors, *Science* **169**:1100–1102.
AGHAJANIAN, G. K., HAIGLER, H. J., and BLOOM, F. E., 1972, Lysergic acid diethylamide and serotonin: Direct actions on serotonin-containing neurons in rat brain, *Life Sci.* **11**:615–622.
AGURELL, S., HOLMSTEDT, B., and LINDGREN, J. E., 1969, Metabolism of 5-methoxy-*N,N*-dimethyltryptamine-¹⁴C in the rat, *Biochem. Pharmacol.* **18**:2771–2781.
AHLBORG, U., HOLMSTEDT, B., and LINDGREN, J. E., 1968, Fate and metabolism of some hallucinogenic indolealkylamines, in: *Advances in Pharmacology* (S. Garattini and P. A. Shores, eds.), Vol. 6B, pp. 213–229, Academic Press, New York.
AHLENIUS, S., ERIKSSON, H., LARSSON, K., MODIGH, K., and SÖDERSTEN, P., 1971, Mating

behavior in the male rat treated with *p*-chlorophenylalanine methyl ester alone and in combination with pargyline, *Psychopharmacologia* **20**:383–388.

AHTEE, L., 1975, Dextromethorphan inhibits 5-hydroxytryptamine uptake by human blood platelets and decreases 5-hydroxyindoleacetic acid content in rat brain, *J. Pharm. Pharmacol.* **27**:117–180.

AHTEE, L., and SAARNIVAARA, L., 1971, The effect of drugs upon the uptake of 5-hydroxytryptamine and metaraminol by human platelets, *J. Pharm. Pharmacol.* **23**:495–501.

AHTEE, L., and SAARNIVAARA, L., 1973, The effect of narcotic analgesics on the uptake of 5-hydroxytryptamine and (−)-metaraminol by blood platelets, *Br. J. Pharmacol.* **47**:808–818.

AIRAKSINEN, M. M., MUSTALA, O., and TORSTI, P., 1966, Effects of some biogenic amines on the blood pressure of pargyline-treated rabbits, *Ann. Med. Exp. Fenn.* **44**:376–381.

ALEXANDER, G. J., and KOPELOFF, L. M., 1970, Metrazol seizures in rats: Effect of *p*-chlorophenylalanine, *Brain Res.* **22**:231–235.

ALLEVA, J. J., and UMBERGER, E. J., 1966, Evidence for neural control of the release of pituitary ovulating hormone in the golden syrian hamster, *Endocrinology* **78**:1125.

ALLEVA, J. J., OVERPECK, J. G., and UMBERGER, E. J., 1966, Effect of tranylcypromine and iproniazid on brain amine levels and ovulation in the golden hamster, *Life Sci.* **5**:1557–1561.

ALPERS, H. S., and HIMWICH, H. E., 1972, The effects of chronic imipramine administration on rat brain levels of serotonin, 5-hydroxyindoleacetic acid, norepinephrine and dopamine, *J. Pharmacol. Exp. Ther.* **180**:531–538.

ALTIER, H., MOLDES, M., and MONTI, J. M., 1975, The actions of dihydroxyphenylalanine and dihydroxyphenylserine on the sleep–wakefulness cycle of the rat after peripheral decarboxylase inhibition, *Br. J. Pharmacol.* **54**:101–106.

ANDÉN, N.-E., CORRODI, H., and FUXE, K., 1972, Effect of neuroleptic drugs on central catecholamine turnover assessed using tyrosine- and dopamine-β-hydroxylase inhibitors, *J. Pharm. Pharmacol.* **24**:177–182.

ANDERSON, E. G., MARKOWITZ, S. D., and BONNYCASTLE, D. D., 1962, Brain 5-hydroxytryptamine and anticonvulsant activity, *J. Pharmacol. Exp. Ther.* **136**:179–182.

ANTONACCIO, M. J., and ROBSON, R. D., 1974, L-Dopa hypotension in dogs: Evidence for mediation through 5-HT release, *Arch. Int. Pharmacodyn. Ther.* **212**:89–102.

ANTONACCIO, M. J., and ROBSON, R. D., 1975, Centrally mediated cardiovascular effects of 5-hydroxytryptophan in MAO-inhibited dogs: Modification by autonomic antagonists, *Arch. Int. Pharmacodyn. Ther.* **213**:200–210.

ANTONACCIO, M. J., and SMITH, C. B., 1967, Effects of chronic pretreatment with pargyline on the contractile responses of isolated guinea-pig left atrial strips to tyramine, *d*-amphetamine and adrenergic nerve stimulation, *Pharmacologist* **9**:211.

ARIOKA, I., and TANIMUKAI, H., 1957, Histochemical studies on monoamine oxidase in the mid-brain of the mouse, *J. Neurochem.* **1**:311–315.

ARNOW, L. E., 1959, Phenelzine: A therapeutic agent for mental depression, *Clin. Med.* **6**:1573–1577.

BLACKWELL, B., MARLEY, E., and MABBIT, L. A., 1965, Effects of yeast extract after monoamine-oxidase inhibition, *Lancet* **1**:940–943.

BLASCHKO, H., 1952, Amine oxidase and amine metabolism, *Pharmacol. Rev.* **4**:415–458.

BLASCHKO, H., 1963, Amine oxidase, in: *The Enzymes* (P. D. Boyer, ed.), pp. 337–351, Academic Press, New York.

BLASCHKO, H., and PHILPOT, F. J., 1953, Enzymic oxidation of tryptamine derivatives, *J. Physiol. (London)* **122**:403–408.

BLOOM, F. E., SIMS, K. L., WEITSEN, H. A., DAVIS, G. A., and HANKER, J. S., 1972, Cytochemical differentiation between monoamine oxidase and other neuronal oxidases, in: *Advances in Biochemical Psychopharmacology*, Vol. 5 (E. Costa and M. Sandler, eds.), pp. 243–262, Raven Press, New York.

Bocknik, S. E., Hingtgen, J. N., Hughes, F. W., and Forney, R. B., 1968, Harmaline effects on tetrabenazine depression of avoidance responding in rats, *Life Sci.* **7**(Pt. I):1189–1201.

Bogdanski, D. F., Weissbach, H., and Udenfriend, S., 1958, Pharmacological studies with the serotonin precursor, 5-hydroxytryptophan, *J. Pharmacol. Exp. Ther.* **122**:188–194.

Boling, J. L., and Blandau, R. J., 1939, The estrogen–progesterone induction of mating responses in the spayed female rat, *Endocrinology* **25**:359–364.

Bolme, P., Corrodi, H., Fuxe, K., Hökfelt, T., Lidbrink, P., and Goldstein, M., 1974, Possible involvement of central adrenaline neurons in vasomotor and respiratory control. Studies with clonidine and its interactions with piperoxane and yohimbine, *Eur. J. Pharmacol.* **28**:89–94.

Bolme, P., Fuxe, K., and Hökfelt, T., 1975, Evidence for a central inhibitory adrenaline and GABA mechanism in the control of arterial blood pressure, 6th International Congress of Pharmacology, July 20–25, Helsinki, Abstract No. 1377, p. 570.

Bond, V. J., Shillito, E. E., and Vogt, M., 1972, Influence of age and of testosterone on the response of male rats to parachlorophenylalanine, *Br. J. Pharmacol.* **46**:46–55.

Bonnycastle, D. D., Giarman, N. J., and Paasonen, M. K., 1957, Anticonvulsant compounds and 5-hydroxytryptamine in rat brain, *Br. J. Pharmacol.* **12**:228–231.

Bouchaud, C., and Jacque, C., 1971, La restauration des monoamine oxydases (MAO) chez le rat après inhibition "irréversible." Étude biochimique et histochimique comparée, *Histochemie* **28**:355–366.

Boulton, A. A., and Baker, G. B., 1975, The subcellular distribution of β-phenylethylamine, p-tyramine and tryptamine in rat brain, *J. Neurochem.* **25**:477–481.

Bowers, M., and Kupfer, D. J., 1971, Central monoamine oxidase inhibition and REM sleep, *Brain Res.* **35**:561–564.

Brachfeld, J., Wirtshafter, A., and Wolfe, S., 1963, Imipramine–tranylcypromine incompatibility. Near-fatal toxic reaction, *J. Am. Med. Assoc.* **186**:1172–1173.

Braestrup, C., Andersen, H., and Randrup, A., 1975, The monoamine oxidase β-inhibitor deprenyl potentiates phenylethylamine behaviour in rat without inhibition of catecholamine metabolite formation, *Eur. J. Pharmacol.* **34**:181–187.

Bramwell, G. J., 1974, The effect of antidepressants on unit activity in the midbrain raphé of rats, *Arch. Intern. Pharmacodyn. Ther.* **211**:24–33.

Brest, A. N., Onesti, G., Heider, C., and Moyer, J. H., 1963, Cardiac and renal hemodynamic response to pargyline, *Ann. N. Y. Acad. Sci.* **107**:1016–1021.

Brodie, B. B., Pletscher, A., and Shore, P. A., 1956, Possible role of serotonin in brain function and in reserpine action, *J. Pharmacol. Exp. Ther.* **116**:9.

Brodie, B. B., Spector, S., and Shore, P. A., 1959, Interaction of monoamine oxidase inhibitors with physiological and biochemical mechanisms in brain, *Ann. N. Y. Acad. Sci.* **80**:609–614.

Brownlee, G., and Williams, G. W., 1963, Potentiation of amphetamine and pethidine by monoamineoxidase inhibitors, *Lancet* **1**:669.

Brunjes, S., Haywood, L. J., and Maronde, R. F., 1963, A controlled study of the antihypertensive response to an MAO inhibitor. B. Urinary excretion of catecholamines and their metabolites, *Ann. N. Y. Acad. Sci.* **107**:982–991.

Buczko, W., De Gaetano, G., and Garattini, S., 1974, Influence of some tricyclic antidepressive drugs on the uptake of 5-hydroxytryptamine by rat blood platelets, *J. Pharm. Pharmacol.* **26**:814–815.

Buus Lassen, J., 1972a, Behavioral effect of tricyclic thymoleptics and chlorpheniramine in mice after pretreatment with 5-hydroxytryptophan (5HTP), *Acta Pharmacol. Toxicol.* **31**(Suppl. I):11.

Buus Lassen, J., 1972b, Potentiation of the anticonvulsant effect of 5-hydroxy-tryptophan (5HTP) in mice by tricyclic thymoleptics and MAO inhibitors, 5th International Congress of Pharmacology, July 23–28 (abstract).

Buus Lassen, J., Squires, R. F., Christensen, J. A., and Molander, L., 1975, Neurochemical and pharmacological studies on a new 5HT-uptake inhibitor, FG 4963, with potential antidepressant properties, *Psychopharmacologia* **42**:21–26.

CARLSSON, A., 1970, Structural specificity for inhibition of [^{14}C]5-hydroxytryptamine uptake by cerebral slices, *J. Pharm. Pharmacol.* **22**:729–732.

CARLSSON, A., and CORRODI, H., 1964, In den Catecholamin-Metabolismus eingreifende Substanzen. 3. 2,3-Dihydroxyphenylacetamide und verwandte Verbindungen, *Helv. Chim. Acta* **47**:1340–1349.

CARLSSON, A., and LINDQVIST, M., 1963, Effect of chlorpromazine or haloperidol on formation of 3-methoxytyramine and normetanephrine in mouse brain, *Acta Pharmacol. Toxicol.* **20**:140–144.

CARLSSON, A., and LINDQVIST, M., 1969, Central and peripheral monoaminergic membrane-pump blockade by some addictive analgesics and antihistamines, *J. Pharm. Pharmacol.* **21**:460–464.

CARLSSON, A., and WALDECK, B., 1963, β-Hydroxylation of tyramine *in vivo*, *Acta Pharmacol. Toxicol.* **20**:371–374.

CARLSSON, A., DAHLSTRÖM, A., FUXE, K., and LINDQVIST, M., 1965, Histochemical and biochemical detection of monoamine release from brain neurons, *Life Sci.* **4**:809–816.

CARLSSON, A., FUXE, K., and UNGERSTEDT, U., 1968, The effect of imipramine on central 5-hydroxytryptamine neurons, *J. Pharm. Pharmacol.* **20**:150–151.

CARLSSON, A., CORRODI, H., FUXE, K., and HÖKFELT, T., 1969*a*, Effect of antidepressant drugs on the depletion of intraneuronal brain 5-hydroxytryptamine stores caused by 4-methyl-α-ethyl-*meta*-tyramine, *Eur. J. Pharmacol.* **5**:357–366.

CARLSSON, A., JONASON, J., LINDQVIST, M., and FUXE, K., 1969*b*, Demonstration of extraneuronal 5-hydroxytryptamine accumulation in brain following membrane-pump blockade by chlorimipramine, *Brain Res.* **12**:456–460.

CHARALAMPOUS, K. D., and TANSEY, L. W., 1967, Metabolic fate of β-(3,4-dimethoxyphenyl)-ethylamine in man, *J. Pharmacol. Exp. Ther.* **155**:318–329.

CHEN, G., and BOHNER, B., 1957, A method for the biological assay of reserpine and reserpine-like activity, *J. Pharmacol. Exp. Ther.* **119**:559–565.

CHEN, G., and BOHNER, B., 1961, The anti-reserpine effects of certain centrally-acting agents, *J. Pharmacol. Exp. Ther.* **131**:179–184.

CHEN, G., ENSOR, C. R., and BOHNER, B., 1954, A facilitation action of reserpine on the central nervous system, *Proc. Soc. Exp. Biol. Med.* **86**:507–510.

CHEN, G., ENSOR, C. R., and BOHNER, B., 1968, Drug effects on the disposition of active biogenic amines in the CNS, *Life Sci.* **7**(Pt. I):1063–1074.

CHESSIN, M., KRAMER, E. R., and SCOTT, C. C., 1957, Modifications of the pharmacology of reserpine and serotonin by iproniazid, *J. Pharmacol. Exp. Ther.* **119**:453–460.

CHOW, M.-I., and HENDLEY, C. D., 1959, Effect of monoamine oxidase inhibitors on experimental convulsions, *Fed. Proc. Fed. Am. Soc. Exp. Biol.* **18**:376.

CHRISTMAS, A. J., COULSON, C. J., MAXWELL, D. R., and RIDDELL, D., 1972, A comparison of the pharmacological and biochemical properties of substrate-selective monoamine oxidase inhibitors, *Br. J. Pharmacol.* **45**:490–503.

CIOFALO, F. R., 1974, Methadone inhibition of ^{3}H-5-hydroxytryptamine uptake by synaptosomes, *J. Pharmacol. Exp. Ther.* **189**:83–89.

CLARKE, D. E., 1970, Restoration of tyramine responses by bretylium, BW 392C60, bethanidine and monoamine oxidase inhibitors in reserpine-treated rats, *Br. J. Pharmacol.* **38**:1–11.

CLEMENT, A. J., and BENAZON, D., 1962, Reactions to other drugs in patients taking monoamine-oxidase inhibitors, *Lancet* **2**:197–198.

CLINESCHMIDT, B. V., 1972, Spinal monoamines and the toxic interaction between monoamine oxidase inhibitors and tricyclic antidepressants, *Eur. J. Pharmacol.* **19**:126–129.

CONSOLO, S., GIACOBINI, E., and KARJALAINEN, K., 1968, Monoamine oxidase in sympathetic ganglia of the cat, *Acta Physiol. Scand.* **74**:513–520.

COPPEN, A., SHAW, D. M., MALLESON, A., ECCLESTON, E., and GUNDY, G., 1965, Tryptamine metabolism in depression, *Br. J. Psychiatry* **3**:993–998.

CORNE, S. J., PICKERING, R. W., and WARNER, B. T., 1963, A method for assessing the effects of drugs on the central actions of 5-hydroxytryptamine, *Br. J. Pharmacol.* **20**:106–120.

CORRODI, H., 1966, Blockade of the psychotic syndrome caused by nialamide in mice, *J. Pharm. Pharmacol.* **18**:197–199.

CORRODI, H., and FUXE, K., 1967, The effect of catecholamine precursors and monoamine oxidase inhibition on the amine levels of central catecholamine neurons after reserpine treatment or tyrosine hydroxylase inhibition, *Life Sci.* **6**:1345–1350.

COWAN, A., and HARRY, E. J. R., 1974, Potentiation of picrotoxin-induced convulsions in mice by antidepressants. Specificity of the effect, *Br. J. Pharmacol.* **52**:432P.

COYLE, J. T., and SNYDER, S. H., 1969a, Catecholamine uptake by synaptosomes in homogenates of rat brain: Stereospecificity in different areas, *J. Pharmacol. Exp. Ther.* **170**:221–231.

COYLE, J. T., and SNYDER, S. H., 1969b, Antiparkinsonian drugs: Inhibition of dopamine uptake in the corpus striatum as a possible mechanism of action, *Science* **166**:899–901.

CRAIG, D. D. ., 1962, Reaction to pethidine in patients on phenelzine, *Lancet* **2**:559.

DAHLSTRÖM, A., 1972, The axonal transport of monoamine oxidases, in: *Advances in Biochemical Psychopharmacology*, Vol. 5 (E. Costa and M. Sandler, eds.), pp. 293–305, Raven Press, New York.

DAHLSTRÖM, A., and FUXE, K., 1964, Evidence for the existence of monoamine-containing neurons in the central nervous system. I. Demonstration of monoamines in the cell bodies of brain stem neurons, *Acta Physiol. Scand.* **62**(Suppl. 232):5–55.

DAHLSTRÖM, A., JONASON, J., and NORBERG, K.-A., 1969, Monoamine oxidase activity in rat sciatic nerves after constriction, *Eur. J. Pharmacol.* **6**:248–254.

DALY, E. C., and APRISON, M. H., 1974, Distribution of serine hydroxymethyltransferase and glycine transaminase in several areas of the central nervous system of the rat, *J. Neurochem.* **22**:877–885.

DA PRADA, M., CARRUBA, M., SANER, A., O'BRIEN, R. A., and PLETSCHER, A., 1973, The action of L-dopa on sexual behaviour of male rats, *Brain Res.* **55**:383–389.

DAVEY, M. J., FARMER, J. B., and REINERT, H., 1963, The effects of nialamide on adrenergic functions, *Br. J. Pharmacol.* **20**:121–134.

DAVIES, G., 1960, Side-effects of phenelzine, *Br. Med. J.* **2**:1019.

DAVIS, J. N., CARLSSON, A., MACMILLIAN, V., and SIESJÖ, B. K., 1973, Brain tryptophan hydroxylation: Dependence on arterial oxygen tension, *Science* **182**:72–74.

DAVISON, A. N., 1958, Physiological role of monoamine oxidase, *Physiol. Rev.* **38**:729–747.

DAY, M. D., and RAND, M. J., 1963, Tachyphylaxis to some sympathomimetic amines in relation to monoamine oxidase, *Br. J. Pharmacol.* **21**:84–96.

DAY, M. D., and ROACH, A. G., 1974a, Central α- and β-adrenoceptors modifying arterial blood pressure and heart rate in conscious cats, *Br. J. Pharmacol.* **51**:325–333.

DAY, M. D., and ROACH, A. G., 1974b, Central adrenoreceptors and the control of arterial blood pressure, *Clin. Exp. Pharmacol. Physiol.* **1**:347–360.

DE JONG, W., 1974, Noradrenaline: Central inhibitory control of blood pressure and heart rate, *Eur. J. Pharmacol.* **29**:179–181.

DE JONG, W., NIJKAMP, F. P., and BOHUS, B., 1975, Role of noradrenaline and serotonin in the central control of blood pressure in normotensive and spontaneously hypertensive rats, *Arch. Intern. Pharmacodyn. Ther.* **213**:272–284.

DE LA LANDE, I. S., HILL, B. D., JELLETT, L. B., and MCNEIL, J. M., 1970, The role of monoamine oxidase in the response of the isolated central artery of the rabbit ear to tyramine, *Br. J. Pharmacol.* **40**:249–256.

DE LA TORRE, J. C., and MULLAN, S., 1970, A possible role for 5-hydroxytryptamine in drug-induced seizures, *J. Pharm. Pharmacol.* **22**:858–859.

DE LA TORRE, J. C., KAWANAGA, H. M., and MULLAN, S., 1970, Seizure susceptibility after manipulation of brain serotonin, *Arch. Intern. Pharmacodyn. Ther.* **188**:298–304.

DEL FIACCO, M., FRATTA, W., GESSA, G. L., and TAGLIAMONTE, A., 1974, Lack of copulatory behaviour in male castrated rats after p-chlorophenylalanine, Br. J. Pharmacol. **51**:249–251.

DELINI-STULA, A., and MAITRE, L., 1975, Effects of psychotropic drugs on the behaviour produced by combined treatment with pargyline and tryptamine, 6th International Congress of Pharmacology, July 20–25, Helsinki (abstract).

DE LORES ARNAIZ, G. R., and DE ROBERTIS, E. D. P., 1962, Cholinergic and non-cholinergic nerve endings in the rat brain. II, J. Neurochem. **9**:503–508.

DELORME, F., JEANNEROD, M., and JOUVET, M., 1965, Effets remarquables de la réserpine sur l'activité EEG phasique ponto-géniculo-occipitale, C. R. Soc. Biol. **159**:900–903.

DENTON, P. H., BORELLI, V. M., and EDWARDS, N. V., 1962, Dangers of monoamine oxidase inhibitors, Br. Med. J. **2**:1752–1753.

DE OLIVEIRA, L. F., and BRETAS, A. D., 1974, Effects of 5-hydroxytryptophan, iproniazid and p-chlorophenylalanine on lidocaine seizure threshold of mice, Eur. J. Pharmacol. **29**:5–9.

DEWSBURY, D. A., DAVIS, H. N., and JANSEN, P. E., 1972, Effects of monoamine oxidase inhibitors on the copulatory behavior of male rats, Psychopharmacologia **24**:209–217.

DIXIT, K. S., DHASMANA, K. M., SINHA, J. N., and BHARGAVA, K. P., 1970, Role of catecholamines in fatal hyperpyrexia induced by imipramine in MAOI treated rabbits, Arch. Intern. Pharmacodyn. Ther. **188**:86–91.

DUBNICK, B., LEESON, G. A., and PHILLIPS, G. E., 1962, An effect of monoamine oxidase inhibitors on brain serotonin of mice in addition to that resulting from inhibition of monoamine oxidase, J. Neurochem. **9**:299–306.

DUBNICK, B., RUCKI, E. W., and SALAMA, A. I., 1973, A comparison of 1-p-acetyldeoxyephed-rine and 4-methyl-α-ethyl-m-tyramine as to lowering of brain serotonin, and their antagonism by antidepressants, Eur. J. Pharmacol. **22**:121–128.

DUNKLEY, B., SANGHVI, I., FRIEDMAN, E., and GERSHON, S., 1972, Comparison of behavioral and cardiovascular effects of L-DOPA and 5-HTP in conscious dogs, Psychopharmacologia **26**:161–172.

DUNLEAVY, D. L. F., 1973, Mood and sleep changes with monoamine-oxidase inhibitors, Proc. R. Soc. Med. **66**:951.

DUNLEAVY, D. L. F., and OSWALD, I., 1973, Phenelzine, mood response, and sleep, Arch. Gen. Psychiatry **28**:353–356.

DYER, D. C., and WEBER, L. J., 1971, 5-Hydroxytryptamine and monoamine oxidase in adult and foetal sheep blood vessels, J. Pharm. Pharmacol. **23**:549–550.

EBLE, J. N., and RUDZIK, A., 1966, The effects of harmine and tranylcypromine on the pressor responses to biogenic amines in the reserpine-pretreated dog, Life Sci. **5**:1125–1131.

ECCLESTON, D., ASHCROFT, G. W., and CRAWFORD, T. B. B., 1965, 5-Hydroxyindole metabolism in rat brain. A study of intermediate metabolism using the technique of tryptophan loading. II. Applications and drug studies, J. Neurochem. **12**:493–503.

ECCLESTON, D., ASHCROFT, G. W., CRAWFORD, T. B. B., and LOOSE, R., 1966, Some observations on the estimation of tryptamine in tissues, J. Neurochem. **13**:93–101.

ELIS, J., LAURENCE, D. R., MATTIE, H., and PRICHARD, B. N. C., 1967, Modification by monoamine oxidase inhibitors of the effect of some sympathomimetics on blood pressure, Br. Med. J. **2**:75–78.

ELTHERINGTON, L. G., and HORITA, A., 1960, Some pharmacological actions of beta-phenylisopropylhydrazine (PIH), J. Pharmacol. Exp. Ther. **128**:7–14.

ENDERSBY, C. A., ROBSON, J. M., SULLIVAN, F. M., and WILSON, C., 1970, The effect of 5-hydroxytryptamine on ovulation in rats, J. Endocrinol. **48**:63–64.

ERNST, A. M., 1972, Relationship of the central effect of dopamine on gnawing compulsion syndrome in rats and the release of serotonin, Arch. Intern. Pharmacodyn. Ther. **199**:219–225.

FAHIM, I., ISMAIL, M., and OSMAN, O. H., 1972, The role of 5-hydroxytryptamine and noradrenaline in the hyperthermic reaction induced by pethidine in rabbits pretreated with pargyline, *Br. J. Pharmacol.* **46**:416–422.

FERGUSON, J., HENRIKSEN, S., COHEN, H., MITCHELL, G., BARCHAS, J., and DEMENT, W., 1970, "Hypersexuality" and behavioral changes in cats caused by administration of *p*-chlorophenylalanine, *Science* **168**:499–501.

FISHER, D. B., and KAUFMAN, S., 1972, The inhibition of phenylalanine and tyrosine hydroxylases by high oxygen levels, *J. Neurochem.* **19**:1359–1365.

FLÓREZ, J., and ARMIJO, J. A., 1974, Effect of central inhibition of the 1-aminoacid decarboxylase on the hypotensive action of 5-HT precursors in cats, *Eur. J. Pharmacol.* **26**:108–110.

FORBES, W. R., 1970, The effects of the monoamine oxidase inhibitor tranylcypromine on the testis weight of the cockerel, *J. Endocrinol.* **47**:387–388.

FUENTES, J. A., and NEFF, N. H., 1975, Selective monoamine oxidase inhibitor drugs as aids in evaluating the role of type A and B enzymes, *Neuropharmacology* **14**:819–825.

FULLER, R. W., 1968, Influence of substrate in the inhibition of rat liver and brain monoamine oxidase, *Arch. Intern. Pharmacodyn. Ther.* **174**:32–37.

FULLER, R. W., 1972, Selective inhibition of monoamine oxidase, in: *Advances in Biochemical Psychopharmacology*, Vol. 5 (E. Costa and M. Sandler, eds.), pp. 339–354, Raven Press, New York.

FULLER, R. W., and ROUSH, B. W., 1972, Substrate-selective and tissue-selective inhibition of monoamine oxidase, *Arch. Intern. Pharmacodyn. Ther.* **198**:270–276.

FULLER, R. W., WARREN, B. J., and MOLLOY, B. B., 1970, Selective inhibition of monoamine oxidase in rat brain mitochondria, *Biochem. Pharmacol.* **19**:2934–2936,

FULLER, R. W., PERRY, K. W., and MOLLOY, B. B., 1974*a*, Effect of an uptake inhibitor on serotonin metabolism in rat brain: Studies with 3-(*p*-trifluoromethylphenoxy)-*N*-methyl-3-phenylpropyl amine (Lilly 110140), *Life Sci.* **15**:1161–1171.

FULLER, R. W., PERRY, K. W., SNODDY, H. D., and MOLLOY, B. B., 1974*b*, Comparison of the specificity of 3-(*p*-trifluoromethylphenoxy)-*N*-methyl-3-phenylpropylamine and chlorimipramine as amine uptake inhibitors in mice, *Eur. J. Pharmacol.* **28**:233–236.

FURCHGOTT, R. F., and GARCIA, P. S., 1968, Effects of inhibition of monoamine oxidase on the actions and interactions of norepinephrine, tyramine and other drugs on guinea-pig left atrium, *J. Pharmacol. Exp. Ther.* **163**:98–122.

FURNESS, J. B., and COSTA, M., 1971, Monoamine oxidase histochemistry of enteric neurones in the guinea-pig, *Histochemie* **28**:324–336.

FUXE, K., and UNGERSTEDT, U., 1967, Localization of 5-hydroxytryptamine uptake in rat brain after intraventricular injection, *J. Pharm. Pharmacol.* **19**:335–337.

FUXE, K., and UNGERSTEDT, U., 1968, Histochemical studies on the effect of (+)-amphetamine, drugs of the imipramine group and tryptamine on central catecholamine and 5-hydroxytryptamine neurons after intraventricular injection of catecholamines and 5-hydroxytryptamine, *Eur. J. Pharmacol.* **4**:135–144.

FUXE, K., HÖKFELT, T., and UNGERSTEDT, U., 1968, Localization of indolealkylamines in CNS, in: *Advances in Pharmacology*, Vol. 6 (S. Garattina and P. A. Shore, eds.), Part A, pp. 235–251, Academic Press, New York and London.

FUXE, K., LIDBRINK, P., HÖKFELT, T., BOLME, P., and GOLDSTEIN, M., 1974, Effects of piperoxane on sleep and waking in the rat. Evidence for increased waking by blocking inhibitory adrenaline receptors on the locus coeruleus, *Acta Physiol. Scand.* **91**:566–567.

GALLAGHER, C. H., KOCH, J. H., MOORE, R. M., and STEEL, J. D., 1964, Toxicity of phalaris tuberosa for sheep, *Nature (London)* **204**:542–545.

GANONG, W. F., 1974, The role of catecholamines and acetylcholine in the regulation of endocrine function, *Life Sci.* **15**:1401–1414.

GAWIENOWSKI, A. M., and HODGEN, G. D., 1971, Homosexual activity in male rats after *p*-chlorophenylalanine: Effects of hypophysectomy and testosterone, *Physiol. Behav.* **7**:551–555.

GEROLD, M., 1968, Wirkung von Tyramin und Käse auf den Blutdruck und deren

Beeinflussung durch DL-Serin-N^2-isopropyl-hydrazid (Ro 4-1038) und wachen intakten Hunden, *Arzneim.-Forsch.* **18:**1198–1200.

GESSA, G. L., and TAGLIAMONTE, A., 1973, Role of brain monoamines in controlling sexual behavior in male animals, in: *Psychopharmacology, Sexual Disorders and Drug Abuse* (T. A. Ban, J. R. Boissier, G. J. Gessa, H. Heimann, L. Hollister, H. E. Lehmann, I. Munkvad, Hannah Steinberg, F. Sulser, A. Sundwall, and O. Vinar, eds.), pp. 451–462, North-Holland Publishing Co., Amsterdam and London; Avicenum Czechoslovak Medical Press, Prague.

GESSA, G. L., and TAGLIAMONTE, A., 1974, Possible role of brain serotonin and dopamine in controlling male sexual behavior, in: *Advances in Biochemical Psychopharmacology* (E. Costa and M. Sandler, eds.), Vol. 11, pp. 217–228, Raven Press, New York.

GESSA, G. L., TAGLIAMONTE, A., TAGLIAMONTE, P., and BRODIE, B. B., 1970, Essential role of testosterone in the sexual stimulation induced by *p*-chlorophenylalanine in male animals, *Nature (London)* **227:**616–617.

GESSNER, P. K., 1973, Antagonism of the tranylcypromine–meperidine interaction by chlorpromazine in mice, *Eur. J. Pharmacol.* **22:**187–190.

GESSNER, P. K., and SOBLE, A. G., 1972, Antagonism by *p*-chlorophenylalanine of late tranylcypromine toxicity, *J. Pharm. Pharmacol.* **24:**825–827.

GESSNER, P. K., and SOBLE, A. G., 1973, A study of the tranylcypromine–meperidine interaction: Effects of *p*-chlorophenylalanine and 1-5-hydroxytryptophan, *J. Pharmacol. Exp. Ther.* **186:**276–287.

GESSNER, P. K., KHAIRALLAH, P. A., McISAAC, W. M., and PAGE, I. H., 1960, The relationship between the metabolic fate and pharmacological actions of serotonin, bufotenine and psilocybin, *J. Pharmacol. Exp. Ther.* **130:**126–133.

GESSNER, P. K., McISAAC, W. M., and PAGE, I. H., 1961, Pharmacological actions of some methoxyindolealkylamines, *Nature (London)* **190:**179–180.

GEY, K. F., and PLETSCHER, A., 1961, Activity of monoamine oxidase in relation to the 5-hydroxytryptamine and norepinephrine content of the rat brain, *J. Neurochem.* **6:**239–243.

GHEZZI, D., SAMANIN, R., BERNASCONI, S., TOGNONI, G., GERNA, M., and GARATTINI, S., 1973, Effect of thymoleptics on fenfluramine-induced depletion of brain serotonin in rats, *Eur. J. Pharmacol.* **24:**205–210.

GIACOBINI, E., and KERPEL-FRONIUS, S., 1970, Histochemical and biochemical correlations of monoamine oxidase activity in autonomic and sensory ganglia of the cat, *Acta Physiol. Scand.* **78:**522–528.

GILLESPIE, J. S., 1973, Uptake of noradrenaline by smooth muscle, *Br. Med. Bull.* **29:**136–141.

GILLESPIE, L., TERRY, L. L., and SJOERDSMA, A., 1959, The application of a monoamine-oxidase inhibitor, 1-phenyl-2-hydrazinopropane (JB-516), to the treatment of primary hypertension, *Am. Heart J.* **58:**1–12.

GLASSMAN, A. H., and PLATMAN, S. R., 1969, Potentiation of a monoamine oxidase inhibitor by tryptophan, *J. Psychiatr. Res.* **7:**83–88.

GLAVAS, E., STOJANOVA, D., TRAJKOV, T., and NIKODIJEVIC, B., 1965, On the hypotensive effect of tranylcypromine, *Arch. Intern. Pharmacodyn. Ther.* **155:**381–387.

GLENNER, G. G., BURTNER, H. J., and BROWN, G. W., 1957, The histochemical demonstration of monoamine oxidase activity by tetrazolium salts, *J. Histochem. Cytochem.* **5:**591–600.

GOLDBERG, L. I., and SJOERDSMA, A., 1959, Effects of several monoamine oxidase inhibitors on the cardiovascular actions of naturally occurring amines in the dog, *J. Pharmacol. Exp. Ther.* **127:**212–218.

GONG, S. N. C., and ROGERS, K. J., 1973, Role of brain monoamines in the fatal hyperthermia induced by pethidine or imipramine in rabbits pretreated with a monoamine oxidase inhibitor, *Br. J. Pharmacol.* **48:**12–18.

GORIDIS, C., and NEFF, N. H., 1971a, Evidence for a specific monoamine oxidase associated with sympathetic nerves, *Neuropharmacology* **10:**557–564.

GORIDIS, C., and NEFF, N. H., 1971b, Monoamine oxidase in sympathetic nerves: A transmitter specific enzyme type, Br. J. Pharmacol. **43**:814–818.

GORIDIS, C., and NEFF, N. H., 1974, Selective localisation of monoamine oxidase forms in rat mesenteric artery, Biochem. Pharmacol. Suppl. (Pt. 1), pp. 106–109.

GORKIN, V. Z., and ROMANOVA, L. A., 1968, On the selective inhibition by some monoamine oxidase inhibitors of deamination of biogenic monoamines in vivo, Biochem. Pharmacol. **17**:855–860.

GOVIER, W. M., HOWES, B. G., and GIBBONS, A. J., 1953, The oxidative deamination of serotonin and other 3-(beta-aminoethyl)-indoles by monoamine oxidase and the effect of these compounds on the deamination of tyramine, Science **118**:596–597.

GRAHAME-SMITH, D. G., 1971a, Studies in vivo on the relationship between brain tryptophan, brain 5-HT synthesis and hyperactivity in rats treated with a monoamine oxidase inhibitor and 1-tryptophan, J. Neurochem. **18**:1053–1066.

GRAHAME-SMITH, D. G., 1971b, Inhibitory effect of chlorpromazine on the syndrome of hyperactivity produced by 1-tryptophan or 5-methoxy-N,N-dimethyltryptamine in rats treated with a monoamine oxidase inhibitor, Br. J. Pharmacol. **43**:856–864.

GRAHAME-SMITH, D. G., 1972, Inhibitory effect of chlorpromazine on the syndrome of hyperactivity produced by 1-tryptophan or 5-methoxy-N,N-dimethyltryptamine in rats treated with a monoamine oxidase inhibitor, Br. J. Pharmacol. **43**:856–864.

GRAHAME-SMITH, D. G., and GREEN, A. R., 1974, The role of brain 5-hydroxytryptamine in the hyperactivity produced in rats by lithium and monoamine oxidase inhibition, Br. J. Pharmacol. **52**:19–26.

GRAY, W. D., and RAUH, C. E., 1967, The anticonvulsant action of inhibitors of carbonic anhydrase: Relation to endogenous amines in brain, J. Pharmacol. Exp. Ther. **155**:127–134.

GRAY, W. D., and RAUH, C. E., 1968, The anticonvulsant action of carbon dioxide: Interaction with reserpine and inhibitors of carbonic anhydrase, J. Pharmacol. Exp. Ther. **163**:431–438.

GRAY, W. D., and RAUH, C. E., 1971, The relation between monoamines in brain and the anticonvulsant action of inhibitors of carbonic anhydrase, J. Pharmacol. Exp. Ther. **177**:206–218.

GRAY, W. D., RAUH, C. E., OSTERBERG, A. C., and LIPCHUCK, L. M., 1958, The anticonvulsant actions of methazolamide (a carbonic anhydrase inhibitor) and diphenylhydantoin, J. Pharmacol. Exp. Ther. **124**:144–160.

GRAY, W. D., RAUH, C. E., and SHANAHAN, R. W., 1963, The mechanism of the antagonistic action of reserpine on the anticonvulsant effect of inhibitors of carbonic anhydrase, J. Pharmacol. Exp. Ther. **139**:350–360.

GREEN, A. R., and GRAHAME-SMITH, D. G., 1974, TRH potentiates behavioural changes following increased brain 5-hydroxytryptamine accumulation in rats, Nature (London) **251**:524–526.

GREEN, A. R., and GRAHAME-SMITH, D. G., 1975, The effect of diphenylhydantoin on brain 5-hydroxytryptamine metabolism and function, Neuropharmacology **14**:107–113.

GREEN, H., and ERICKSON, R. W., 1962, Further studies with tranylcypromine (monoamine oxidase inhibitor) and its interaction with reserpine in rat brain, Arch. Intern. Pharmacodyn. Ther. **135**:407–425.

GREEN, H., and SAWYER, J. L., 1960, Correlation of tryptamine-induced convulsions in rats with brain tryptamine concentration (25762), Proc. Soc. Exp. Biol. Med. **104**:153–155.

GREEN, H., and SAWYER, J. L., 1966, Demonstration, characterization, and assay procedure of tryptophan hydroxylase in rat brain, Anal. Biochem. **15**:53–64.

GREENAWALT, J. W., 1972, Localization of monoamine oxidase in rat liver mitochondria, in: Advances in Biochemical Psychopharmacology, Vol. 5 (E. Costa and M. Sandler, eds.), pp. 207–226, Raven Press, New York.

GUNN, J. A., 1935, Relations between chemical constitution, pharmacological actions, and therapeutic uses, in harmine group of alkaloids, *Arch. Intern. Pharmacodyn. Ther.* **50:**379–396.

GUNN, J. A., and GURD, M. R., 1940, Action of some amines related to adrenaline. Cyclohexylalkylamines, *J. Physiol.* **97:**453–470.

GYLYS, J. A., MUCCIA, P. M. R., and TAYLOR, M. K., 1963, Pharmacological and toxicological properties of 2-methyl-3-piperidinopyrazine, a new antidepressant, *Ann. N. Y. Acad. Sci.* **107:**899–911.

HAEUSLER, G., 1973, Activation of the central pathway of the baroreceptor reflex, a possible mechanism of the hypotensive action of clonidine, *Naunyn-Schmiedebergs Arch. Pharmakol.* **278:**231–246.

HAIGLER, H. J., and AGHAJANIAN, G. K., 1974, Lysergic acid diethylamide and serotonin: A comparison of effects on serotonergic neurons and neurons receiving a serotonergic input, *J. Pharmacol. Exp. Ther.* **188:**688–699.

HALARIS, A. E., LOVELL, R. A., and FREEDMAN, D. X., 1973, Effect of chlorimipramine on the metabolism of 5-hydroxytryptamine in the rat brain, *Biochem. Pharmacol.* **22:**2200–2202.

HALL, D. W. R., LOGAN, B. W., and PARSONS, G. H., 1969, Further studies on the inhibition of monoamine oxidase M and B 9302 (clorgyline). I. Substrate specificity in various mammalian species, *Biochem. Pharmacol.* **18:**1447–1454.

HALLIDAY, R. P., DAVIS, C. S., HEOTIS, J. P., PALS, D. T., WATSON, E. J., and BICKERTON, R. K., 1968, Allenic amines: A new class of nonhydrazine MAO inhibitors, *J. Pharm. Sci.* **57:**430–433.

HAMBERGER, B., MALMFORS, T., NORBERG, K.-A., and SACHS, C., 1964, Uptake and accumulation of catecholamines in peripheral adrenergic neurons of reserpinized animals, studied with a histochemical method, *Biochem. Pharmacol.* **13:**841–844.

HAMON, M., BOURGOIN, S., MOROT-GAUDRY, Y., and GLOWINSKI, J., 1972, End product inhibition of serotonin synthesis in the rat striatum, *Nature (London)* **237:**184–187.

HAMON, M., BOURGOIN, S., and GLOWINSKI, J., 1973, Feedback regulation of 5-HT synthesis in rat striatal slices, *J. Neurochem.* **20:**1727–1745.

HARTMANN, E., 1968, On the pharmacology of dreaming sleep (the D state), *J. Nerv. Ment. Dis.* **146:**165–173.

HARTMANN, E., BRIDWELL, T. J., and SCHILDKRAUT, J. J., 1971, Alpha-methylparatyrosine and sleep in the rat, *Psychopharmacologia* **21:**157–164.

HEISE, G. A., and BOFF, E., 1960, Behavioral determination of time and dose parameters of monoamine oxidase inhibitors, *J. Pharmacol. Exp. Ther.* **129:**155–162.

HENNING, M., and RUBENSON, A., 1970, Central hypotensive effect of L-3,4-dihydroxyphenylalanine in the rat, *J. Pharm. Pharmacol.* **22:**553–560.

HENNING, M., and RUBENSON, A., 1971, Effects of 5-hydroxytryptophan on arterial blood pressure, body temperature and tissue monoamines in the rat, *Acta Pharmacol. Toxicol.* **29:**145–154.

HENNING, M., RUBENSON, A., and TROLIN, G., 1972, On the localization of the hypotensive effect of L-dopa, *J. Pharm. Pharmacol.* **24:**447–451.

HENRIKSEN, S., GONDA, W., COHEN, H., BARCHAS, J., and DEMENT, W., 1970, The effect of monoamine oxidase inhibitor (Pargyline) on the central monoamine levels and sleep in the PCPA cat, *Psychophysiology* **7:**321.

HESS, S. M., and DOEPFNER, W., 1961, Behavioral effects and brain amine content in rats, *Arch. Intern. Pharmacodyn. Ther.* **134:**89–99.

HESS, S. M., REDFIELD, B. G., and UDENFRIEND, S., 1959, The effect of monoamine oxidase inhibitors and tryptophan on the tryptamine content of animal tissues and urine, *J. Pharmacol. Exp. Ther.* **127:**178–181.

HIMWICH, W. A., DAVIS, J. M., FORBES, D. J., GLISSON, S. N., MAGNUSSON, T., STOUT, M. A., and TRUSTY, D. W., 1972, Indole metabolism and behavior in dog, *Biol. Psychiatr.* **4:**51–63.

HO, B. T., TANSEY, L. W., BALSTER, R. L., AN, R., MCISAAC, W. M., and HARRIS, R. T., 1970, Amphetamine analogs. II. Methylated phenethylamines, *J. Med. Chem.* **13:**134–135.

HODGE, J. V., OATES, J. A., and SJOERDSMA, A., 1964, Reduction of the central effects of tryptophan by a decarboxylase inhibitor, *Clin. Pharmacol. Ther.* **5**:149–155.

HÖKFELT, T., FUXE, K., GOLDSTEIN, M., and JOHANSSON, O., 1974, Immunohistochemical evidence for the existence of adrenaline neurons in the rat brain, *Brain Res.* **66**:235–251.

HOLLISTER, L. E., and FRIEDHOFF, A. J., 1966, Effects of 3,4-dimethoxyphenylethylamine in man, *Nature (London)* **210**:1377–1378.

HORITA, A., 1958, Beta-phenylisopropylhydrazine, a potent and long acting monoamine oxidase inhibitor, *J. Pharmacol. Exp. Ther.* **122**:176–181.

HORITA, A., 1967, Biochemistry and pharmacology of the monoamine oxidase inhibitors (hydrazines): Addendum, in: *Psychopharmacological Agents*, Vol. II (M. Gordon, ed.), pp. 523–532, Academic Press, New York and London.

HORITA, A., and CARINO, M. A., 1970, Modification of the toxic actions of 1-tryptophan by pargyline and *p*-chlorophenylalanine, *Biochem. Pharmacol.* **19**:1521–1524.

HORITA, A., and GOGERTY, J. H., 1958, The pyretogenic effect of 5-hydroxytryptophan and its comparison with that of LSD, *J. Pharmacol. Exp. Ther.* **122**:195–200.

HORN, A. S., and TRACE, R. C. A. M., 1974, Structure–activity relations for the inhibition of 5-hydroxytryptamine uptake by tricyclic antidepressants into synaptosomes from serotoninergic neurones in rat brain homogenates, *Br. J. Pharmacol.* **51**:399–403.

HORWITZ, D., LOVENBERG, W., ENGELMAN, K., and SJOERDSMA, A., 1964, Monoamine oxidase inhibitors, tyramine, and cheese, *J. Am. Med. Assoc.* **188**:1108–1110.

HOYLAND, V. J., SHILLITO, E. E., and VOGT, M., 1970, The effect of parachlorophenylalanine on the behaviour of cats, *Br. J. Pharmacol.* **40**:659–667.

HYTTEL, J., 1974, Effect of neuroleptics on the disappearance rate of [¹⁴C] labelled catecholamines formed from [¹⁴C] tyrosine in mouse brain, *J. Pharm. Pharmacol.* **26**:588–596.

ITO, A., and SCHANBERG, S. M., 1972, Central nervous system mechanisms responsible for blood pressure elevation induced by *p*-chlorophenylalanine, *J. Pharmacol. Exp. Ther.* **181**:65–74.

IWATA, H., OKAMOTO, H., and KURAMOTO, I., 1974, Effect of lithium on serum tryptophan and brain serotonin in rats, *Jpn. J. Pharmacol.* **24**:235–240.

JACOB, J., and SIMON, P., 1968, Effets pharmacologiques des inhibiteurs des monoamine oxidases, in: *Monoamine Oxidase Inhibitors: Relationship Between Pharmacological and Clinical Effects* (J. Cheymol and J. R. Boissier, eds.), pp. 33–47, Pergamon Press, London.

JACOBS, B. L., 1974a, Effect of two dopamine receptor blockers on a serotonin-mediated behavioral syndrome in rats, *Eur. J. Pharmacol.* **27**:363–366.

JACOBS, B. L., 1974b, Evidence for the functional interaction of two central neurotransmitters, *Psychopharmacologia* **39**:81–86.

JACOBS, B. L., HENRIKSEN, S. J., and DEMENT, W. C., 1972, Neurochemical bases of the PGO wave, *Brain Res.* **48**:406–411.

JACOBS, B. L., EUBANKS, E. E., and WISE, W. D., 1974, Effect of indolealkylamine manipulations on locomotor activity in rats, *Neuropharmacology* **13**:575–583.

JACOBS, B. L., MOSKO, S. S., and TRULSON, M. E., 1975, The investigation of the role of serotonin in mammalian behavior, in: *Neurobiology of Sleep and Memory* (J. L. McGaugh, ed.), Academic Press, New York (in press).

JAITLY, K. D., ROBSON, J. M., SULLIVAN, F. M., and WILSON, C., 1968a, The effects of amine oxidase inhibitors on ovulation, implantation and pregnancy, *J. Reprod. Fertil. Suppl. 4*, pp. 75–79.

JAITLY, K. D., ROBSON, J. M., SULLIVAN, F. M., and WILSON, C., 1968b, Maintenance of pregnancy after implantation in hypophysectomized or ovariectomized mice treated with phenelzine derivatives, *J. Endocrinol.* **41**:519–530.

JALFRE, M., RUCH-MONACHON, M.-A., and HAEFELY, W., 1974, Methods for assessing the interaction of agents with 5-hydroxytryptamine neurons and receptors in the brain, in: *Advances in Biochemical Psychopharmacology*, Vol 10 (E. Costa and M. Sandler, eds.), pp. 121–134, Raven Press, New York.

JANSEN, G. S. I. M., VRENSEN, G. F. J. M., and VAN KEMPEN, G. M. J., 1974, Intracellular localization of phenol sulphotransferase in rat brain, *J. Neurochem.* **23**:329–335.

JARROTT, B., 1971, Occurrence and properties of monoamine oxidase in adrenergic neurons, *J. Neurochem.* **18**:7–16.

JARROTT, B., and LANGER, S. Z., 1971, Changes in monoamine oxidase and catechol-*o*-methyl transferase activities after denervation of the nictitating membrane of the cat, *J. Physiol.* **212**:549–559.

JAVOY, F., AGID, Y., BOUVET, D., and GLOWINSKI, J., 1972, Feedback control of dopamine synthesis in dopaminergic terminals of the rat striatum, *J. Pharmacol. Exp. Ther.* **182**:454–463.

JAVOY, F., YOUDIM, M. B. H., AGID, Y., and GLOWINSKI, J., 1973, Early effects of monoamine oxidase inhibitors on dopamine metabolism and monoamine oxidase activity in the neostriatum of the rat, *J. Neural Transm.* **34**:279–289.

JENNER, F. A., JUDD, A., and PARKER, J., 1975, The effects of lithium, rubidium and caesium on the response of rats to tranylcypromine and α-methyl-*p*-tyrosine given separately or in combination, *Br. J. Pharmacol.* **54**:233P–234P.

JOBE, P. C., PICCHIONI, A. L., and CHIN, L., 1973a, Role of brain norepinephrine in audiogenic seizure in the rat, *J. Pharmacol. Exp. Ther.* **184**:1–10.

JOBE, P. C., PICCHIONI, A. L., and CHIN, L., 1973b, Role of brain 5-hydroxytryptamine in audiogenic seizure in the rat, *Life Sci.* **13**:1–13.

JOBE, P. C., STULL, R. E., and GEIGER, P. F., 1974, The relative significance of norepinephrine, dopamine and 5-hydroxytryptamine in electroshock seizure in the rat, *Neuropharmacology* **13**:961–968.

JOHNSON, D. N., FUNDERBURK, W. H., and WARD, J. W., 1971, Effects of fenfluramine on sleep–wakefulness in cats, *Psychopharmacologia* **20**:1–9.

JOHNSTON, J. P., 1968, Some observations upon a new inhibitor of monoamine oxidase in brain tissue, *Biochem. Pharmacol.* **17**:1285–1297.

JONASON, J., and RUTLEDGE, C. O., 1969, Effects of reserpine, dopamine and nialamide on the synthesis of α-methylnoradrenaline, *Eur. J. Pharmacol.* **6**:24–28.

JONES, B. E., 1972, The respective involvement of noradrenaline and its deaminated metabolites in waking and paradoxical sleep: A neuropharmacological model, *Brain Res.* **39**:121–136.

JORI, A., BONACCORSI, A., VALZELLI, L., and GARATTINI, S., 1963, New orally active monoamine oxidase (MAO) inhibitors, *Life Sci.* **8**:611–617.

JOUNELA, A. J., 1970, Influence of phenelzine on the toxicity of some analgesics in mice, *Ann. Med. Exp. Fenn.* **48**:261–265.

JOUNELA, A. J., and MATTILA, M. J., 1975, Effect of selective MAO inhibitors on the pethidine toxicity in rabbits, 6th International Congress of Pharmacology, July 20–25, Helsinki (Abstract).

JOUVET, M., 1967, Mechanisms of the states of sleep: A neuropharmacological approach, in: *Sleep and Altered States of Consciousness*, Vol. 45, pp. 86–126, Williams & Wilkins, Baltimore.

JOUVET, M., 1969, Biogenic amines and the states of sleep. Pharmacological and neurophysiological studies suggest a relationship between brain serotonin and sleep, *Science* **163**:32–41.

JOUVET, M., 1972, The role of monoamines and acetylcholine-containing neurons in the regulation of the sleep–waking cycle, *Rev. Physiol.* **64**:166–307.

JOUVET, M., and MICHEL, F., 1959, Corrélations électromyographiques du sommeil chez le chat décortique et mésencephalique chronique, *C. R. Soc. Biol.* **153**:422–425.

JOUVET, M., VIMONT, P., and DELORME, F., 1965, Suppression élective du sommeil paradoxal chez le chat par les inhibiteurs de la monoamineoxydase, *C. R. Soc. Biol.* **159**:1595–1599.

JUDD, A., PARKER, J., and JENNER, F. A., 1975, The role of noradrenaline, dopamine and 5-hydroxytryptamine in the hyperactivity response resulting from the administration of tranylcypromine to rats pretreated with lithium or rubidium, *Psychopharmacologia* **42:**73–77.

KAKIMOTO, Y., and ARMSTRONG, M. D., 1962, On the identification of octopamine in mammals, *J. Biol. Chem.* **237:**422–427.

KALBERER, F., KREIS, W., and RUTSCHMANN, J., 1962, The fate of psilocin in rat, *Biochem. Pharmacol.* **11:**261–269.

KALNINS, I., and RUF, K. B., 1971, The role of hypothalamic monoamines in the central control of ovulation, *Schweiz. Z. Gynaekol. Geburtshilfe* **2:**255–263.

KAMBERI, I. A., and DE VELLIS, J., 1975, Brain neurotransmitters and the secretions of gonadotropins and gonadotropin-releasing hormones, 6th International Congress of Pharmacology, July 20–25, Helsinki.

KANNENGIESSER, M. H., HUNT, P., and RAYNAUD, J.-P., 1973, An *in vitro* model for the study of psychotropic drugs and as a criterion of antidepressant activity, *Biochem. Pharmacol.* **22:**73–84.

KATIC, F., LAVERY, H., and LOWE, R. D., 1972, The central action of clonidine and its antagonism, *Br. J. Pharmacol.* **44:**779–787.

KAUL, C. L., and GREWAL, R. S., 1972, Antihypertensive and monoamine oxidase inhibitory activity of 3-amino-2-oxazolidinone (3AO) and its condensation product with 2-substituted-3-formyl-4-oxo-(4H)pyridol (1,2-a) pyrimidines, *Biochem. Pharmacol.* **21:**303–316.

KAYAALP, S. O., KAYMEKCALAN, S., and ÖZER, A., 1968, Interaction between some cheeses and monoamine oxidase inhibitors, *Arzneim.-Forsch.* **18:**1195–1198.

KHAZAN, N., and BROWN, P., 1970, Differential effects of three tricyclic antidepressants on sleep and REM sleep in the rat, *Life Sci.* **9**(Pt. 1):279–284.

KHAZAN, N., and SAWYER, C. H., 1964, Mechanisms of paradoxical sleep as revealed by neurophysiologic and pharmacologic approaches in the rabbit, *Psychopharmacologia* **5:**457–466.

KING, C. D., and JEWETT, R. E., 1968, Sleep in cats treated with α-methyl-p-tyrosine, *Pharmacologist* **10:**160.

KLINGMAN, G. I., 1966, Monoamine oxidase activity of peripheral organs and sympathetic ganglia of the rat after immunosympathectomy, *Biochem. Pharmacol.* **15:**1729–1736.

KNAPP, S., and MANDELL, A. J., 1973, Short- and long-term lithium administration: Effects on the brain's serotonergic biosynthetic systems, *Science* **180:**645–647.

KNOLL, J., and MAGYAR, K., 1972, Some puzzling pharmacological effects of monoamine oxidase inhibitors, in: *Advances in Biochemical Psychopharmacology*, Vol. 5 (E. Costa and M. Sandler, eds.), pp. 393–408, Raven Press, New York.

KOBINGER, W., 1958, Beeinflussung der Cardiazolkrampfschwelle durch veränderten 5-Hydroxytryptamingehalt des Zentralnervensystems, *Arch. Exp. Pathol. Pharmakol.* **233:**559–566.

KOE, B. K., and WEISSMAN, A., 1968, The pharmacology of parachlorophenylalanine, a selective depletor of serotonin stores, in: *Advances in Pharmacology*, Vol. 6B (S. Garattini and P. A. Shore, eds.), pp. 29–47, Academic Press, New York and London.

KOELLE, G. B., and VALK, A. DE T., 1954, Physiological implications of the histochemical localization of monoamine oxidase, *J. Physiol.* **126:**434–447.

KOPIN, I. J., 1966, Biochemical aspects of release of norepinephrine and other amines from sympathetic nerve endings, *Pharmacol. Rev.* **18:**513–523.

KOPIN, I. J., FISCHER, J. E., MUSACCHIO, J., and HORST, W. D., 1964, Evidence for a false neurochemical transmitter as a mechanism for the hypotensive effect of monoamine oxidase inhibitors, *Proc. Natl. Acad. Sci. U.S.A.* **52:**716–721.

KOPIN, I. J., FISCHER, J. E., MUSACCHIO, J. M., HORST, W. D., and WEISE, V. K., 1965, "False neurochemical transmitters" and the mechanism of sympathetic blockade by monoamine oxidase inhibitors, *J. Pharmacol. Exp. Ther.* **147:**186–193.

KORDON, C., 1969, Effects of selective experimental changes in regional hypothalamic monoamine levels on superovulation in the immature rat, *Neuroendocrinology* **4:**129–138.

KORDON, C., and GLOWINSKI, J., 1972, Role of hypothalamic monoaminergic neurones in the gonadotrophin release-regulating mechanisms, *Neuropharmacology* **11**:153–162.

KORDON, C., and VASSENT, G., 1968, Effet de micro-injections intrahypothalamiques et intrahypophysaires d'un inhibiteur de la monoamine-oxydase sur l'ovulation provoquée chez la ratte impubere, *C. R. Acad. Sci.* **266**:2473–2476.

KORDON, C., JAVOY, F., VASSENT, G., and GLOWINSKI, J., 1968, Blockade of superovulation in the immature rat by increased brain serotonin, *Eur. J. Pharmacol.* **4**:169–174.

KORDUBA, C. A., VEALS, J., and SYMCHOWICZ, S., 1973, The effect of pheniramine and its structural analogues on 5-hydroxytryptamine in rat and mouse brain, *Life Sci.* **13**:1557–1564.

KOSLOW, S. H., and SCHLUMPF, M., 1974, Quantitation of adrenaline in rat brain nuclei and areas by mass fragmentography, *Nature (London)* **251**:530–531.

LABHSETWAR, A. P., 1971*a*, Effects of serotonin on spontaneous ovulation: A theory for the dual hypothalamic control of ovulation, *Acta Endocrinol.* **68**:334–344.

LABHSETWAR, A. P., 1971*b*, Effects of serotonin on spontaneous ovulation in rats, *Nature (London)* **229**:203–204.

LABHSETWAR, A. P., 1972, Role of monoamines in ovulation: Evidence for a serotoninergic pathway for inhibition of spontaneous ovulation, *J. Endocrinol.* **54**:269–275.

LADER, M. H., SAKALIS, G., and TANSELLA, M., 1970, Interactions between sympathomimetic amines and a new monoamine oxidase inhibitor, *Psychopharmacologia* **18**:118–123.

LANDS, A. M., and GRANT, J. I., 1952, The vasopressor action and toxicity of cyclohexylethylamine derivatives, *J. Pharmacol. Exp. Ther.* **106**:341–345.

LARSSON, K., and SÖDERSTEN, P., 1971, Lordosis behavior in male rats treated with estrogen in combination with tetrabenazine and nialamide, *Psychopharmacologia* **21**:13–16.

LAUER, J. W., INSKIP, W. M., BERNSOHN, J., and ZELLER, A., 1958, Observations on schizophrenic patients after iproniazid and tryptophan, *Arch. Neurol. Psychiatry* **80**:122–130.

LAVERTY, R., 1973, The mechanisms of action of some antihypertensive drugs, *Br. Med. Bull.* **29**:152–157.

LEE, F. I., 1961, Imipramine overdosage—report of a fatal case, *Br. Med. J.* **1**:338–339.

LEHMANN, A., 1967, Audiogenic seizures data in mice supporting new theories of biogenic amines mechanisms in the central nervous system,*Life Sci.* **6**:1423–1431.

LESSIN, A. W., and PARKES, M. W., 1959, The effects of reserpine and other agents upon leptazol convulsions in mice, *Br. J. Pharmacol.* **14**:108–111.

LICHTENSTEIGER, W., MUTZNER, U., and LANGEMANN, H., 1967, Uptake of 5-hydroxytryptamine and 5-hydroxytryptophan by neurons of the central nervous system normally containing catecholamines,*J. Neurochem.* **14**:489–497.

LIDBRINK, P., JONSSON, G., and FUXE, K., 1971, The effect of imipramine-like drugs and antihistamine drugs on uptake mechanisms in the central noradrenaline and 5-hydroxytryptamine neurons, *Neuropharmacology* **10**:521–536.

LIN, R. C., NEFF, N. H., NGAI, S. H., and COSTA, E., 1969, Turnover rates of serotonin and norepinephrine in brain of normal and pargyline-treated rats, *Life Sci.* **8**:1077–1084.

LINDSAY, D., POULSON, E., and ROBSON, J. M., 1963, The effect of 5-hydroxytryptamine on pregnancy,*J. Endocrinol.* **26**:85–96.

LINDSTRÖM, L. H., 1970, The effect of pilocarpine in combination with monoamine oxidase inhibitors, imipramine or desmethylimipramine on oestrous behaviour in female rats, *Psychopharmacologia* **17**:160–168.

LIPPMANN, W., 1968, Relationship between hypothalamic norepinephrine and serotonin and gonadotrophin secretion in the hamster, *Nature (London)* **218**:173–174.

LOEW, D., and TAESCHLER, M., 1965, Der Einfluss von tricyclischen Antidepressiva und Thioridazin auf das 5-Hydroxytryptophan (5-HTP)-Fieber des Kaninchens, *Arch. Exp. Pathol. Pharmakol.* **251**:139.

LOVELESS, A. H., and MAXWELL, D. R., 1965, A comparison of the effects of imipramine, trimipramine, and some other drugs in rabbits treated with a monoamine oxidase inhibitor, *Br. J. Pharmacol.* **25:**158–170.

Lu, L. W., Wilson, A., Moore, R. H., and Domino, E. F., 1974, Correlation between brain *N,N*-dimethyltryptamine (DMT) levels and bar pressing behavior in rats: Effect of MAO inhibition, *Pharmacologist* **16:**237.

Luby, E. D., and Domino, E. F., 1961, Toxicity from large doses of imipramine and an MAO inhibitor in suicidal intent, *J. Am. Med. Assoc.* **177:**68–69.

Luttge, W. G., 1975, Stimulation of estrogen induced copulatory behavior in castrate male rats with the serotonin biosynthesis inhibitor *p*-chlorophenylalanine, *Behav. Biol.* **14:**373–378.

Lynes, T. E., 1966, Pargyline on blood pressure in spinal and decerebrate cats, *J. Pharm. Pharmacol.* **18:**759–760.

Macon, J. B., Sokoloff, L., and Glowinski, J., 1971, Feedback control of rat brain 5-hydroxytryptamine synthesis, *J. Neurochem.* **18:**323–331.

Malmnäs, C. O., 1973, Monoamine precursors and copulatory behavior in the male rat, *Acta Physiol. Scand.* (Suppl.) **395:**47–68.

Malmnäs, C. O., 1974, Opposite effects of serotonin and dopamine on copulatory activation in castrated male rats, in: *Advances in Biochemical Psychopharmacology* (E. Costa and P. Greengard, eds.) Vol. 11, pp. 243–248, Raven Press, New York.

Malmnäs, C. O., and Meyerson, B. J., 1970, Monoamines and testosterone activated copulatory behaviour in the castrated male rat, *Acta Pharmacol.* **28:**67.

Malmnäs, C. O., and Meyerson, B. J., 1971, *p*-Chlorophenylalanine and copulatory behaviour in the male rat, *Nature (London)* **232:**398–400.

Mannisto, P., Nikki, P., and Rissanen, A., 1971, The toxicity of two MAO inhibitors combined with 5-HTP or L-DOPA in anaesthetized mice, *Acta Pharmacol. Toxicol.* **29:**441–448.

Mantegazzini, P., 1966, Pharmacological actions of indolealkylamines and precursor aminoacids on the central nervous system, in: *Handbuch der experimentellen Pharmakologie*, Vol. 19 (O. Eichler and A. Farah, eds.), pp. 424–436, Springer-Verlag, Berlin—Heidelberg—New York.

Marderosian, A. H. der, Pinkley, H. V., and Dobbins, M. F., 1968, Native use and occurrence of *N,N*-dimethyltryptamine in the leaves of *Banisteriopsis rusbyana*, *Am. J. Pharm.* **140:**137–147.

Maronde, R. F., and Haywood, L. J., 1963, Evaluation of the monoamine oxidase inhibitor, pargyline, as an antihypertensive agent. A. Clinical results, *Ann. N. Y. Acad. Sci.* **107:**975–979.

Marsden, C. A., and Curzon, G., 1974, Effects of lesions and drugs on brain tryptamine, *J. Neurochem.* **23:**1171–1176.

Martin, W. R., and Eades, C. G., 1970, The action of tryptamine on the dog spinal cord and its relationship to the agonistic actions of LSD-like psychotogens, *Psychopharmacologia* **17:**242–257.

Martin, W. R., and Sloan, J. W., 1970, Effects of infused tryptamine in man, *Psychopharmacologia* **18:**231–237.

Martin, W. R., Sloan, J. W., Christian, S. T., and Clements, T. H., 1972, Brain levels of tryptamine, *Psychopharmacologia* **24:**331–346.

Martin, W. R., Sloan, J. W., Buchwald, W. F., and Bridges, S. R., 1974, The demonstration of tryptamine in regional perfusates of the dog brain, *Psychopharmacologia* **37:**189–198.

Martin, W. R., Sloan, J. W., Buchwald, W. F., and Clements, T. H., 1975, Neurochemical evidence for tryptaminergic ascending and descending pathways in the spinal cord of the dogs, *Psychopharmacologia* **43:**131–134.

Matsumoto, J., and Jouvet, M., 1964, Effets de réserpine, DOPA et 5 HTP sur les deux états de sommeil, *C. R. Soc. Biol.* **158:**2137–2140.

MATTILA, M. J., and JOUNELA, A. J., 1973, Effect of p-chlorophenylalanine on the interaction between phenelzine and pethidine in conscious rabbits, *Biochem. Pharmacol.* **22:**1674–1676.

MAXWELL, D. R., GRAY, W. R., and TAYLOR, E. M., 1961, Relative activity of some inhibitors of mono-amine oxidase in potentiating the action of tryptamine *in vitro* and *in vivo*, *Br. J. Pharmacol.* **17:**310–320.

MAXWELL, M. H., 1963, Observations pertinent to antihypertensive mechanisms of MAO inhibitors using *dl*-serine isopropylhydrazine, *Ann. N. Y. Acad. Sci.* **107:**993–1004.

McCANN, S. M., 1970, Neurohormonal correlates of ovulation, *Fed. Proc. Fed. Am. Soc. Exp. Biol.* **29:**1888–1894.

McCANN, S. M., and Moss, R. L., 1975, Putative neurotransmitters involved in discharging gonadotropin-releasing neurohormones and the action of LH-releasing hormone on the CNS, *Life Sci.* **16:**833–852.

McCAULEY, R., and RACKER, E., 1973, Separation of two monoamine oxidases from bovine brain, *Mol. Cell. Biochem.* **1:**73–81.

McKEARNEY, J. W., 1968, The relative effects of *d*-amphetamine, imipramine and harmaline on tetrabenazine suppression of schedule-controlled behavior in the rat, *J. Pharmacol. Exp. Ther.* **159:**429–440.

MEEK, J. L., FUXE, K., and CARLSSON, A., 1971, Blockade of p-chloromethamphetamine induced 5-hydroxytryptamine depletion by chlorimipramine, chlorpheniramine and meperidine, *Biochem. Pharmacol.* **20:**707–709.

MEYER, H., and FREY, H.-H., 1973, Dependence of anticonvulsant drug action on central monoamines, *Neuropharmacology* **12:**939–947.

MEYERSON, B. J., 1964a, Estrus behaviour in spayed rats after estrogen or progesterone treatment in combination with reserpine or tetrabenazine, *Psychopharmacologia* **6:**210–218.

MEYERSON, B. J., 1964b, The effect of neuropharmacological agents on hormone-activated estrus behaviour in ovariectomised rats, *Arch. Int. Pharmacodyn. Ther.* **150:**4–33.

MEYERSON, B. J., 1966, The effect of imipramine and related antidepressive drugs on estrus behaviour in ovariectomised rats activated by progesterone, reserpine or tetrabenazine in combination with estrogen, *Acta Physiol. Scand.* **67:**411–422.

MEYERSON, B. J., 1968, Amphetamine and 5-hydroxytryptamine inhibition of copulatory behaviour in the female rat, *Ann. Med. Exp. Fenn.* **46:**394–398.

MEYERSON, B. J., and LEWANDER, T., 1970, Serotonin synthesis inhibition and estrous behavior in female rats, *Life Sci.* **9**(Pt. 1):661–671.

MEYERSON, B. J., and SAWYER, C. H., 1967, Monoamines and ovulation in the rat, *Acta Pharmacol. Toxicol.* **25**(Suppl. 4):18–19.

MEYERSON, B. J., and SAWYER, C. H., 1968, Monoamines and ovulation in the rat, *Endocrinology* **83:**170–176.

MEYERSON, B. J., ELIASSON, M., LINDSTRÖM, L., MICHANEK, A., and SÖDERLUND, A. CH., 1973, Monoamines and female sexual behaviour, in: *Psychopharmacology, Sexual Disorders and Drug Abuse* (T. A. Ban, J. R. Boissier, G. J. Gessa, H. Heimann, L. Hollister, H. E. Lehmann, I. Munkvad, H. Steinberg, F. Sulser, A. Sundwall, and O. Vinar, eds.), pp. 463–472, North-Holland Publishing Co., Amsterdam and London; Avicenum, Czechoslovak Medical Press, Prague.

MEYERSON, B. J., CARRER, H., and ELIASSON, M., 1974, 5-Hydroxytryptamine and sexual behavior in the female rat, in: *Advances in Biochemical Psychopharmacology*, Vol. 11 (E. Costa and P. Greengard, eds.), pp. 229–242, Raven Press, New York.

MILLARD, S. A., COSTA, E., and GAL, E. M., 1972, On the control of brain serotonin turnover rate by end product inhibition, *Brain Res.* **40:**545–551.

MITCHELL, R. S., 1955, Fatal toxic encephalitis occurring during iproniazid therapy in pulmonary tuberculosis, *Ann. Intern. Med.* **42:**417–424.

MODIGH, K., 1972, Central and peripheral effects of 5-hydroxytryptophan on motor activity in mice, *Psychopharmacologia* **23**:48–54.

MODIGH, K., 1973, Effects of chlorimipramine and protriptyline on the hyperactivity induced by 5-hydroxytryptophan after peripheral decarboxylase inhibition in mice, *J. Neural Transm.* **34**:101–109.

MODIGH, K., and SVENSSON, T. H., 1972, On the role of central nervous system catecholamines and 5-hydroxytryptamine in the nialamide-induced behavioural syndrome, *Br. J. Pharmacol.* **46**:32–45.

MOLINOFF, P., and AXELROD, J., 1969, Octopamine: Normal occurrence in sympathetic nerves of rats, *Science* **164**:428–429.

MOLINOFF, P. B., and AXELROD, J., 1972, Distribution and turnover of octopamine in tissues, *J. Neurochem.* **19**:157–163.

MOLINOFF, P. B., LANDSBERG, L., and AXELROD, J., 1969, An enzymatic assay for octopamine and other β-hydroxylated phenylethylamines, *J. Pharmacol. Exp. Ther.* **170**:253–261.

MONACHON, M.-A., BURKARD, W. P., JALFRE, M., and HAEFELY, W., 1972, Blockade of central 5-hydroxytryptamine receptors by methiothepin, *Naunyn-Schmiedebergs Arch. Pharmacol.* **274**:192–197.

MOORE, R. H., DEMETRIOU, S. K., and DOMINO, E. F., 1975, Effects of iproniazid, chlorpromazine and methiothepin on DMT-induced changes in body temperature, pupillary dilatation, blood pressure and EEG in the rabbit, *Arch. Intern. Pharmacodyn. Ther.* **213**:64–72.

MOSER, M., BRODOFF, B., MILLER, A., and GOLDMAN, A. G., 1964, Pargyline treatment of hypertension: Experience with a nonhydrazine amine oxidase inhibitor, *J. Am. Med. Assoc.* **187**:192–195.

MOURET, J., VILPPULA, A., FRANCHON, N., and JOUVET, M., 1968, Effets d'un inhibiteur de la monoamine oxydase sur le sommeil du rat, *C. R. Soc. Biol.* **162**:914–917.

MUSTALA, O. O., and JOUNELA, A. J., 1966, Influence of pargyline on the toxicity of morphine and pethidine in mice, *Ann. Med. Exp. Fenn.* **44**:395–396.

NAGATSU, T., LEVITT, M., and UDENFRIEND, S., 1964, Tyrosine hydroxylase: The initial step in norepinephrine biosynthesis, *J. Biol. Chem.* **239**:2910–2917.

NEFF, N. H., and COSTA, E., 1966, The influence of monoamine oxidase inhibition on catecholamine syntheses, *Life Sci.* **5**:951–959.

NEFF, N. H., and GORIDIS, C., 1972, Neuronal monoamine oxidase: Specific enzyme types and their rates of formation, in: *Advances in Biochemical Psychopharmacology*, Vol. 5 (E. Costa and P. Greengard, eds.), pp. 307–323, Raven Press, New York.

NEFF, N. H., YANG, H.-Y. T., and GORIDIS, C., 1974, Degradation of the transmitter amines by specific types of monoamine oxidase, *Biochem. Pharmacol. Suppl.*, pp. 86–90.

NEIDLE, A., VAN DEN BERG, C. J., and GRYNBAUM, A., 1969, The heterogeneity of rat brain mitochondria isolated on continuous sucrose gradients, *J. Neurochem.* **16**:225–234.

NYBÄCK, H., SEDVALL, G., and KOPIN, I. J., 1967, Accelerated synthesis of dopamine-C^{14} from tyrosine-C^{14} in rat brain after chlorpromazine, *Life Sci.* **6**:2307–2312.

NYBÄCK, H., BORZECKI, Z., and SEDVALL, G., 1968, Accumulation and disappearance of catecholamines formed from tyrosine-^{14}C in mouse brain: Effect of some psychotropic drugs, *Eur. J. Pharmacol.* **4**:395–403.

NYBÄCK, H., SCHUBERT, J., and SEDVALL, G., 1970, Effect of apomorphine and pimozide on synthesis and turnover of labelled catecholamines in mouse brain, *J. Pharm. Pharmacol.* **22**:622–624.

NYMARK, M., and MØLLER NIELSEN, I., 1963, Reactions due to the combination of monoamineoxidase inhibitors with thymoleptics, pethidine, or methylamphetamine, *Lancet* **2**:524–525.

OATES, J. A., and SJOERDSMA, A., 1960, Neurologic effects of tryptophan in patients receiving a monoamine oxidase inhibitor, *Neurology* **10**:1076–1078.

OBIANWU, H. O., 1969, Possible functional differentiation between the stores from which adrenergic nerve stimulation, tyramine and amphetamine release noradrenaline, *Acta Physiol. Scand.* **75**:92–101.

O'DEA, K., and RAND, M. J., 1969, Interaction between amphetamine and monoamine oxidase inhibitors, *Eur. Pharmacol. J.* **6**:115–120.

OLSSON, S. O., and SCHROLD, J., 1971, A comparison of FG 5310, a new selective monoamine oxidase inhibitor, and other MAO inhibitors on the blood pressure response to tyramine, *Acta Pharmacol. Toxicol.* **29**(Suppl. 4):51.

ORVIS, H. H., TAMAGNA, I. G., and THOMAS, R. E., 1959, Evaluation of 2 monoamine oxidase inhibitors (iproniazid and JB 516) in the therapy of arterial hypertension, *Am. J. Med. Sci.* **238**:336–342.

ORVIS, H. H., TAMAGNA, I. G., HORWITZ, D., and THOMAS, R., 1963, Correlation of hypotensive effects and urinary tryptamine levels during pargyline therapy, *Ann. N. Y. Acad. Sci.* **107**:958–963.

O'STEEN, W. K., 1964, Serotonin suppression of luteinization in gonadotrophin-treated, immature rats, *Endocrinology* **74**:885–888.

O'STEEN, W. K., 1965, Suppression of ovarian activity in immature rats by serotonin, *Endocrinology* **77**:937–939.

OSUMI, S., and FUJIWARA, M., 1969, Tissue distribution of exogenously administered, and endogenously accumulated octopamine in rats, *Jpn. J. Pharmacol.* **19**:185–193.

OSWALD, I., 1968, Drugs and sleep, *Pharmacol. Rev.* **20**:273–303.

OSWALD, I., 1969, Human brain protein, drugs and dreams, *Nature (London)* **223**:893–897.

OWMAN, C., and ROSENGREN, E., 1967, Dopamine formation in brain capillaries—an enzymic blood–brain barrier mechanism, *J. Neurochem.* **14**:547–550.

OXENKRUG, G. F., 1973, Similarity between the effects of dimethyl and monomethyl tricyclic drugs on reserpine effects in the frog and 5-hydroxytryptamine uptake by human blood platelets, *J. Pharm. Pharmacol.* **25**:1013–1015.

PACHTER, I. J., ZACHARIAS, D. E., and RIBEIRO, O., 1959, Indole alkaloids of *Acer saccharinum* (the silver maple), *Dictyoloma incanescens, Piptadenia colubrina*, and *Mimosa hostilis, J. Org. Chem.* **24**:1285–1287.

PALM, D., and MAGNUS, U., 1967, Hemmung der Monoaminoxydase (MAO) und Diaminoxydase (DAO) durch Furazolidon (Furoxon) im Tier- und Selbstversuch, *Naunyn-Schmiedebergs Arch. Pharmakol. Exp. Pathol.* **257**:319–320.

PALMER, H., 1960, Potentiation of pethidine, *Br. Med. J.* **2**:944.

P'AN, S. Y., FUNDERBURK, W. H., and FINGER, K. F., 1961, Anticonvulsant effect of nialamide and diphenylhydantoin, *Proc. Soc. Exp. Biol. Med.* **108**:680–683.

PAPP, C., and BENAIM, S., 1958, Toxic effects of iproniazid in a patient with angina, *Br. Med. J.* **2**:1070–1072.

PASSOUANT, P., CADILHAC, J., BILLIARD, M., and BESSET, A., 1973, La suppression du sommeil paradoxal par la clomipramine, *Therapie* **28**:379–392.

PATANE, S., and ARRIGO REINA, R., 1970, Azione inibente di alcuni derivati del pirazolinone sulla inattivazione metabolica della 5-idrossitriptamina. Azione di alcuni derivati del pirazolinone sull "attivita" pressoria della tiramina, *Boll. Soc. Ital. Biol. Sper.* **45**:1079–1083.

PENN, R. G., and ROGERS, K. J., 1971, Comparison of the effects of morphine, pethidine and pentazocine in rabbits pretreated with a monoamine oxidase inhibitor, *Br. J. Pharmacol.* **42**:485–492.

PENNES, H. H., and HOCH, P. H., 1957, Psychotomimetics, clinical and theoretical considerations: Harmine, win-2299 and nalline, *Am. J. Psychiatry* **113**:887–892.

PEREZ-CRUET, J., TAGLIAMONTE, A., TAGLIAMONTE, P., and GESSA, G. L., 1971, Stimulation of serotonin synthesis by lithium, *J. Pharmacol. Exp. Ther.* **178**:325–330.

PETTINGER, W. A., and OATES, J. A., 1968, Supersensitivity to tyramine during monoamine oxidase inhibition in man. Mechanism at the level of the adrenergic neuron, *Clin. Pharmacol. Ther.* **9**:341–344.

PFEIFER, A. K., and GALAMBOS, E., 1967, The effect of reserpine α-methyl-m-tyrosine, prenylamine, and guanethidine on metrazol-convulsions and the brain monoamine level in mice, *Arch. Intern. Pharmacodyn. Ther.* **165**:201–211.

PHILIPS, S. R., DURDEN, D. A., and BOULTON, A. A., 1974, Identification and distribution of tryptamine in the rat, *Can. J. Biochem.* **52**:447–451.

PLETSCHER, A., 1957, Wirkung von Isopropyl-isonicotinsäure-hydrazid auf den Stoffwechsel von Catecholaminen und 5-Hydroxytryptamin im Gehirn, *Schweiz. Med. Wochenschr.* **87**:1532–1534.

PLETSCHER, A., BESENDORF, H., BÄCHTOLD, H. P., and GEY, K. F., 1959, Über pharmakologische Beeinflussung des Zentralnervensystems durch kurzwirkende Monoaminoxydasehemmer aus der Gruppe der Harmala-Alkaloide, *Helv. Physiol. Acta* **17**:202–214.

PLOTNIKOFF, N., HUANG, J., and HAVENS, P., 1963, Effect of monoamino oxidase inhibitors on audiogenic seizures, *J. Pharm. Sci.* **52**:172–173.

PLUMMER, A. J., and FURNESS, P. A., 1963, Biological estimation of the intensity and duration of action of monoamine oxidase inhibitors, *Ann. N. Y. Acad. Sci.* **107**:865–877.

POITOU, P., GUERINOT, F., and BOHUON, C., 1974, Effect of lithium on central metabolism of 5-hydroxytryptamine, *Psychopharmacologia* **38**:75–80.

POULSON, E., and ROBSON, J. M., 1963, The effect of amine oxidase inhibitors on pregnancy, *J. Endocrinol.* **27**:147–152.

POULSON, E., and ROBSON, J. M., 1964, Effect of phenelzine and some related compounds on pregnancy and on sexual development, *J. Endocrinol.* **30**:205–215.

PROCKOP, D. J., SHORE, P. A., and BRODIE, B. B., 1959a, An anticonvulsant effect of monoamine oxidase inhibitors, *Experientia* **15**:145–147.

PROCKOP, D. J., SHORE, P. A., and BRODIE, B. B., 1959b, Anticonvulsant properties of monoamine oxidase inhibitors, *Ann. N. Y. Acad. Sci.* **80**:643–651.

PRZUNTEK, H., GUIMARÃES, S., and PHILIPPU, A., 1971, Importance of adrenergic neurons of the brain for the rise of blood pressure evoked by hypothalamic stimulation, *Naunyn-Schmiedebergs Arch. Pharmakol.* **271**:311–319.

PSCHEIDT, G. R., 1964, Monoamine oxidase inhibitors, in: *International Review of Neurobiology*, Vol. 7 (Carl C. Pfeiffer and J. R. Smythies, eds.), pp. 191–229, Academic Press, New York and London.

PUJOL, J.-F., BUGUET, A., FROMENT, J.-L., JONES, B., and JOUVET, M., 1971, The central metabolism of serotonin in the cat during insomnia. A neurophysiological and biochemical study after administration of p-chlorophenylalanine or destruction of the raphé system, *Brain Res.* **29**:195–212.

RAND, M. J., and TRINKER, F. R., 1968, The mechanism of the augmentation of responses to indirectly acting sympathomimetic amines by monoamine oxidase inhibitors, *Br. J. Pharmacol. Chemother.* **33**:287–303.

RANDALL, L. O., and BAGDON, R. E., 1959, Pharmacology of iproniazid and other amine oxidase inhibitors, *Ann. N. Y. Acad. Sci.* **80**:626–636.

RANDRUP, A., and MUNKVAD, I., 1966, Dopa and other naturally occurring substances as causes of stereotypy and rage in rats, *Acta Psychiatr. Scand. Suppl. 191*, pp. 193–199.

RANDRUP, A., and MUNKVAD, I., 1970, Biochemical, anatomical and psychological investigations of stereotyped behavior induced by amphetamines, in: *Amphetamines and Related Compounds* (E. Costa and S. Garattini, eds.), pp. 695–713, Raven Press, New York.

REITE, M., INGRAM, G. V., STEPHENS, L. M., BIXLER, E. C., and LEWIS, O. L., 1969, The effect of reserpine and monoamine oxidase inhibitors on paradoxical sleep in the monkey, *Psychopharmacologia* **14**:12–17.

RENTON, K. W., and EADE, N. R., 1972, Microsomal enzymes and potentiation of tyramine pressor response, *Biochem. Pharmacol.* **21**:1393–1402.

ROBINSON, N., 1967, Histochemistry of monoamine oxidase in the developing rat brain, *J. Neurochem.* **14**:1083–1089.

ROBINSON, N., 1968, Histochemistry of rat brain stem monoamine oxidase during maturation, *J. Neurochem.* **15**:1151–1158.

ROBINSON, N., 1972, Enzyme histochemistry of the rat hypothalamus during early development, *J. Neurochem.* **19:**1577–1585.

ROBSON, J. M., and BOTROS, M., 1961, The effect of 5-hydroxytryptamine and of monoamine oxidase inhibitors on sexual maturity, *J. Endocrinol.* **22:**165–175.

ROGERS, K. J., 1971, Role of brain monoamines in the interaction between pethidine and tranylcypromine, *Eur. J. Pharmacol.* **14:**86–88.

ROGERS, K. J., and THORNTON, J. A., 1969, The interaction between monoamine oxidase inhibitors and narcotic analgesics in mice, *Br. J. Pharmacol.* **36:**470–480.

ROSS, S. B., and RENYI, A. L., 1975, Tricyclic antidepressant agents. I. Comparison of the inhibition of the uptake of ^{3}H-noradrenaline and ^{14}C-5-hydroxytryptamine in slices and crude synaptosome preparations of the midbrain–hypothalamus region of the rat brain, *Acta Pharmacol. Toxicol.* **36:**382–394.

ROSS, S. B., RENYI, A. L., and ÖGREN, S.-O., 1972, Inhibition of the uptake of noradrenaline and 5-hydroxytryptamine by chlorphentermine and chlorimipramine, *Eur. J. Pharmacol.* **17:**107–112.

ROTH, R. H., and STONE, E. A., 1968, The action of reserpine on noradrenaline biosynthesis in sympathetic nerve tissue, *Biochem. Pharmacol.* **17:**1581–1590.

RUCH-MONACHON, M.-A., JALFRE, M., and HAEFELY, W. E., 1975a, Drugs and PGO waves in the lateral geniculate body of the curarized cat. I. PGO wave activity induced by Ro 4-1284 and by *p*-chlorophenylalanine (PCPA) as a basis for neuropharmacological studies, *Arch. Int. Pharmacodyn. Ther.* **219:**251–268.

RUCH-MONACHON, M.-A., JALFRE, M., and HAEFELY, W., 1975b, Drugs and PGO waves in the lateral geniculate body of the curarized cat. II. PGO wave activity and brain 5-hydroxytryptamine, *Arch. Int. Pharmacodyn. Ther.* **219:**269–286.

RUCH-MONACHON, M.-A., JALFRE, M., and HAEFELY, W., 1975c, Drugs and PGO waves in the lateral geniculate body of the curarized cat. III. PGO wave activity and brain catecholamines, *Arch. Int. Pharmacodyn. Ther.* **219:**287–307.

RUCH-MONACHON, M.-A., JALFRE, M., and HAEFELY, W., 1975d, Drugs and PGO waves in the lateral geniculate body of the curarized cat. IV. The effects of acetylcholine, GABA, and benzodiazepines on PGO wave activity, *Arch. Int. Pharmacodyn. Ther.* **219:**308–325.

RUCH-MONACHON, M.-A., JALFRE, M., and HAEFELY, W., 1975e, Drugs and PGO waves in the lateral geniculate body of the curarized cat. V. Miscellaneous compounds. Synopsis of the role of central neurotransmitters on PGO wave activity, *Arch. Int. Pharmacodyn. Ther.* **219:**326–346.

RUDZIK, A. D., and MENNEAR, J. H., 1965, The mechanism of action of anticonvulsants. I. Diphenylhydantoin, *Life Sci.* **4:**2373–2382.

RUDZIK, A. D., and MENNEAR, J. H., 1966, The mechanism of action of anticonvulsants. II. Acetazolamide, *Life Sci.* **5:**747–756.

SAAVEDRA, J. M., 1974, Enzymatic–isotopic method for octopamine at the picogram level, *Anal. Biochem.* **59:**628–633.

SAAVEDRA, J. M., and AXELROD, J., 1973, Effect of drugs on the tryptamine content of rat tissues, *J. Pharmacol. Exp. Ther.* **185:**523–529.

SAAVEDRA, J. M., and AXELROD, J., 1974a, Brain tryptamine and the effects of drugs, in: *Advances in Biochemical Psychopharmacology* (E. Costa and P. Greengard, eds.), Vol. 10, pp. 135–139, Raven Press, New York.

SAAVEDRA, J. M., and AXELROD, J., 1974b, Developmental characteristics of phenylethanolamine and octopamine in the rat brain, *J. Neurochem.* **23:**511–515.

SAAVEDRA, J. M., PALKOVITS, M., BROWNSTEIN, M. J., and AXELROD, J., 1974, Localisation of phenylethanolamine *N*-methyl transferase in the rat brain nuclei, *Nature (London)* **248:**695–696.

SABELLI, H. C., and MOSNAIM, A. D., 1974, Phenylethylamine hypothesis of affective behavior, *Am. J. Psychiatry* **131:**695–699.

SABELLI, H. C., VAZQUEZ, A. J., and FLAVIN, D., 1975, Behavioral and electrophysiological effects of phenylethanolamine and 2-phenylethylamine, *Psychopharmacologia* **42:**117–125.

SACHS, C., 1970, *Noradrenaline Uptake Mechanisms. A Biochemical and Histochemical Study,* Department of Histology, Karolinske Institutet, Stockholm, Sweden.

SALIS, P. J., and DEWSBURY, D. A., 1971, *p*-Chlorophenylalanine facilitates copulatory behaviour in male rats, *Nature (London)* **232:**400–401.

SANDERS, F., and BUSH, M. T., 1967, Distribution, metabolism and excretion of bufotenine in the rat with preliminary studies of its *o*-methyl derivative, *J. Pharmacol. Exp. Ther.* **158:**340–352.

SANGHVI, I., and GERSHON, S., 1970, Similarities between behavioral and pharmacological actions of yohimbine and 5-hydroxytryptophan in the conscious dog, *Eur. J. Pharmacol.* **11:**125–129.

SANSONE, M., and DELL'OMODARME, G., 1963, Influence de l'isocarboxazide (marplan) et de deux nouveaux inhibiteurs de la MAO sur les convulsions cloniques et sur la mortalité per métrazol, *Arch. Intern. Pharmacodyn. Ther.* **144:**392–398.

SCHEEL-KRÜGER, J., and JONAS, W., 1973, Pharmacological studies on tetrabenazine-induced excited behaviour of rats pretreated with amphetamine or nialamide, *Arch. Intern. Pharmacodyn. Ther.* **206:**47–65.

SCHLESINGER, K., BOGGAN, W., and FREEDMAN, D. X., 1968*a*, Genetics of audiogenic seizures. II. Effects of pharmacological manipulation of brain serotonin, norepinephrine and gamma-aminobutyric acid, *Life Sci.* **7**(Pt. I):437–447.

SCHLESINGER, K., BOGGAN, W. O., and GRIEK, B. J., 1968*b*, Pharmacogenetic correlates of pentylenetetrazol and electroconvulsive seizure thresholds in mice, *Psychopharmacologia* **13:**181–188.

SCHMITT, H., SCHMITT, H., and FENARD, S., 1971, Evidence for an α-sympathomimetic component in the effects of catapresan on vasomotor centres: Antagonism by piperoxane, *Eur. J. Pharmacol.* **14:**98–100.

SCHNAITMAN, C., and GREENAWALT, J. W., 1968, Enzymatic properties of the inner and outer membranes of rat liver mitochondria, *J. Cell Biol.* **38:**158–175.

SCHOEPKE, H. G., and SWETT, L. R., 1967, Chemistry and pharmacology of monoamine oxidase inhibitors, in: *Antihypertensive Agents* (E. Schlittler, ed.), pp. 393–428, Academic Press, New York and London.

SCHOEPKE, H. G., and WIEGAND, R. G., 1963, Relation between norepinephrine accumulation or depletion and blood pressure responses in the cat and rat following pargyline administration, *Ann. N. Y. Acad. Sci.* **107:**924–934.

SCHUBERT, J., 1973, Effect of chronic lithium treatment on monoamine metabolism in rat brain, *Psychopharmacologia* **32:**301–311.

SCHWEITZER, J. W., and FRIEDHOFF, A. J., 1968, The metabolism of dimethoxyphenethylamine, a compound found in the urine of schizophrenics, *Am. J. Psychiatry* **124:**1249–1253.

SHASKAN, E. G., and SNYDER, S. H., 1970, Kinetics of serotonin accumulation into slices from rat brain: Relationship to catecholamine uptake, *J. Pharmacol. Exp. Ther.* **175:**404–418.

SHEARD, M. H., 1969, The effect of *p*-chlorophenylalanine on behavior in rats: Relation to brain serotonin and 5-hydroxyindoleacetic acid, *Brain Res.* **15:**524–528.

SHEARD, M. H., 1974, The effect of *p*-chloroamphetamine on single raphe neurons, in: *Advances in Biochemical Psychopharmacology,* Vol. 10 (E. Costa and P. Greengard, eds.), pp. 179–184, Raven Press, New York.

SHEARD, M. H., and AGHAJANIAN, G. K., 1970, Neuronally activated metabolism of brain serotonin: Effect of lithium, *Life Sci.* **9**(Pt. I):285–290.

SHEARD, M. H., ZOLOVICK, A., and AGHAJANIAN, G. K., 1972, Raphe neurons: Effect of tricyclic antidepressant drugs, *Brain Res.* **43:**690–694.

SHEE, J. C., 1960, Dangerous potentiation of pethidine by iproniazid, and its treatment, *Br. Med. J.* **2:**507–509.

SHILLITO, E. E., 1970, The effect of parachlorophenylalanine on social interaction of male rats, Br. J. Pharmacol. **38**:305–315.

SHIMIZU, N., MORIKAWA, N., and OKADA, M., 1959, Histochemical studies of monoamine oxidase of the brain of rodents, Z. Zellforsch. **49**:389–400.

SHORE, P. A., and BRODIE, B. B., 1957, LSD-like effects elicited by reserpine in rabbits pretreated with iproniazid (22968), Proc. Soc. Exp. Biol. Med. **94**:433–435.

SHULGIN, A. T., SARGENT, T., and NARANJO, C., 1966, Role of 3,4-dimethoxyphenethylamine in schizophrenia, Nature (London) **212**:1606–1607.

SHULGIN, A. T., SARGENT, T., and NARANJO, C., 1969, Structure–activity relationships of one-ring psychotomimetics, Nature (London) **221**:537–541.

SHULGIN, A. T., SARGENT, T., and NARANJO, C., 1971, 4-Bromo-2,5-dimethoxyphenylisopropylamine, a new centrally active amphetamine analog, Pharmacology **5**:103–107.

SINCLAIR, J. G., 1972a, The effects of meperidine and morphine in rabbits pretreated with phenelzine, Toxicol. Appl. Pharmacol. **22**:231–240.

SINCLAIR, J. G., 1972b, Ethoheptazine–monoamine oxidase inhibitor interaction in rabbits, Can. J. Physiol. Pharmacol. **50**:923–926.

SINCLAIR, J. G., 1972c, Antihistamine–monoamine oxidase inhibitor interaction in rabbits, J. Pharm. Pharmacol. **24**:955–961.

SINCLAIR, J. G., 1973, Dextromethorphan–monoamine oxidase inhibitor interaction in rabbits, J. Pharm. Pharmacol. **25**:803–808.

SINGH, H., 1960, Atropine-like poisoning due to tranquilizing agents, Am. J. Psychiatry **117**:360–361.

SINHA, J. N., DHASMANA, K. M., DIXIT, K. S., and BHARGAVA, K. P., 1969, Antagonism of imipramine induced fatal hyperpyrexia in MAO inhibitor treated rabbits, Jpn. J. Pharmacol. **19**:623–625.

SJOERDSMA, A., GILLESPIE, L., and UDENFRIEND, S., 1959a, A method for measurement of monoamine oxidase inhibition in man: Application to studies on hypertension, N. Y. Acad. Sci. **80**:969–980.

SJOERDSMA, A., LOVENBERG, W., OATES, J. A., CROUT, J. R., and UDENFRIEND, S., 1959b, Alterations in the pattern of amine excretion in man produced by a monoamine oxidase inhibitor, Science **130**:225.

SJOERDSMA, A., OATES, J. A., ZALTZMAN, P., and UDENFRIEND, S., 1959c, Identification and assay of urinary tryptamine: Application as an index of monoamine oxidase inhibition in man, J. Pharmacol. Exp. Ther. **126**:217–222.

SLATER, I. H., JONES, G. T., and MOORE, R. A., 1974, Sleep studies with the specific inhibitor of serotonin uptake, 3-(p-trifluoromethylphenoxy)-n-methyl-3-phenylpropylamine hydrochloride, Lilly 110140, Association for the Psychophysiological Study of Sleep, June 6–9, Jackson Hole, Wyoming, 14th Annual meeting (Abstract).

SLOAN, J. W., MARTIN, W. R., CLEMENTS, T. H., BUCHWALD, W. F., and BRIDGES, S. R., 1975, Factors influencing brain and tissue levels of tryptamine: Species, drugs and lesions, J. Neurochem. **24**:523–532.

SMYTHIES, J. R., JOHNSTON, V. S., BRADLEY, R. J., BENINGTON, F., MORIN, R. D., and CLARK, L. C., 1967, Some new behaviour-disrupting amphetamines and their significance, Nature (London) **216**:128–129.

SNODGRASS, S. R., and HORN, A. S., 1973, An assay procedure for tryptamine in brain and spinal cord using its (^{3}H) dansyl derivative, J. Neurochem. **21**:687–696.

SNODGRASS, S. R., and IVERSEN, L. L., 1974, Formation and release of ^{3}H-tryptamine from ^{3}H-tryptophan in rat spinal cord slices, in: Advances in Biochemical Psychopharmacology, Vol. 10 (E. Costa and P. Greengard, eds.), pp. 141–150, Raven Press, New York.

SNYDER, S. H., FISCHER, J., and AXELROD, J., 1965, Evidence for the presence of monoamine oxidase in sympathetic nerve endings, Biochem. Pharmacol. **14**:363–365.

SNYDER, S. H., WEINGARTNER, H., and FAILLACE, L. A., 1971, DOET (2,5-dimethoxy-4-ethylamphetamine), a new psychotropic drug. Effects of varying doses in man, Arch. Gen. Psychiatry **24**:50–55.

SPANO, P. F., 1966, Potentiation of the noradrenaline-releasing action of tyramine by monoamine oxidase inhibitors, *J. Pharm. Pharmacol.* **18**:548–549.

SPECTOR, S., 1963, Monoamine oxidase in control of brain serotonin and norepinephrine content, *Ann. N. Y. Acad. Sci.* **107**:856–864.

SPECTOR, S., PROCKOP, D., SHORE, P. A., and BRODIE, B. B., 1958, Effect of iproniazid on brain levels of norepinephrine and serotonin, *Science* **127**:704.

SPECTOR, S., SHORE, P. A., and BRODIE, B. B., 1960*a*, Biochemical and pharmacological effects of the monoamine oxidase inhibitors, iproniazid, 1-phenyl-2-hydrazinopropane (JB 516) and 1-phenyl-3-hydrazinobutane (JB 835), *J. Pharmacol. Exp. Ther.* **128**:15–21.

SPECTOR, S., KUNTZMAN, R., SHORE, P. A., and BRODIE, B. B., 1960*b*, Evidence for release of brain amines by reserpine in presence of monoamine oxidase inhibitors: Implication of monoamine oxidase in norepinephrine metabolism in brain, *J. Pharmacol. Exp. Ther.* **130**:256–261.

SPENCER, J. N., PORTER, M., FROEHLICH, H. L., and WENDEL, H., 1960, Observations on the cardiovascular effects of tranylcypromine, *Fed. Proc. Fed. Am. Soc. Exp. Biol.* **19**:277.

SPOERLEIN, M. T., and ELLMAN, A. M., 1961, Facilitation of metrazol-induced seizures by iproniazid and betaphenylisopropylhydrazine in mice, *Arch. Intern. Pharmacodyn. Ther.* **133**:193–199.

SPRINCE, H., PARKER, C. M., JAMESON, D., and ALEXANDER, F., 1963, Urinary indoles in schizophrenic and psychoneurotic patients after administration of tranylcypromine (parnate) and methionine or tryptophan, *J. Nerv. Ment. Dis.* **137**:246–251.

SQUIRES, R. F., 1968, Additional evidence for the existence of several forms of mitochondrial monoamine oxidase in the mouse, *Biochem. Pharmacol.* **17**:1401–1409.

SQUIRES, R. F., 1971, On the decrease in concentration of 5-HIAA in rat brain by imipramine and related substances, *Acta Pharmacol. Toxicol.* **29**(Suppl. 4):56.

SQUIRES, R., 1972*a*, Antagonism of *p*-chloroamphetamine (PCA) induced depletion of 5-HT from rat brain by some thymoleptics and other psychotropic drugs, *Acta Pharmacol. Toxicol.* **31**(Suppl. 1):35.

SQUIRES, R. F., 1972*b*, Multiple forms of monoamine oxidase in intact mitochondria as characterized by selective inhibitors and thermal stability: A comparison of eight mammalian species, in: *Advances in Biochemical Psychopharmacology*, Vol. 5 (E. Costa and P. Greengard, eds.), pp. 355–370, Raven Press, New York.

SQUIRES, R. F., 1974, Effects of noradrenaline pump blockers on its uptake by synaptosomes from several regions; additional evidence for dopamine terminals in the frontal cortex, *J. Pharm. Pharmacol.* **26**:364–367.

SQUIRES, R. F., 1975, Evidence that 5-methoxy-*N,N*-dimethyltryptamine is a specific substrate for MAO-A in the rat: Implications for the indolamine dependent behavioural syndrome, *J. Neurochem.* **24**:47–50.

SQUIRES, R. F., and BUUS LASSEN, J., 1968, Some pharmacological and biochemical properties of γ-morpholino-butyrophenone (NSD 2023), a new monoamine oxidase inhibitor, *Biochem. Pharmacol.* **17**:369–384.

SQUIRES, R. F., and BUUS LASSEN, J., 1975, The inhibition of A and B forms of MAO in the production of a characteristic behavioural syndrome in rats after L-tryptophan loading, *Psychopharmacologia* **41**:145–151.

STEIN, D., JOUVET, M., and PUJOL, J.-F., 1974, Effects of α-methyl-*p*-tyrosine upon cerebral amine metabolism and sleep states in the cat, *Brain Res.* **72**:360–365.

STRUYKER BOUDIER, H. A. J., and BEKERS, A., 1975, Adrenaline-induced cardiovascular changes after intrahypothalamic administration to rats, *Eur. J. Pharmacol.* **31**:153–155.

STRUYKER BOUDIER, H., SMEETS, G., BROUWER, G., and VAN ROSSUM, J. M., 1975, Central nervous system α-adrenergic mechanisms and cardiovascular regulation in rats, *Arch. Intern. Pharmacodyn. Ther.* **213**:285–293.

SZARA, S., 1956, Dimethyltryptamine: Its metabolism in man: the relation of its psychotic effect to the serotonin metabolism, *Experientia* **12**:441–442.

SZARA, S., ROCKLAND, L. H., ROSENTHAL, D., and HANDLON, J. H., 1966, Psychological effects and metabolism of *N,N*-diethyltryptamine in man, *Arch. Gen. Psychiatry* **15**:320–329.

TABAKOFF, B., MEYERSON, L., and ALIVISATOS, S. G. A., 1974, Properties of monoamine oxidase in nerve endings from two bovine brain areas, *Brain Res.* **66**:491–508.

TABORSKY, R. G., and MCISAAC, W. M., 1964, The relationship between the metabolic fate and pharmacological action of 5-methoxy-*N*-methyltryptamine, *Biochem. Pharmacol.* **13**:531–552.

TAGLIAMONTE, A., TAGLIAMONTE, P., GESSA, G. L., and BRODIE, B. B., 1969, Compulsive sexual activity induced by *p*-chlorophenylalanine in normal and pinealectomized male rats, *Science* **166**:1433–1435.

TAGLIAMONTE, A., TAGLIAMONTE, P., PEREZ-CRUET, J., and GESSA, G. L., 1971a, Increase of brain tryptophan caused by drugs which stimulate serotonin synthesis, *Nature (London) New Biol.* **229**:125–126.

TAGLIAMONTE, A., TAGLIAMONTE, P., PEREZ-CRUET, J., STERN, S., and GESSA, G. L., 1971b, Effect of psychotropic drugs on tryptophan concentration in the rat brain, *J. Pharmacol. Exp. Ther.* **177**:475–480.

TAGLIAMONTE, A., TAGLIAMONTE, P., and GESSA, G. L., 1971c, Reversal of pargyline-induced inhibition of sexual behaviour in male rats by *p*-chlorophenylalanine, *Nature (London)* **230**:244–245.

TARVER, J., BERKOWITZ, B., and SPECTOR, S., 1971, Alterations in tyrosine hydroxylase and monoamine oxidase activity in blood vessels, *Nature (London) New Biol.* **231**:252–253.

TAYLOR, D. C., 1962, Antidepressives in chronic schizophrenics, *Lancet* **2**:401–402.

TEDESCHI, D. H., and FELLOWS, E. J., 1964, Monoamine oxidase inhibitors: Augmentation of pressor effects of peroral tyramine, *Science* **144**:1225–1226.

TEDESCHI, D. H., TEDESCHI, R. E., and FELLOWS, E. J., 1959, The effects of tryptamine on the central nervous system, including a pharmacological procedure for the evaluation of iproniazid-like drugs, *J. Pharmacol. Exp. Ther.* **126**:223–232.

TEDESCHI, D. H., TEDESCHI, R. E., and FELLOWS, E. J., 1960, *In vivo* monoamine oxidase inhibition measured by potentiation of tryptamine convulsions in rats (25633), *Proc. Soc. Exp. Biol. Med.* **103**:680–682.

TEDESCHI, D. H., TEDESCHI, R. E., and FELLOWS, E. J., 1961, Central serotonin antagonist activity of a number of phenothiazines, *Arch. Intern. Pharmacodyn. Ther.* **132**:172–179.

TEDESCHI, R. E., TEDESCHI, D. H., AMES, P. L., COOK, L., MATTIS, P. A., and FELLOWS, E. J., 1959, Some pharmacological observations on tranylcypromine (SKF trans-385); A potent inhibitor of monoamine oxidase, *Proc. Soc. Exp. Biol. Med.* **102**:380–381.

TISSARI, A. H., and SUURHASKO, B. V. A., 1971, Transport of 5HT in synaptosomes of developing rat brain, *Acta Pharmacol. Toxicol.* **29**(Suppl. 4):59.

TODA, N., YAMAWAKI, T., and MISU, Y., 1962, The sympathomimetic effects of SKF-385 on blood pressure in dog, *Jpn. J. Pharmacol.* **12**:166–179.

TODRICK, A., and TAIT, A. C., 1969, The inhibition of human platelet 5-hydroxy-tryptamine uptake by tricyclic antidepressive drugs. The relation between structure and potency, *J. Pharm. Pharmacol.* **21**:751–762.

TOYODA, J., 1964, The effects of chlorpromazine and imipramine on the human nocturnal sleep electroencephalogram, *Folia Psychiatr. Neurol. Jpn.* **18**:198–221.

TUCHMANN-DUPLESSIS, H., and MERCIER-PAROT, L., 1962, Influence de la niamide sur la sphere sexuelle et la fertilité du rat, *Chemotherapia* **4**:304–313.

TUOMISTO, J., 1974, A new modification for studying 5-HT uptake by blood platelets: A re-evaluation of tricyclic antidepressants as uptake inhibitors, *J. Pharm. Pharmacol.* **26**:92–100.

UCHIDA, T., and O'BRIEN, R. D., 1964, The effects of hydrazines on rat brain 5-hydroxytryptamine, norepinephrine, and gamma-aminobutyric acid, *Biochem. Pharmacol.* **13**:725–730.

UDENFRIEND, S., WEISSBACH, H., and BOGDANSKI, D. F., 1957a, Increase in tissue serotonin following administration of its precursor 5-hydroxytryptophan, *J. Biol. Chem.* **224**:803–810.

UDENFRIEND, S., WEISSBACH, H., and BOGDANSKI, D. F., 1957*b*, Biochemical findings relating to the action of serotonin, *Ann. N. Y. Acad. Sci.* **66**:602–608.

URRY, R. L., and DOUGHERTY, K. A., 1975, Inhibition of rat spermatogenesis and seminiferous tubule growth after short-term and long-term administration of a monoamine oxidase inhibitor, *Fertil. Steril.* **26**:232–239.

VALZELLI, L., and GARATTINI, S., 1968, Biogenic amines in discrete brain areas after treatment with monoamineoxidase inhibitors, *J. Neurochem.* **15**:259–261.

VAN DER ZEE, P., and HESPE, W., 1973, Influence of orphenadrine HCl and its *N*-demethylated derivatives on the *in vitro* uptake of noradrenaline and 5-hydroxytryptamine by rat brain slices, *Neuropharmacology* **12**:843–851.

VANE, J. R., COLLIER, H. O. J., CORNE, S. J., MARLEY, E., and BRADLEY, P. B., 1961, Tryptamine receptors in the central nervous system, *Nature (London)* **191**:1068–1069.

VANOV, S., 1962, Effect of monoamine oxidase inhibitors and pyrogallol on the pressor response to adrenaline, noradrenaline, normetanephrine and tyramine in the rat, *Arch. Intern. Pharmacodyn. Ther.* **138**:51–61.

VAN ZWIETEN, P. A., 1973, The central action of antihypertensive drugs, mediated via central α-receptors, *J. Pharm. Pharmacol.* **25**:89–95.

VASKO, M. R., LUTZ, M. P., and DOMINO, E. F., 1974, Structure activity relations of some indolealkylamines in comparison to phenethylamines on motor activity and acquisition of avoidance behavior, *Psychopharmacologia* **36**:49–58.

VOGEL, W. H., 1967, Physiological disposition and metabolism of 3,4-dimethoxyphenylethylamine (DMPEA) in the rat, *Pharmacologist* **9**:238.

VOGEL, W. H., 1968, Physiological disposition and metabolism of 3,4-dimethoxyphenylethylamine in the rat, *Int. J. Neuropharmacol.* **7**:373–381.

VOGEL, W. H., and HORWITT, M. K., 1967, Brain levels of 3,4-dimethoxyphenylethylamine (DMPEA) and climbing performance of rats, *Psychopharmacologia* **11**:265–269.

WEBER, L. J., 1966, Influence of monoamine oxidase inhibitors on 5-hydroxytryptamine synthesis in the brain (31395), *Proc. Soc. Exp. Biol. Med.* **123**:35–38.

WENGER, G. R., STITZEL, R. E., and CRAIG, C. R., 1973, The role of biogenic amines in the reserpine-induced alteration of minimal electroshock seizure thresholds in the mouse, *Neuropharmacology* **12**:693–703.

WESTHEIMER, R., and KLAWANS, H. L., 1974, The role of serotonin in the pathophysiology of myoclonic seizures associated with acute imipramine toxicity, *Neurology* **24**:1175–1177.

WHALEN, R. E., and LUTTGE, W. G., 1970, *p*-Chlorophenylalanine methyl ester: An aphrodisiac?, *Science* **169**:1000–1001.

WIEGAND, R. G., and PERRY, J. E., 1961, Effect of L-dopa and *n*-methyl-benzyl-2-propynylamine-HCl on DOPA, dopamine, norepinephrine, epinephrine and serotonin levels in mouse brain, *Biochem. Pharmacol.* **7**:181–186.

WILSON, C. A., 1974, Hypothalamic amines and the release of gonadotrophins and other anterior pituitary hormones, in: *Advances in Drug Research*, Vol. 8 (N. J. Harper and A. B. Simmonds, eds.), pp. 119–204, Academic Press, London—New York—San Francisco.

WINTER, C. H., and FLATAKER, L., 1951, The effect of antihistaminic drugs upon the performance of trained rats, *J. Pharmacol. Exp. Ther.* **101**:156–162.

WU, P. H., and BOULTON, A. A., 1975, Metabolism, distribution, and disappearance of injected β-phenylethylamine in the rat, *Can. J. Biochem.* **53**:42–50.

WYATT, R. J., KUPFER, D. J., SCOTT, J., ROBINSON, D. S., and SNYDER, F., 1969, Longitudinal studies on the effect of monoamine oxidase inhibitors on sleep in man, *Psychopharmacologia* **15**:236–244.

WYATT, R. J., CHASE, T. N., SCOTT, J., SNYDER, F., and ENGLEMAN, K., 1970, Effect of L-dopa on the sleep of man, *Nature (London)* **228**:999–1001.

WYATT, R. J., FRAM, D. H., KUPFER, D. J., and SNYDER, F., 1971*a*, Total prolonged drug-induced REM sleep suppression in anxious-depressed patients, *Arch. Gen. Psychiatry* **24:**145–155.

WYATT, R. J., FRAM, D. H., BUCHBINDER, R., and SNYDER, F., 1971*b*, Treatment of intractable narcolepsy with a monoamine oxidase inhibitor, *N. Engl. J. Med.* **285:**987–991.

YAMORI, Y., LOVENBERG, W., and SJOERDSMA, A., 1970, Norepinephrine metabolism in brainstem on spontaneously hypertensive rats, *Science* **170:**544–546.

YAMORI, Y., DE JONG, W., YAMABE, H., LOVENBERG, W., and SJOERDSMA, A., 1972, Effects of L-dopa and inhibitors of decarboxylase and monoamine oxidase on brain noradrenaline levels and blood pressure in spontaneously hypertensive rats, *J. Pharm. Pharmacol.* **24:**690–695.

YANG, H.-Y. T., and NEFF, N. H., 1973, β-Phenylethylamine: A specific substrate for type B monoamine oxidase of brain, *J. Pharmacol. Exp. Ther.* **187:**365–371.

YANG, H.-Y. T., and NEFF, N. H., 1974, The monoamine oxidases of brain: Selective inhibition with drugs and the consequences for the metabolism of the biogenic amines, *J. Pharmacol. Exp. Ther.* **189:**733–740.

YATES, C. M., TODRICK, A., and TAIT, A. C., 1964, Effect of imipramine and some analogues on the uptake of 5-hydroxytryptamine by human blood platelets *in vitro*, *J. Pharm. Pharmacol.* **16:**460–463.

YEN, H. C. Y., SALVATORE, A. T., SILVERMAN, A. J., and KING, T. O., 1962, A study of the effect of iproniazid on anticonvulsants in mice, *Arch. Intern. Pharmacodyn. Ther.* **140:**631–645.

ZBINDEN, G., and STUDER, A., 1959, Experimental pathology of iproniazid and related compounds, *Ann. N. Y. Acad. Sci.* **80:**873–884.

ZELLER, E. A., 1951, Oxidation of amines, in: *The Enzymes,* Vol. II (J. B. Sumner and K. Myrbäck, eds.), Pt. 1, pp. 536–544.

ZEMLAN, F. P., WARD, I. L., CROWLEY, W. R., and MARGULES, D. L., 1973, Activation of lordotic responding in female rats by suppression of serotonergic activity, *Science* **179:**1010–1011.

ZIRKLE, C. L., and KAISER, C., 1964, Monoamine oxidase inhibitors (nonhydrazines), in: *Psychopharmacological Agents,* Vol. I (M. Gordon, ed.), pp. 445–554, Academic Press, New York and London.

ZIRKLE, C. L., KAISER, C., TEDESCHI, D. H., and TEDESCHI, R. E., 1962, 2-Substituted cyclopropylamines. II. Effect of structure upon monoamine oxidase-inhibitory activity as measured *in vivo* by potentiation of tryptamine convulsions, *J. Med. Pharm. Chem.* **5:**1265–1284.

ZOLOVICK, A., and LABHSETWAR, A. P., 1973, Evidence for the theory of dual hypothalamic control of ovulation, *Nature (London)* **245:**158–159.

ZOR, U., DIKSTEIN, S., and SULMAN, F. G., 1965*a*, The effect of monoamine oxidase inhibitors on growth and the rat tibia test, *J. Endocrinol.* **32:**35–43.

ZOR, U., DIKSTEIN, S., and SULMAN, F. G., 1965*b*, The effect of monoamine oxidase inhibitors on growth: Mechanism of the potentiating effect on corticosteroids, *J. Endocrinol.* **33:**211–222.

ZOR, U., AILABOUNI, H., and SULMAN, F. G., 1966, The combined effect of monoamine oxidase inhibitors and corticosteroids on the pituitary–gonadal system of male rats, *J. Endocrinol.* **35:**217–222.

ZOR, U., LOCKER, D., SCHLEIDER, M., and SULMAN, F. G., 1968, Metabolic and enzymatic effects of monoamine oxidase inhibitors with and without hydrocortisone of the accessory sex glands of the rat, *Eur. J. Pharmacol.* **3:**81–83.

2

MONOAMINE OXIDASE, MONOAMINE-OXIDASE-INHIBITING DRUGS, AND HUMAN BEHAVIOR

Dennis L. Murphy

1. INTRODUCTION

Monoamine-oxidase- (MAO)-inhibiting drugs, which reduce the oxidative deamination of the brain biogenic amine neurotransmitters, were the first effective antidepressant agents used in medicine. Although there have been many studies of the clinical efficacy of these agents, there have been only a handful of reports examining their other effects on human behavior and psychological function. There are also only a small number of studies of the effects of *in vivo* treatment with MAO-inhibiting drugs on human monoamine oxidase activity.

Recently, a number of investigations of human platelet MAO activity have reported altered activity of this enzyme in individuals with some psychiatric syndromes. Correlations between platelet MAO activity and individual differences in spontaneous behavior in the rhesus monkey (Redmond *et al.*, 1975) and in human personality characteristics measured by psychological testing (Murphy *et al.*, 1977a) have also been observed.

This chapter reviews the evidence suggesting some associations between monoamine oxidase activity and human behavior. It examines the small portion of the MAO-inhibiting drug literature which provides some hypotheses about the behavioral effects of these drugs. It surveys the few

Dennis L. Murphy • Clinical Neuropharmacology Branch, National Institute of Mental Health, Bethesda, Maryland.

studies of human brain monoamine oxidase. It focuses in greatest detail on the recent studies of human platelet monoamine oxidase and the evidence indicating that drugs as well as genetic, nutritional, and hormonal factors can influence the activity of this enzyme and possibly its relationships with human behavior.

2. MAO-INHIBITING DRUGS: BIOLOGIC, PHYSIOLOGIC, AND BEHAVIORAL EFFECTS IN MAN

Among the monoamine oxidase-inhibiting drugs used clinically, all of those studied (phenelzine, tranylcypromine, isocarboxazid, clorgyline, pargyline, nialamide, and iproniazid) have been demonstrated to markedly reduce human MAO activity during the continued administration of usual clinical dosages (Ganrot et al., 1962; Murphy et al., 1977b; Robinson et al., 1968; Youdim et al., 1972). Treatment with an irreversible hydrazine MAO-inhibitor such as phenelzine (60 mg/day) leads to maximum inhibition of the platelet and plasma enzymes after 7–10 days, with a delayed period of recovery after cessation of treatment (Fig. 1) (Murphy et al., 1977b).

2.1. Monoamine Changes during MAO-Inhibitor Administration to Man

Treatment with MAO-inhibiting drugs is associated with changes in monoamine metabolism as indicated by altered levels of monoamines or their metabolites in cerebrospinal fluid, autopsy brain samples, and urine. Brain serotonin is increased (Ganrot et al., 1962; MacLean et al., 1965), and there are a number of changes in urinary and cerebrospinal fluid levels of indoleamine and catecholamine metabolites (Gjessing, 1964; Kupfer and Bowers, 1973; Sjoerdsma et al., 1959a,b) as well as platelet amine level changes (Anthony and Lance, 1969; Murphy et al., 1977b). Whether any of these changes are involved in or are indirectly related to the behavioral effects of the MAO-inhibiting drugs is not known, but they have nonetheless been the subject of much analysis and speculation (Himwich, 1970; Schildkraut and Kety, 1967). One of the earliest observed correlates of MAO-inhibitor administration, the marked increase in urinary tryptamine excretion (Sjoerdsma et al., 1959a), has remained of interest because of reports of correlations of tryptamine excretion with changes in psychopathology or psychophysiology in some patient groups (Herkert and Keup, 1969; Himwich, 1970) and normals (Marjerisson, 1966). In addition, the occurrence of an enzyme, indoleamine N-methyl transferase, which converts tryptamine to the psychotomimetic substance dimethyltryptamine has been demonstrated in man (Wyatt et al., 1973). Tryptamine is rapidly and primarily degraded by

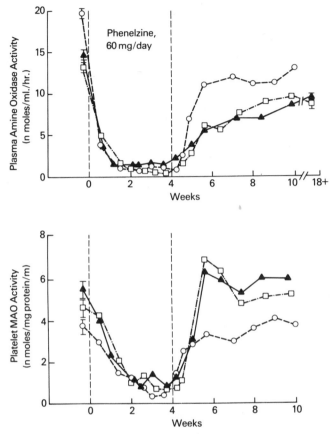

FIG. 1. Time course of the inhibition of human platelet and plasma amine oxidases by phenelzine, 60 mg/day, given to three patients with depression.

MAO, and in the presence of MAO inhibition, unusually large amounts of tryptamine may become available to this enzyme for conversion to dimethyltryptamine. The occurrence of increased amounts of tyramine (Sjoerdsma *et al.*, 1959*b*) and octopamine (Murphy *et al.*, 1975) during periods of MAO inhibition may also be of some relevance to the behavioral changes observed with MAO-inhibiting drugs, via direct effects and also possible "false neurotransmitter" effects (Murphy, 1972*a*).

2.2. Physiological Changes during MAO-Inhibitor Treatment

A marked reduction or obliteration of rapid eye movement (REM) sleep occurs during MAO-inhibitor administration in man (Akindele *et al.*, 1970; Dunleavy and Oswald, 1973; Wyatt *et al.*, 1971). Blood pressure and other physiologic functions are also altered in conjunction with MAO-inhibitor treatment (Stockley, 1973).

Most evidence points towards attribution of the behavioral and physiological consequences of these drugs to reduced monoamine oxidase activity and its sequelae (Pletcher et al., 1966). These agents, however, have other direct effects on neurotransmitter synaptic functions (Hendley and Snyder, 1968) as well as on other neurochemical events (Pletcher et al., 1966). Several forms of monoamine oxidase exist (Sandler and Youdim, 1972), and there are several other amine oxidases in different species which have overlapping substrate affinities and which are affected by some MAO-inhibiting drugs (Blaschko, 1974). MAO has indirect, regulatory effects on biogenic amine storage and synthesis which are impaired by MAO-inhibiting drugs, rendering the organism more vulnerable to other events which alter amine function (Murphy, 1972a; Murphy et al., 1974). These multiple, interactive effects of MAO-inhibiting drugs have made it very difficult to attribute with confidence a specific behavioral or physiological consequence of their use to any one biochemical or biological change (Murphy et al., 1974).

2.3. Behavioral Changes during MAO-Inhibitor Administration to Man

MAO-inhibiting drugs are best known for their antidepressant behavioral effects. There is substantial evidence establishing the efficacy of several of these drugs, including phenelzine, tranylcypromine, isocarboxazid, and iproniazid in the treatment of depression (Klein and Davis, 1969). Iproniazid was the first of these agents used extensively, although it has been supplanted by other less toxic drugs.

Other behavioral effects or side effects of these drugs (in addition to their antidepressant effects) include overstimulation, irritability, restlessness, and insomnia. A recent review of the behavioral side effects of MAO-inhibiting antidepressants reported average incidence figures of 11%, 13%, and 27% for phenelzine, tranylcypromine, and iproniazid, respectively, although methodologic problems in the assessment and reporting of side effects render these figures useful only as gross estimates (Murphy, 1977). The incidence of behavioral side effects is proportional to drug dosage and to duration of treatment. The most common severe side effects were hypomania, mania, paranoid episodes, and confusional behavior. Patients with prior psychiatric symptoms (e.g., mania) tended to be more prone to the recurrence of such symptoms during drug treatment. However, over-elation, hypomanic behavior, and paranoid psychotic episodes as well as lesser behavioral changes also developed in normals and medical patients with tuberculosis, hypertension, and cancer treated with these drugs (Murphy, 1977).

There are only a few studies of MAO-inhibiting drugs which have quantitatively assessed specific psychological effects of the drugs. Wittenborn *et al.* (1961) reported that iproniazid in comparison to placebo produced increased psychomotor speed, increased externally directed motivation, an enhancement in a number of cognitive and perceptual test performances, and Clyde mood-scale elevations in "friendly," "energetic," and "clear-thinking" scores and reductions in the "jittery" factor scores. These changes were interpreted as representing an overall psychomotor stimulant effect of the drug (Cole, 1964; Wittenborn *et al.*, 1961), an effect not evident in a similarly detailed study of the non-MAO-inhibiting antidepressant imipramine, conducted by the same investigators (Wittenborn *et al.*, 1962). In another study, Marjerrison (1966) compared visual imagery production in individuals receiving either placebo or the MAO-inhibiting drug pheniprazine. An increase in the intensity and the structural detail of visual imagery occurred in the pheniprazine-treated group. Increased urinary tryptamine excretion was positively correlated with both the intensity ($r = 0.56$, $P < 0.05$) and the amount ($r = 0.52$, $P < 0.05$) of visual imagery reported. EEG measures and psychological test score changes also discriminated those individuals with the greatest changes in imagery and suggested that there was an association between drug-induced imagery production and increased attentiveness or vigilance reflected in the psychological and EEG changes (Marjerrison, 1966).

3. MONOAMINE OXIDASE IN HUMAN BRAIN AND OTHER TISSUES

Although most of the comprehensive studies of MAO as an enzyme have used nonhuman tissues, there are a few reports describing some characteristics of human brain MAO. MAO specific activities varied approximately one- to threefold in different brain areas, depending both upon the specific brain areas investigated and the substrates studied (tryptamine, β-phenylethylamine, or serotonin) (Collins *et al.*, 1970; Domino *et al.*, 1973; Gottfries *et al.*, 1974; Schwartz *et al.*, 1974*a,b*; Vogel *et al.*, 1969). Comparisons between substrates (studied at concentrations proportionate to their K_ms) yielded the following order of specific activities: dopamine > tryptamine > norepinephrine > serotonin for a solubilized preparation of human cortex or hypothalamus (Jain and Sands, 1974) and dopamine > serotonin > tryptamine > norepinephrine for a crude mitochondrial preparation of human pons/medulla (Jain *et al.*, 1974).

The existence of multiple forms of MAO in human brain was suggested by electrophoretic studies identifying four or five different protein bands with enzyme activity (Collins *et al.*, 1970), which were also found to be differentially sensitive to a series of MAO-inhibiting drugs (clorgyline, tranylcypromine, and isocarboxazid) used *in vivo* (Youdim *et al.*, 1972).

However, it has been suggested that changes in the enzyme as a result of preparation procedures (Houslay and Tipton, 1972), specifically the presence of varying amounts of lipids and other mitochondrial membrane fragments (Oreland, 1971), may account for the apparent multiplicity of MAO forms since they have not been observed in studies using different preparation procedures (Houslay *et al.,* 1974; Jain and Sands, 1974).

Following evidence suggesting that tyramine was deaminated by two forms of the enzyme designated MAO A and MAO B (Johnston, 1968), studies of the inhibition by clorgyline of tyramine deamination revealed a plateau-shaped curve and suggested that MAO A and B forms also existed in human brain (Hall *et al.*, 1969). Investigations of substrate competition offer further support for two or more catalytically independent MAO sites in human brain, with the clearest differences revealed between a serotonin-specific site and a phenylethylamine-specific site (White and Wu, 1975). Along the lines of evidence from other species (Squires, 1972; Yang and Neff, 1973), tyramine, tryptamine and, to some extent, dopamine, were substrates for both the serotonin and the phenylethylamine sites. Norepinephrine deamination was less sensitive to inhibition by both phenylethylamine and serotonin, suggesting the possibility that it is deaminated at another site, as had been previously suggested by Huszti (1972). Whether these different MAO catalytic sites represent different enzyme proteins or are located on the same molecule can only be answered after better solubilization procedures for this membrane-bound enzyme are developed.

Human brain MAO activity has been suggested to increase with age when measured in a small number of individuals with benzylamine (Robinson *et al.*, 1971) or β-phenylethylamine, but not tryptamine (Gottfries *et al.*, 1974). Females had slightly (7.5%) but not significantly higher hindbrain MAO activities than males in one study (Robinson *et al.*, 1971).

Human brain MAO is sensitive to MAO-inhibiting drugs given clinically. Iproniazid (75–125 mg/day for 1–3 weeks) produced a 95% inhibition of brain MAO measured with tyramine as substrate (Ganrot *et al.*, 1962). Isocarboxazid (30 mg/day) reduced brain MAO 40–95%, depending on brain area and substrate used; dopamine deamination, for example, was relatively less inhibited than was that of tyramine, tryptamine, or kynuramine (Youdim *et al.*, 1972). Clorgyline (20 mg/day) produced a 0–50% inhibition of human brain MAO, while tranylcypromine (30 mg/day), produced a 30–70% inhibition with all substrates (Youdim *et al.*, 1972).

Human brain MAO has been measured in a small number of psychiatric patients and suicides. Several studies of schizophrenic patients reveal either no differences (Domino *et al.*, 1973; Schwartz *et al.*, 1974*a,b*; Wise *et al.*, 1974) or slight reductions (Birkhauser, 1941; Utena *et al.*, 1968) in comparisons of patients and controls. Using both serotonin and phenylethylamine as substrates, Schwartz *et al.* (1974*b*) found no differences in three brain areas, although the ratio of serotonin to phenylethylamine deamination was reduced 23–32% in these three brain areas in chronic schizophrenic patients. Brain MAO activity measured with both β-phenylethylamine and tryptamine was found to be reduced an average of 28% in all 13 brain regions studied in 15 suicides compared to 20 controls (Gottfries *et al.*, 1974). Nonsignificant MAO reductions of 13% in four depressive suicides and 18% in three alcoholic suicides compared to seven controls were reported in a study using kynuramine as substrate (Grote *et al.*, 1974).

4. HUMAN PLATELET MONOAMINE OXIDASE

Platelets constitute a readily available tissue source for the measurement of MAO activity in man. Those cells appear to be specialized for biogenic amine-related functions more so than other blood cells, as they contain not only MAO but also amine storage vesicles and amine transport mechanisms very similar to those found in brain (Murphy, 1973; Murphy and Costa, 1975). MAO activity has also been measured directly in a number of human tissues other than postmortem brain samples, including liver (McEwen *et al.*, 1968, 1969*a,b*; Takahashi, 1955), sympathetic ganglia (Goridis and Neff, 1972; Harkonen and Penttila, 1971), pineal gland (Goridis and Neff, 1972), fetal para-aortic tissue (Gennser and Studnitz, 1969), placenta (Sandler and Coveney, 1962; Thompson and Tickner, 1949), uterus (Grant and Pryse-Davies, 1968), intestine and kidney during early development (Epps, 1945), retina (Kojima *et al.*, 1961), skin (Lovenberg *et al.*, 1968), and vas deferens (Miura *et al.*, 1973). Attempts have also been made to assess MAO-inhibitor drug effects or individual differences in MAO activity using such indirect methods as measurement of urinary or cerebrospinal amine or amine metabolite levels, especially tryptamine (Kupfer and Bowers, 1973; Levine and Sjoerdsma, 1963; Murphy *et al.*, 1977*b*; Sjoerdsma *et al.*, 1959*a,b*), as well as by the measurement of the conversion of radioactively labeled amines to their deaminated metabolites (Feldstein *et al.*, 1964; Rosenblatt *et al.*, 1969). Although amine metabolite levels in urine or cerebrospinal fluid may represent the summation of many different processes ranging from dietary intake through non-MAO-related metabolism to renal or cerebrospinal transport processes, some of these measures are sensitive to MAO-inhibitor drug effects (Murphy *et al.*, 1977*b*) and deserve further investigation to determine how well they correlate with direct measures of enzyme activity.

4.1. Characteristics of Human Platelet Monoamine Oxidase

Platelet monoamine oxidase is thought to be localized in mitochondria (Paasonen and Solatunturi, 1965), as is the case with most other tissue monoamine oxidases. However, the small size of platelet mitochondria and the consequent problems in isolating them by differential centrifugation

from other platelet constituents such as alpha granules and amine storage
vesicles have made definitive localization studies difficult. Platelet MAO has
been solubilized and purified 12-fold by Collins and Sandler (1971), who
reported an estimated molecular weight of 235,000 daltons, a value considerably lower than that reported for human brain MAO (Nagatsu *et al.*, 1970;
Tipton, 1973).

In contrast to brain, liver, and other tissues where multiple forms of
MAO have been demonstrated, most evidence suggests that the platelet
possesses only one molecular form of MAO. Studies with the MAO-inhibiting
drugs clorgyline and deprenyl, which in other tissues have suggested the
presence of two enzyme forms, MAO A and MAO B, on the basis of biphasic
log inhibition plots with tyramine as substrate (Johnston, 1968), have
revealed only simple sigmoid curves with tyramine, tryptamine, and benzylamine for the platelet enzyme (Donnelly and Murphy, 1976; Murphy and
Donnelly, 1974). Polyacrylamide gel electrophoresis of the platelet enzyme
has revealed either a single tetrazolium-stained band (Collins and Sandler,
1971) or two bands which had the same relative activity for each of four
substrates (Edwards and Chang, 1975).

The 200-fold greater sensitivity of the platelet MAO to inhibition by
deprenyl compared to clorgyline suggests that platelet MAO is an MAO B
form (Murphy and Donnelly, 1974). This conclusion is supported by the
high activity of the platelet enzyme with the relatively specific MAO B
substrate, β-phenylethylamine, in contrast to its markedly lower activity with
serotonin and norepinephrine, which are MAO A substrates (Donnelly and
Murphy, 1977; Murphy and Donnelly, 1974; Robinson *et al.*, 1968).

Patient subgroup differences in platelet MAO activities measured with
different substrates have been reported in several studies (Meltzer and Stahl,
1974; Nies *et al.*, 1974; Sandler *et al.*, 1974*a*; Zeller *et al.*, 1975). Although
the only reported statistical comparison of platelet MAO activities in different
individuals measured with tryptamine and benzylamine yielded a very high
correlation coefficient ($r = 0.89, P < 0.001, N = 75$) (Murphy and Donnelly,
1974), the question of whether moderate differences in MAO activities
measured with phenylethylamine, dopamine (Sandler *et al.*, 1974*b*), octopamine, tryptamine (Meltzer and Stahl, 1974), or substituted benzylamine
substrates (Zeller *et al.*, 1975) are indicative of platelet MAO heterogeneity
still remains an open possibility.

4.2. Genetic Basis for Individual Differences in Platelet MAO Activity

Platelet MAO activity differences range over tenfold in normal individuals. Studies comparing enzyme activity differences between monozygotic and
dizygotic twins have been used to determine the magnitude of genetic
contributions to individual variations in platelet MAO. Nies *et al.* (1973) and

Murphy (1973) have reported significantly higher intraclass correlation coefficients for normal monozygotic compared to dizygotic twins, and these differences have been confirmed by nonparametric statistical measures as well (Murphy and Costa, 1975). In addition, comparisons of sib pairs vs. nonrelated pairs matched for age and sex have also confirmed a large genetic contribution to MAO activity differences (Murphy and Donnelly, 1974). Similarly high intraclass correlation coefficients have also been observed in monozygotic twins with bipolar manic-depressive disorders (Murphy et al., 1974) and monozygotic twins discordant for schizophrenia (Wyatt et al., 1973). The latter finding not only supported a major genetic contribution to the enzyme activities measured in schizophrenic patients but also suggested that being schizophrenic itself did not appreciably alter platelet MAO activity, since the nonschizophrenic twins had MAO values similar to those in the schizophrenic twins.

Nies et al. (1973) observed a bimodal distribution pattern in platelet MAO activities of 80 normal subjects. This was, of course, of interest since it directly suggested that two enzyme forms might exist. However, other studies of 167 normals (Murphy et al., 1974) and of 680 normals (Murphy et al., 1977a) did not yield a bimodal distribution pattern, but rather a typical unimodal pattern (Fig. 2). It is possible that these differing results are due to the different substrates and assay methods used. Furthermore, the occurrence of a unimodal distribution pattern does not eliminate the possibility of more than one enzyme form existing. For example, erythrocyte acid phosphatase activities are distributed in a unimodal pattern, but electrophoretic studies have revealed five different enzyme proteins contributing in an overlapping fashion to the unimodal pattern (Harris, 1971).

4.3. Factors Influencing Platelet MAO Activity

In addition to genetically based differences, there are a number of other factors which may affect platelet MAO activity. Of particular concern in evaluating the possible relationship between platelet and brain MAO activities are the factors which may be specifically important to blood cell enzymes but not to enzymes in other tissues, including for example, issues related to cell age and turnover and to the use of anticoagulant drugs in obtaining blood cell samples.

4.3.1. Assay Duplicability and Reliability

High correlation coefficients have been reported for MAO activities measured in the same assay ($r = 0.98, P < 0.001, N = 52$) (Murphy et al., 1976a). As noted above, high correlations ($r = 0.89, P < 0.001, N = 75$) were also obtained for comparisons of the same platelet pellets with two

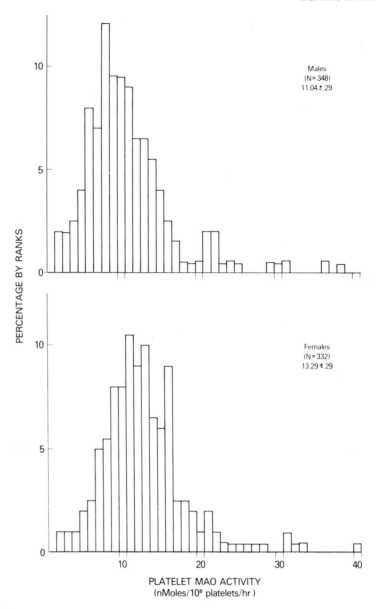

Fɪɢ. 2. Means and frequency distributions for platelet MAO activity in 680 normal subjects.

different substrates, tryptamine and benzylamine (Murphy and Donnelly, 1974). Normal individuals studied 1–2 weeks and 8–10 weeks after an initial study yielded highly correlated results for both time periods ($r = 0.94$ and $r = 0.86$, respectively, both $P < 0.001$) (Murphy *et al.*, 1976a).

4.3.2. Sex

Females have somewhat higher (10–20%) MAO activities than males (Friedman *et al.*, 1974; Murphy *et al.*, 1976*a*; Robinson *et al.*, 1971; Zeller *et al.*, 1975) (Fig. 3). Most other studies of platelet MAO have not separated subjects by sex.

4.3.3. Age

Moderately increasing activity with increasing age has been observed in one study of platelet MAO (Robinson *et al.*, 1971). Our data from a large number of normal subjects, however, does not indicate any significant increase in MAO activity with age after puberty, although insufficient information is available for subjects over age 60 (Murphy *et al.*, 1977*a*; Fig. 2).

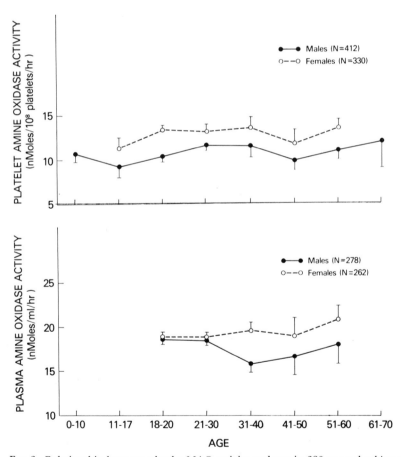

FIG. 3. Relationship between platelet MAO activity and age in 680 normal subjects.

4.3.4. Hormone, Nutritional, and Stress Effects

Menstrual-cycle-related changes in platelet MAO activity occur during the human and nonhuman primate menstrual cycle (Belmaker *et al.*, 1974; Redmond *et al.*, 1975), with the highest enzyme activity occurring just prior to ovulation and the lowest activity during the postovulatory period. Peak-to-trough alterations averaged approximately 20%. Ovariectomy was associated with elevations in platelet MAO activity in the rhesus monkey (Redmond *et al.*, 1975). In male rhesus monkeys, MAO activity was observed to vary between mating and nonmating seasons, in association with marked changes in plasma testosterone levels (Redmond *et al.*, 1976).

Platelet MAO activity was not altered by food ingestion (Belmaker *et al.*, 1974). Iron-deficiency anemia was associated with a marked reduction in platelet MAO activity, which was reversed by treatment with iron (Youdim *et al.*, 1975). On the basis of animal data (Youdim and Sourkes, 1972), it would be expected that riboflavin-deficiency states might also affect the activity of platelet MAO. Marked clinical changes accompanied by alterations in physical activity and psychological "stress," as in patients studied during periods of severe depression, mania, and normality, do not seem to be associated with changes in MAO activity (Murphy and Wyatt, 1975). However, epinephrine administration raised platelet MAO activity in one study (Gentil *et al.*, 1975). The synthetic corticosteroid, prednisone (60 mg/day), did not affect platelet MAO activity (Murphy *et al.*, 1974).

4.4. Drug Effects on Platelet MAO Activity

Human platelet MAO is markedly inhibited both *in vitro* and *in vivo* by a number of drugs used clinically as antidepressant and antihypertensive agents including tranylcypromine, phenelzine, isocarboxazid, and pargyline (Robinson *et al.*, 1968). In our studies, phenelzine in 60-mg/day doses produced approximately 80% inhibition of pletelet MAO, with steady-state inhibition levels reached after 5–14 days of treatment (Fig. 1, Murphy *et al.*, 1977*b*). Phenelzine treatment in this study was associated with changes in monoamine metabolism, including an increased urinary excretion of tryptamine and the *O*-methylated catecholamine metabolites, normetanephrine and metanephrine, and decreased excretion of 3-methoxy, 4-hydroxyphenylglycol and vanylmandelic acid. Other drugs given clinically including lithium carbonate, L-tryptophan, L-dopa, prednisone, and phenothiazine antipsychotic agents were not observed to be associated with altered platelet MAO activity in our studies (Murphy and Wyatt, 1975). Two other reports, however, have described both increased (Bockar *et al.*, 1974) and decreased (Pandey *et al.*, 1975) platelet MAO activity during lithium carbonate treatment.

In vitro, a wide range of inhibitory effects was observed with both typical

MAO-inhibiting drugs and some other psychoactive drugs (Donnelly and Murphy, 1976). Deprenyl, pargyline, and tranylcypromine were among the drugs with highest inhibitory potency for the platelet enzyme, with ID_{50}'s of 0.02, 0.04 and 0.2 μM, respectively, when 10^{-3} M tyramine was used as substrate. The tricyclic antidepressant drugs also inhibit the platelet enzyme, although higher drug concentrations, 60–400 μM, were required, as Edwards and Burns (1974) have recently observed. *d*- and *l*-Amphetamine and chlorpromazine are among the drugs requiring extremely high concentrations (500–790 μM) to produce platelet MAO inhibition.

4.5. Associations between Platelet MAO Activity and Various Human Disorders

Alterations in platelet MAO activity have been described in some patients with affective disorders and schizophrenia, as well as in some patients with other medical disorders. Information available at the present time does not indicate that any more than a small proportion of these differences can be explained by general factors such as age or sex, iron deficiency, abnormalities in thyroid or testosterone states, or drug treatment (Murphy *et al.*, 1977*c*). While it may be that genetically based differences in MAO activity are responsible for these associations with psychiatric disorders, continued caution is necessary in reaching this conclusion, as we have repeatedly indicated (Murphy and Wyatt, 1972; Murphy *et al.*, 1974).

4.5.1. Platelet MAO Activity in Affective Disorders

While platelet MAO activity was no different in 57 patients hospitalized for depression compared to 52 normal controls, a subgroup of the depressed patients who had histories of mania and had been identified as bipolar manic-depressive individuals had significantly reduced MAO levels compared to both the controls and the nonbipolar depressed patients (Murphy and Weiss, 1972). This conclusion was based on the mean of 2–5 platelet MAO measurements per patient obtained during a drug-free interval of a minimum of two weeks. In fact, only three of the bipolar patients had received phenothiazines and/or butyrophenones, and only four had received tricyclic antidepressant drugs during the preceding three months.

Somewhat contrasting data was presented in preliminary form by Nies *et al.* (1974) from a study of a large number of inpatient and outpatient depressed patients, including some bipolar patients. They observed a small but significant increase in platelet MAO activity in the depressed patients as a group. They also suggested that the higher incidence of depression in females and in older individuals might be associated with the higher platelet and brain MAO activity observed by them in females and in association with increasing age (Robinson *et al.*, 1971).

4.5.2. Platelet MAO Activity in Schizophrenia

Reduced platelet MAO activity has also been observed in some patients with schizophrenia. Thirty-three chronically hospitalized schizophrenic patients were reported to have markedly reduced mean MAO activities in comparison to controls of similar age and sex (Murphy and Wyatt, 1972). Patients who had not received phenothiazines for an average of 30 days had equally marked MAO activity differences as did those receiving drugs. Chronicity, severity of impairment, or diagnostic subclass of schizophrenia were not correlated with MAO activity differences within this patient group.

In contrast, a study of 44 individuals hospitalized because of an acute schizophrenic episode revealed no differences in platelet MAO activity compared to controls (Carpenter et al., 1975). This difference from the results in chronic schizophrenic patients was considered of some interest because of the recently reported lack of an increased incidence of schizophrenia and the schizophrenic spectrum disorders in the families of acute schizophrenic patients compared to chronic schizophrenic females (Rosenthal, 1971). The acute schizophrenic patients in the platelet MAO study were evaluated after a 2-week drug-free period; most patients had been receiving antipsychotic drugs for variable but generally brief periods prior to hospitalization. A small number of patients with diagnoses other than acute schizophrenia or schizoaffective schizophrenia (i.e., paranoid, catatonic, and chronic schizophrenia, total $N = 13$) had significantly reduced platelet MAO activity compared to the controls (Carpenter et al., 1975). A comparison of the six patients with the lowest MAO activity vs. 15 with the highest MAO activity from the entire group of 44 patients did not reveal any significant discriminatory variables. There were some trends, however, for the low-MAO group to have more severely impaired reality testing, more paranoid and grandiose delusions, better prognostic scores, and less restlessness.

Reduced platelet MAO activity in schizophrenic patients compared to controls was also observed by Meltzer and Stahl (1974), who studied four substrates, tryptamine, tyramine, metaiodobenzylamine, and octopamine. Female patients had significant MAO reductions with all four substrates, while in male schizophrenic patients only MAO activities measured with tyramine and metaiodobenzylamine were significantly different from controls. When the patients were divided into chronic vs. acute groups, the chronic group manifested reduced MAO activity with all four substrates, while in the acute group only tyramine and metaiodobenzylamine, again, were discriminatory. While the patients in this study were receiving antipsychotic drugs, no significant correlation between phenothiazine drug dosage and platelet MAO activity was observed.

Nies et al. (1974) studied a small number of schizophrenic patients who had experienced at least two schizophrenic episodes but who had been hospitalized for no more than four months in any one year and no more than a total of one year out of the preceding five years. They also observed substrate differences in the platelet MAO comparisons, with the schizophrenic patients having a statistically significant reduction in MAO activity when tryptamine but not benzylamine was used as the substrate. However, it is noteworthy that the controls in this study had MAO activities with benzylamine of 22.1 nM/mg protein/hr, while age-matched control values from a large number of individuals previously reported by the same investigators were 37 nM/mg protein/hr (Nies *et al.*, 1974). This raises the question of whether an atypical control population was obtained by chance.

Friedman *et al.* (1974) also studied a small mixed group of schizophrenic patients, most experiencing an acute re-exacerbation of symptoms, and did not observe a significant mean difference from age- and sex-matched normal controls in platelet MAO activity using tryptamine as the substrate. Schizoaffective, chronic undifferentiated, and paranoid subtypes also did not show any tendency to differ in MAO activity. The female schizophrenic patients had 32% less platelet MAO activity than the female controls, although this difference was not quite statistically significant.

Shaskan and Becker (1975) reported preliminary data from anergic, depressed, schizophrenic outpatients indicating that there were no differences in platelet MAO activity in these patients compared to eight alcoholic and seven normal staff controls. Unfortunately, this study is severely limited by the few normal controls studied, and by the observations of an unusual biphasic distribution of MAO activities in all three of the subject groups, with no overlap between high- vs. low-activity subgroups—a finding in contrast to that observed in our studies of large numbers of normals and patient groups. Their observation that platelet MAO activity remained stable over five weeks' observation which included a drug-free baseline period and then treatment for four weeks with either chlorpromazine (100–1200 mg/day) plus imipramine (150 mg/day) or thiothixene (5–60 mg/day) is of interest in providing further information indicating that phenothiazine-related drugs in clinically used amounts do not appear to alter platelet MAO activity.

Zeller *et al.* (1975) examined platelet MAO activity in 37 patients consisting of men (average age 42) with chronic schizophrenia and a smaller group of younger men and women (average age 22) with acute and subacute forms of schizophrenia. The 102 controls ranged in age from 18 to 50. The 27 male patients and 10 female patients had significantly reduced platelet MAO activity compared to the sex-matched controls with all three of the substrates studied (tyramine, *m*-iodobenzylamine, and *p*-methoxybenzylamine). The latter substrate yielded a significantly smaller differentiation between the patients and the controls than did tyramine. On the basis that the active site of the platelet MAO from schizophrenics appears less capable of accommodating tyramine and *m*-iodobenzylamine than *p*-methoxybenzylamine, Zeller *et al.* (1975) suggested that the platelet MAO of schizophrenics is structurally different from that of nonschizophrenics.

Domino and Khanna (1976) studied platelet MAO activity in 13 chronic schizophrenic patients and observed a statistically significant reduction in

MAO activity in the patient group, with no overlap between the schizo-phrenic patients' values and the controls. These patients were all chronically hospitalized, but as they had not shown therapeutic responses to drug treatment, they had all been drug-free for a minimum of six months. This study provides explicit evidence that the reduction in platelet MAO activity is not a concomitant of antipsychotic drug treatment.

4.5.3. Evaluation of Platelet MAO Activity Differences in Psychiatric Patient Groups

At the present time, it is not clear precisely how the apparent association between reduced platelet MAO activity and psychiatric sympto-mology can best be understood. The majority of studies on this question do point toward some relationship, most clearly exemplified in the chronic schizophrenic patient group (Meltzer and Stahl, 1974; Murphy and Wyatt, 1972; Wyatt *et al.*, 1973) and also in the bipolar subgroup of patients with affective disorders (Murphy and Weiss, 1972). The direct study of known nongenetic factors affecting platelet MAO [including age, sex, clinical state, and such nutritional and hormonal elements as are reflected in plasma levels of iron, triiodothyronine, testosterone (Murphy *et al.*, 1977c)] has not yielded any evidence to explain the reduced platelet MAO activity in these patient groups. In addition, the study of monozygotic twins discordant for schizo-phrenia (Wyatt *et al.*, 1973) suggests that the reduced MAO activity observed in schizophrenic patients is not a consequence of being schizophrenic (or being treated for schizophrenia) but rather may represent or correlate with some vulnerability factor for psychopathology.

The lack of understanding of the molecular basis for reduced MAO activity in those psychiatric patient groups with reduced MAO activity cautions against attributing these differences to a genetic basis at present. Studies of kinetic parameters (Friedman *et al.*, 1974; Murphy and Weiss, 1972; Murphy and Wyatt, 1972; Murphy *et al.*, 1976b) and of possible dialyzable inhibitors (Murphy and Weiss, 1972; Murphy *et al.*, 1976b) have not revealed any differences associated with reduced MAO activity. In addition, schizophrenic patients have not been identified as having reduc-tions in either total MAO or MAO type B activity in brain (Domino *et al.*, 1973; Nies *et al.*, 1974; Schwartz *et al.*, 1974b; Wise *et al.*, 1974). Since the localization and function of MAO type B in brain and other tissues are not known, however, continued efforts to determine the basis for platelet MAO activity differences in patient groups are still required.

4.5.4. Platelet MAO Activity in Other Medical Disorders

Platelet MAO activity was reduced from 37 to 52% of normal in patients with iron-deficiency anemia, who had hemoglobin levels 63% of controls and serum iron levels 17% of controls; elevated iron levels in response to treatment with iron were associated with a return of platelet MAO activities to normal, although hemoglobin changes did not necessarily follow (Youdim *et al.*, 1975). Patients with recurrent migraine headaches had a 41–67% reduction in platelet MAO activity compared to controls (Sandler *et al.*, 1974*a*). Patients with chocolate-sensitive migraine, who had a threefold higher incidence of headaches in response to phenylethylamine than to lactose placebo, had a similarly significant reduction in platelet MAO when compared to unselected migraine patients. The reduction in MAO activity was not marked when phenylethylamine was used as the substrate (41% reduction) compared to tyramine (48%), dopamine (67%) and 5-hydroxy-tryptamine (67%) (Sandler *et al.*, 1974*a*). Platelet MAO activity was found to be increased in a small number of uremic patients compared to controls (Jain *et al.*, 1974). In individuals with Down's syndrome, both reduced (Benson and Southgate, 1971) and normal (Paasonen *et al.*, 1964; Lott *et al.*, 1972) platelet MAO activities have been observed.

5. POSSIBLE ASSOCIATION BETWEEN PLATELET MAO ACTIVITY AND GENERAL PERSONALITY AND BEHAVIORAL FACTORS

Studies of platelet monoamine oxidase in psychiatric patients, medical patients, and normals have clearly indicated that there is no simple one-to-one relationship between a particular psychiatric entity or behavioral syndrome and reduced MAO activity. Although it is still possible that there may be more similarities between the bipolar manic-depressive patient and the chronic schizophrenic patient than Kraepelin and some subsequent psychiatric diagnosticians have suspected (Murphy, 1972*b*), there are certainly many differences in overt behavior between these patient groups which share the most marked reductions in platelet MAO activity. Furthermore, there is very definite overlap between patients and controls in MAO activity, with 10% of normals having platelet MAO activities as low as the mean of the chronic schizophrenic group. Thus, it is possible to have fairly marked reductions in platelet MAO activity either endogenously or in association with diseases like iron-deficiency anemia (Youdim *et al.*, 1975) and migraine (Sandler *et al.*, 1974*a*) without having a psychiatric disorder. This point was also evident from our study of identical twins discordant for schizophrenia, which demonstrated that the nonschizophrenic twins had MAO activities as low as the schizophrenic twins (Wyatt *et al.*, 1973).

On the basis of the above information, we have suggested that reduced MAO activity might be associated with a predisposition or vulnerability to psychopathology (Murphy and Weiss, 1972; Murphy *et al.*, 1974; Wyatt *et al.*, 1973). Consequently, we have begun studies attempting to determine whether any psychological features of normal individuals might be correlated with, or might be predicted from, platelet MAO activity differences.

Our initial results from a study of 95 normal young adult volunteers demonstrated a greater number of significant correlations than expected on a chance basis between platelet MAO activity and scale scores from the Minnesota Multiphasic Personality Inventory (MMPI) and the Zuckerman Sensation Seeking Scale (SSS) (Murphy *et al.*, 1977*a*). In addition, sex-related differences were present in the correlational patterns. A subgroup of male subjects with quite low platelet MAO activities demonstrated a definite increase in many of the MMPI and SSS scales.

To more directly evaluate the possible relationship between platelet MAO activity and the range of psychological differences, including psychopathology, present in normal young adults, a prospective study was carried out by Buchsbaum *et al.* (1976). After screening 375 college-student volunteers for platelet MAO activity, the lower and upper 10% in MAO activity were interviewed and family history obtained. Low MAO probands reported more frequent psychiatric or psychologic counseling experiences and more frequent problems with the law. Three past psychiatric hospitalizations were reported in the low MAO group and none in the high group. More extremely low MAO values were found in male volunteers than female volunteers, and low MAO males had an overall higher incidence of psychosocial problems and of suicide in their relatives. A suicide rate of 3.93% was found in the relatives of low MAO males, which was eight times that of the 0.45% rate in high MAO males. These findings constitute further evidence indicating that reduced MAO levels are predictive of a higher risk for psychiatric disorders.

Redmond *et al.* (1975) have also been pursuing a similar approach, using quantitative behavioral measures obtained over several months' time in both free-ranging and corralled rhesus monkeys as variables for correlational studies with platelet MAO activity. In preliminary results from this study (Redmond and Murphy, 1975) the highest positive correlation with platelet MAO activity in both sexes was with "time spent alone" ($r = 0.49, P < 0.001$, $N = 43$). Moderately high positive correlations were also found for inactivity ($r = 0.32, P < 0.05$) and passivity ($r = 0.31, P < 0.05$) measures. Significant negative correlations were found for some corresponding behaviors, including ambulatory movement ($r = -0.33, P < 0.05$), social contact ($r = -0.31$, $P < 0.05$), and play in males ($r = -0.66, P < 0.01$).

These three studies in normal populations all demonstrate that platelet MAO activity may reflect not only some proclivity to psychopathology, but also some aspects of personality function and behavior in normal young adults and in nonhuman primates studied under natural conditions. It clearly seems possible that some "normal" personality characteristics and behavior may be related to the consequences of genetically and nongenetically based differences in monoamine oxidase activity as they affect the function of biogenic amines at synapses.

6. REFERENCES

AKINDELE, M. O., EVANS, J. I., and OSWALD, I., 1970, Mono-amine oxidase inhibitors, sleep and mood, *Electroenceph. Clin. Neurophysiol.* **29**:447–456.

ANTHONY, M., and LANCE, J. W., 1969, Monoamine oxidase inhibition in the treatment of migraine, *Arch. Neurol.* **21**:263–268.

BENSON, P. F., and SOUTHGATE, J., 1971, Diminished activity of platelet monoamine oxidase in Down's syndrome, *Am. J. Hum. Genet.* **23**:211–214.

BELMAKER, R. H., MURPHY, D. L., WYATT, R. J., and LORIAUX, D. L., 1974, Human platelet monoamine oxidase changes during the menstrual cycle, *Arch. Gen. Psychiatry* **31**:553–556.

BIRKHAUSER, V. H., 1941, Cholinesterase und mono-aminoxydase in zetralen nervensystem, *Schweiz. Med. Wochenschr.* **22**:750–752.

BLASCHKO, H., 1974, The natural history of amine oxidases, *Rev. Physiol. Biochem. Pharmacol.* **70**:83–148.

BOCKAR, J., ROTH, R., and HENINGER, G., 1974, Increased human platelet monoamine oxidase during lithium carbonate therapy, *Life Sci.* **15**:2109–2118.

BUCHSBAUM, M., COURSEY, R. D., and MURPHY, D. L., 1976, The biochemical high risk paradigm: Behavioral and familial correlates of low platelet monoamine oxidase activity, *Science* **194**:339–341.

CARPENTER, W. T., MURPHY, D. L., and WYATT, R. J., 1975, Platelet monoamine oxidase activity in acute schizophrenia, *Am. J. Psychiatry* **132**:438–441.

COLE, J. O., 1964, Therapeutic efficacy of antidepressant drugs, *J. Am. Med. Assoc.* **190**:448–455.

COLLINS, G. G. S., and SANDLER, M., 1971, Human blood platelet monoamine oxidase, *Biochem. Pharmacol.* **20**:289–296.

COLLINS, G. G. S., SANDLER, M., WILLIAMS, E. D., and YOUDIM, M. B. H., 1970, Multiple forms of human brain mitochondrial monoamine oxidase, *Nature* **225**:817–819.

DOMINO, E. F., and KHANNA, S. S., 1976, Decreased blood platelet MAO activity in unmedicated chronic schizophrenic patients, *Am. J. Psychiatry* **133**:323–326.

DOMINO, E. F., KRAUSE, R. R., and BOWERS, J., 1973, Various enzymes involved with putative transmitters, *Arch. Gen. Psychiatry* **29**:195–201.

DONNELLY, C. H., and MURPHY, D. L., 1977, Substrate- and inhibitor-related characteristics of human platelet monoamine oxidase, *Biochem. Pharmacol.* **26**:853–858.

DUNLEAVY, D. L. F., and OSWALD, I., 1973, Phenelzine, mood response, and sleep, *Arch. Gen. Psychiatry* **28**:353–396.

EDWARDS, D. J., and BURNS, M. O., 1974, Effects of tricyclic antidepressants upon platelet monoamine oxidase, *life Sci.* **15**:2045–2058.

EDWARDS, D. J., and CHANG, S-S., 1975, Evidence for interacting catalytic sites of human platelet monoamine oxidase, *Biochem. Biophys. Res. Commun.* **65**:1018–1025.

EPPS, H. M. R., 1945, The development of amine oxidase activity by human tissues after birth, *Biochem. J.* **39**:37–42.

FELDSTEIN, A., HOAGLAND, H., WONG, K. K., OKTEM, M. R., and FREEMAN, H., 1964, MAO activity in relation to depression, *Am. J. Psychiatry* **131**:1392–1394.

FRIEDMAN, E., SHOPSIN, B., SATHANANTHAN, G., and GERSHON, S., 1974, Blood platelet MAO activity in psychiatric patients, *Am. J. Psychiatry* **131**:1392–1394.

GANROT, P. O., ROSENGREN, E., and GOTTFRIES, C. G., 1962, Conversion of β-mercaptopyruvate to 2-mercaptoethanol by yeast enzymes, *Experientia* **18**:260–261.

GENNSER, G., and STUDNITZ, W. V., 1969, Monoamine oxidase, catechol-*O*-methyltransferase and phenylethanolamine-*N*-methyltransferase activity in para-aortic tissue of the human fetus, *Scand. J. Clin. Lab. Invest.* **24**:169–171.

GENTIL, V., GREENWOOD, M. H., and LADER, M. H., 1975, The effect of adrenaline on human platelet MAO, *Psychopharmacologia* **44**:187–194.

GJESSING, L. R., 1964, Studies of periodic catatonia—II The urinary excretion of phenolic amines and acids with and without loads of different drugs, *J. Psychiatr. Res.* **2:**149–162.

GORIDIS, C., and NEFF, N. H., 1972, Evidence for specific monoamine oxidases in human sympathetic nerve and pineal gland, *Proc. Soc. Exp. Biol. Med.* **140:**573–574.

GOTTFRIES, C.-G., ORELAND, L., WIBERG, A., and WINBLAD, B., 1974, Brain levels of monoamine oxidase in depression, *Lancet* **2:**360–361.

GRANT, E. C. G., and PRYSE-DAVIES, J., 1968, Effect of oral contraceptives on depressive mood changes and on endometrial monoamine oxidase and phosphatases, *Br. Med. J.* **3:**777–780.

GROTE, S. S., MOSES, S. G., ROBINS, E., HUDGENS, R. W., and CRONINGER, A. B., 1974, A study of selected catecholamine metabolizing enzymes: A comparison of depressive suicides and alcoholic suicides with controls, *J. Neurochem.* **23:**791–802.

HALL, D. W. R., LOGAN, B. W., and PARSONS, G. H., 1969, Further studies on the inhibition of monoamine oxidase by M & B 9302 (clorgyline)—I.Substrate specificity in various mammalian species, *Biochem. Pharmacol.* **18:**1447–1454.

HARKONEN, M., and PENTTILA, A., 1971, Catecholamines, monoamine oxidase and cholinesterase activity in the human sympathetic ganglion, *Acta Physiol. Scand.* **82:**310–321.

HARRIS, H., 1971, *The Principles of Human Biochemical Genetics*, p. 140, American Elsevier, New York.

HENDLEY, E. D., and SNYDER, S. H., 1968, Relationship between the action of monoamine oxidase inhibitors on the noradrenaline uptake system and their antidepressant efficacy, *Nature* **220:**1330–1331.

HERKERT, E. E., and KEUP, W., 1969, Excretion patterns of tryptamine, indole-acetic acid, and their correlation with mental changes in schizophrenia patients under medication with alpha-methyldopa, *Psychopharmacologia* **15:**48–59.

HIMWICH, H. E., 1970, Indoleamines and the schizophrenias, in: *Biochemistry Schizophrenias, and Affective Illnesses* (H. E. Himwich, ed.), pp. 79–122, Williams and Wilkins, Baltimore.

HOUSLAY, M. D., and TIPTON, K. F., 1973, The nature of the electrophoretically separable multiple forms of rat liver monoamine oxidase, *Biochem. J.* **135:**173–186.

HOUSLAY, M. D., GARRETT, N. J., and TIPTON, K. F., 1974, Mixed substrate experiments with human brain monoamine oxidase, *Biochem. Pharmacol.* **23:**1937–1944.

HUSZTI, Z., 1972, Kinetic studies on rat brain monoamine oxidase, *Mol. Pharmacol.* **8:**385–397.

JAIN, M. L., and SANDS, F. L., 1974, Electrophoretic homogeneity of solubilized human brain monoamine oxidase, *J. Neurochem.* **23:**1291–1293.

JAIN, M., BAKUTIS, E., GAYLE, T., and LANSKY, P., 1974, Some kinetic and inhibition properties of human brain mitochondrial monoamine oxidase (EC 1.4.3.4), *Neurobiology* **4:**180–190.

JOHNSTON, J. P., 1968, Some observations upon a new inhibitor of monoamine oxidase in brain tissue, *Biochem. Pharmacol.* **17:**1285–1297.

KLEIN, D. F., and DAVIS, J. M., 1969, *Diagnosis and Drug Treatment of Psychiatric Disorders,* pp. 205–211, Williams and Wilkins, Baltimore.

KOJIMA, K., IIDA, M., MAJIMA, Y., and OKADA, S., 1961, Histochemical studies on monoamine oxidase (MAO) of the human retina, *Jpn. J. Opthalmol.* **5:**205–210.

KUPFER, D., and BOWERS, M. B., 1973, REM sleep and central monoamine oxidase inhibition, *Psychopharmacologia* **27:**183–190.

LEVINE, R. J., and SJOERDSMA, A., 1963, Estimation of monoamine oxidase activity in man: Techniques and applications, *Ann. N.Y. Acad. Sci.* **107:**966–974.

LOTT, I. T., CHASE, T. H., and MURPHY, D. L., 1972, Down's syndrome: Transport, storage and metabolism of serotonin in blood platelets, *Pediatr. Res.* **6:**730–735.

LOVENBERG, W., DIXON, E., KEISER, H. R., and SJOERDSMA, A., 1968, A comparison of amine oxidase activity in human skin, rat skin and rat liver: Relevance to collagen cross-linking, *Biochem. Pharmacol.* **17:**1117–1120.

MacLean, R., Nicholson, W. J., Pare, C. M., and Stacey, R. S., 1965, Effect of monoamine-oxidase inhibitors on the concentrations of 5-hydroxytryptamine in the human brain, *Lancet* **2**:205–208.

Marjerrison, G., 1966, The effects of pheniprazine on visual imagery in perceptual deprivation, *J. Nerv. Ment. Dis.* **142**:254–264.

McEwen, C. M., Jr., Sasaki, G., and Lenz, W. R., 1968, Human liver mitochondrial monoamine oxidase. I. Kinetic studies of model interactions, *J. Biol. Chem.* **243**:5217–5225.

McEwen, C. M., Jr., Sasaki, G., and Jones, D. C., 1969*a*, Human liver mitochondrial monoamine oxidase. II. Determinants of substrate and inhibitor specificities, *Biochemistry* **8**:3952–3962.

McEwen, C. M., Jr., Sasaki, G., and Jones, D. C., 1969*b*, Human liver mitochondrial monoamine oxidase. III. Kinetic studies concerning time-dependent inhibitions, *Biochemistry* **8**:3963–3972.

Meltzer, H. Y., and Stahl, S. M., 1974, Platelet monoamine oxidase activity and substrate preferences in schizophrenic patients, *Res. Commun. Chem. Pathol. Pharmacol.* **7**:419–431.

Miura, Y., Mendez, R., and DeQuattro, V., 1973, Norepinephrine (NE) content and activities of enzymes regulating NE biosynthesis and metabolism in human vas deferens, *Fed. Proc.* **32**:770.

Murphy, D. L., 1972*a*, Amine precursors, amines and false neurotransmitters in depressed patients, *Am. J. Psychiatry* **129**:141–148.

Murphy, D. L., 1972*b*, L-Dopa, behavioral activation and psychopathology, in: *Neurotransmitters* (I. J. Kopin, ed.), *Res. Publ. Assoc. Res. Nerv. Ment. Dis.* **50**:472–493.

Murphy, D. L., 1973, Technical strategies for the study of catecholamines in man, in: *Frontiers in Catecholamine Research* (F. Usdin and S. Snyder, eds.), pp. 1077–1082, Pergamon Press, Oxford.

Murphy, D. L., 1977, The behavioral toxicity of monoamine oxidase-inhibiting antidepressants, *Adv. Pharmacol. Chemother.* **14**:72–105.

Murphy, D. L., and Costa, J. L., 1975, Utilization of cellular studies of neurotransmitter-related enzymes and transport processes in man for the investigation of biological factors in behavioral disorders, in: *Recent Biological Studies of Depressive Illness* (J. Mendels, ed.), pp. 223–236, Spectrum Publications, New York.

Murphy, D. L., and Donnelly, C. H., 1974, Monoamine oxidase in man: Enzyme characteristics in platelets, plasma and other human tissues, in: *Neuropsychopharmacology of Monoamines and Their Regulatory Enzymes* (E. Usdin, ed.), pp. 71–85, Raven Press, New York.

Murphy, D. L., and Weiss, R., 1972, Reduced monoamine oxidase activity in blood platelets from bipolar depressed patients, *Am. J. Psychiatry* **128**:1351–1357.

Murphy, D. L., and Wyatt, R. J., 1972, Reduced monoamine oxidase activity in blood platelets from schizophrenic patients, *Nature* **238**:225–226.

Murphy, D. L., and Wyatt, R. J., 1975, Enzyme studies in the major psychiatric disorders: I. Catechol-*O*-methyl-transferase, monoamine oxidase in the affective disorders, and factors affecting some behavior-related enzyme activities, in: *The Biology of the Major Psychoses: A Comparative Analysis* (D. X. Freedman, ed.), pp. 289–296, Raven Press, New York.

Murphy, D. L., Belmaker, R., and Wyatt, R. J., 1974, Monoamine oxidase in schizophrenia and other behavioral disorders, *J. Psychiatr. Res.* **11**:221–247.

Murphy, D. L., Cahan, D. H., and Molinoff, P. B., 1975, Occurrence, transport and storage of octopamine in human blood platelets. *Clin. Pharmacol. Ther.* **18**:587–593.

Murphy, D. L., Wright, C., Buchsbaum, M., Costa, J., Nichols, A., and Wyatt, R. J., 1976*a*, Platelet and plasma amine oxidase activity in 680 normals: Sex and age differences and stability over time *Biochem. Med.* **16**:254–265.

Murphy, D. L., Donnelly, C. H., Miller, L., and Wyatt, R. J., 1976*b*, Platelet monoamine oxidase in chronic schizophrenia: Some enzyme characteristics relevant to reduced activity *Arch. Gen. Psychiat.* **33:**1377–1381.

MURPHY, D. L., BELMAKER, R. H., BUCHSBAUM, M., WYATT, R. J., MARTIN, N. F., and CIARANELLO, R., 1977*a*, Biogenic amine-related enzymes and personality variations in normals, *Psychol. Med.* **7:**149–157.

MURPHY, D. L., BRAND, E., GOLDMAN, T., BAKER, M., WRIGHT, C., VAN KAMMEN, D., |and GORDON, E., 1977*b*, Platelet and plasma amine oxidase inhibition and urinary amine excretion changes during phenelzine treatment, *J. Nerv. Ment. Dis.* **164:**129–134.

MURPHY, D. L., BELMAKER, R., CARPENTER, W. T., and WYATT, R. J., 1977*c*, Monoamine oxidase in chronic schizophrenia: Studies of hormonal and other factors affecting enzyme activity. *Brit. J. Psychiat.* **130:**151–158.

NAGATSU, T., YAMAMOTO, T., and HARADA, M., 1970, Purification and properties of human brain mitochondrial monoamine oxidase, *Enzymologia* **39:**15–25.

NIES, A., ROBINSON, D. S., LAMBORN, K. R., and LAMBERT, R. P., 1973, Genetic control of platelet and plasma monoamine oxidase activity, *Arch. Gen. Psychiatry* **28:**834–838.

NIES, A., ROBINSON, D. S., HARRIS, L. S., and LAMBORN, K. R., 1974, Comparison of monoamine oxidase substrate activities in twins, schizophrenics, depressives, and controls, in: *Neuropsychopharmacology of Monoamines and Their Regulatory Enzymes* (E. Usdin, ed.), pp. 59–70, Raven Press, New York.

ORELAND, L., 1971, Purification and properties of pig liver mitochondrial monoamine oxidase, *Arch. Biochem. Biophys.* **146:**410–421.

PAASONEN, M. K., and SOLATUNTURI, E., 1965, Monoamine oxidase in mammalian blood platelets. *Ann. Med. Exp. Biol. Fenn.* **43:**98–100.

PAASONEN, M. K., SOLATUNTURI, E., and KIYALO, E., 1964, Monoamine oxidase activity of blood platelets and their ability to store 5-hydroxytryptamine in some mental deficiencies, *Psychopharmacologia* **6:**120–124.

PANDEY, G. N., DORUS, E. B., DEKIRMENJIAN, H., and DAVIS, J. M., 1975, Effect of lithium treatment on blood COMT and platelet MAO in normal human subjects, *Fed. Proc.* **34:**778.

PLETCHER, A., GEY, F. K., and BURKAND, W. P., 1966, Inhibitors of monoamine oxidase and decarboxylase of aromatic amine acids, *Handb. Exp. Pharmacol.* **19:**953–1047.

REDMOND, D. E., JR., and MURPHY, D. L., 1975, Behavioral correlates of platelet monoamine oxidase (MAO) activity in rhesus monkeys, *Psychosom. Med.* **37:**80.

REDMOND, D. E., MURPHY, D. L., ZIEGLER, M. G., LAKE, C. R., and BAULU, J., 1975, Menstrual cycle and ovarian hormone effects on plasma and platelet monoamine oxidase (MAO) and plasma dopamine-beta-hydroxylase (DBH) activities in the rhesus monkey. *Psychosom. Med.* **37:**417–428.

REDMOND, D. E., BAULU, J., MURPHY, D. L., LORIAUX, D. L., ZIEGLER, M. G., and LAKE, C. R., 1976, Effects of testosterone on plasma and platelet monoamine oxidase and plasma dopamine β-hydroxylase activities in the male rhesus monkey, *Psychosom. Med.* **38:**315–326.

ROBINSON, D. S., LOVENBERG, W., KEISER, H., and SJOERDSMA, J., 1968, Effects of drugs on human blood platelet and plasma amine oxidase activity *in vitro* and *in vivo*, *Biochem. Pharmacol.* **17:**109–119.

ROBINSON, D. S., DAVIS, J. M., NIES, A., RAVARIS, C. L., and SYLWESTER, D., 1971, Relation of sex and aging to monoamine oxidase activity of human brain, plasma, and platelets, *Arch. Gen. Psychiatry* **24:**536–539.

ROSENBLATT, S., CHANLEY, J. D., and LEIGHTON, W. P., 1969, The investigation of adrenergic metabolism with 7H³-norepinephrine in psychiatric disorders, *J. Psychiatr. Res.* **6:**320–333.

ROSENTHAL, D., 1971, Two adoption studies of heredity in the schizophrenic disorders, in: *The Origin of Schizophrenia* (M. Bleuler and J. Angst, eds.), pp. 21–34, Verlag Hans Huber, Berlin.

SANDLER, M., and COVENEY, J., 1962, Placental monoamine-oxidase activity in toxemia of pregnancy, *Lancet* **1:**1096–1098.

SANDLER, M., and YOUDIM, M. B. H., 1972, Multiple forms of monoamine oxidase: Functional significance, *Pharmacol. Rev.* **24:**331–348.

SANDLER, M., CARTER, S. B., GOODWIN, B. L., RUTHVEN, C. R. J., YOUDIM, M. B. H., HANINGTON, E., CUTHBERT, M. F., and PARE, C. M. B., 1974a, Multiple forms of monoamine oxidase: Some *in vivo* correlations, in: *Neuropsychopharmacology of Monoamines and Their Regulatory Enzymes* (E. Usdin, ed.), pp. 3–10, Raven Press, New York.

SANDLER, M., YOUDIM, M. B. H., and HANINGTON, E., 1974b, A phenylethylamine oxidizing defect in migraine, *Nature* **250:**335–337.

SCHILDKRAUT, J. J., and KETY, S. S., 1967, Biogenic amines and emotion, *Science* **156:**21–30.

SCHWARTZ, M. A., AIKENS, A. M., and WYATT, R. J., 1974a, Monoamine oxidase activity in brains from schizophrenic and mentally normal individuals, *Psychopharmacologia* **38:**319–328.

SCHWARTZ, M. A., WYATT, R. J., YANG, H-Y. T., and NEFF, N. H., 1974b, Multiple forms of brain monoamine oxidase in schizophrenic and normal individuals, *Arch. Gen. Psychiatry* **31:**557–560.

SHASKAN, E. G., and BECKER, R. E., 1975, Platelet monoamine oxidase in schizophrenics, *Nature* **253:**659–660.

SJOERDSMA, A., OATES, J. A., ZALTZMAN, P., and UDENFRIEND, S., 1959a, Identification and assay of urinary tryptamine: Application as an index of monoamine oxidase inhibition in man, *J. Pharmacol. Exp. Ther.* **126:**217–222.

SJOERDSMA, A., LOVENBERG, W., OATES, J. A., CROUT, J. R., and UDENFRIEND, S., 1959b, Alterations in the pattern of amine excretion in man produced by a monoamine oxidase inhibitor, *Science* **130:**225.

SQUIRES, R. J., 1972, Multiple forms of monoamine oxidase in intact mitochondria as characterized by selective inhibitors and thermal stability; a comparison of eight mammalian species, in: *Advances in Biochemical Psychopharmacology* (E. Costa and P. Greengard, eds.), p. 335, Raven Press, New York.

STOCKLEY, I. H., 1973, Monoamine oxidase inhibitors Part 1: Interactions with sympathomimetic amines, *Pharm. J.* **210:**590–594; Part 2: Interactions with antihypertensive agents, hypoglycaemics, CNS depressants, narcotics and antiParkinsonian agents, *Pharm. J.* **211:**95–98.

TAKAHASHI, Y., 1955, Amine oxidase activity of liver tissues obtained by needle biopsy together with other liver function tests on schizophrenic patients. A preliminary report, *Folia Psychiatr. Neurol. Jpn.* **10:**263–278.

THOMPSON, R. H. S., and TICKNER, A., 1949, Observations on the mono-amine oxidase activity of platelet and uterus, *Biochem. J.* **45:**125–130.

TIPTON, K. F., 1973, Biochemical aspects of monoamine oxidase, *Br. Med. Bull.* **29:**116–119.

UTENA, H., KANAMURA, H., SUDA, S., NAKAMURA, R., MACHIYAMA, Y., and TAKAHASHI, R., 1968, Studies on the regional distribution of the monoamine oxidase activity in the brains of schizophrenic patients, *Proc. Jpn. Acad.* **44:**1078–1083.

VOGEL, W. H., ORFEL, V., and CENTURY, B., 1969, Activities of enzymes involved in the formation and destruction of biogenic amines in various areas of human brain, *J. Pharmacol. Exp. Ther.* **165:**196–203.

WHITE, H. L., and WU, J. C., 1975, Multiple binding sites of human brain monoamine oxidase as indicated by substrate competition, *J. Neurochem.* **25:**21–26.

WISE, C. D., BADEN, M. H., and STEIN, L., 1974, Postmortem measurements of enzymes in human brain: Evidence of a central noradrenergic deficit in schizophrenia, *J. Psychiatr. Res.* **11:**221–248.

WITTENBORN, J. R., PLANTE, M., BURGESS, F., and LIVERMORE, N., 1961, The efficacy of electroconvulsive therapy, iproniazid and placebo in the treatment of young depressed women, *J. Nerv. Ment. Dis.* **133:**316–332.

WITTENBORN, J. R., PLANTE, M., BURGESS, F., and MAURER, H. A., 1962, A comparison of imipramine, electroconvulsive therapy and placebo in the treatment of depressions, *J. Nerv. Ment. Dis.* **135:**131–137.

WYATT, R. J., FRAM, D. H., KUPFER, D. J., and SNYDER, F., 1971, Total prolonged drug-induced REM sleep suppression in anxious-depressed patients, *Arch. Gen. Psychiatry* **24:**145–155.

WYATT, R. J., SAAVEDRA, J. M., and AXELROD, J., 1973, A dimethyltryptamine (DMT) forming enzyme in human blood, *Am. J. Psychiatry* **130:**754–760.

YANG, H-Y. T., and NEFF, N. H., 1973, β-Phenylethylamine: A specific substrate for type B monoamine oxidase of brain, *J. Pharmacol. Exp. Ther.* **187:**365–371.

YOUDIM, M. B. H., and SOURKES, T. L., 1972, The flavin prosthetic group of purified rat liver mitochondrial monoamine oxidase, *Adv. Biochem. Psychopharmacol.* **5:**45–54.

YOUDIM, M. B. H., COLLINS, G. G. S., SANDLER, M., BEVAN JONES, A. B., PARE, C. M. B., and NICHOLSON, W. J., 1972, Human brain monoamine oxidase: Multiple forms and selective inhibitors, *Nature* **236:**225–227.

YOUDIM, M. B. H., WOODS, H. F., MITCHELL, B., GRAHAME-SMITH, D. G., and CALLENDER, S., 1975, Human platelet monoamine oxidase activity in iron-deficiency anaemia, *Clin. Sci. Mol. Med.* **48:**289–295.

ZELLER, E. A., BOSHES, B., DAVIS, J. M., and THORNER, M., 1975, Molecular aberration in platelet monoamine oxidase in schizophrenia, *Lancet* **1:**1385.

3

TRICYCLIC AND MONOAMINE OXIDASE INHIBITOR ANTIDEPRESSANTS: STRUCTURE–ACTIVITY RELATIONSHIPS

Robert A. Maxwell and Helen L. White

1. INTRODUCTION

1.1. Background

Tricyclic and monoamine oxidase inhibitor (MAOI) antidepressants are the two classes of drugs most frequently used in the treatment of moderate to severe depression. Their efficacy in depression has been known for nearly two decades (Crane, 1957; Loomer *et al.*, 1957; Kuhn, 1958). The tricyclic inhibitors tend to increase concentrations of certain biogenic amines in synaptic clefts in peripheral organs and brain by preventing their reuptake into the nerve endings from which they were secreted. MAOIs block the catabolism of biogenic amines within presynaptic nerve terminals, and thus provide that greater amounts of these transmitters accumulate within nerve terminals and are released into the synaptic cleft. Therefore, both drug classes can be expected to accomplish a similar effect—an increase in amine concentration in the synaptic cleft and a consequent greater excitation of postsynaptic receptors. This common effect of MAOIs and of tricyclic antidepressants as exerted in brain is generally considered to be the basis for

Robert A. Maxwell and Helen L. White • Department of Pharmacology, Wellcome Research Laboratories, Burroughs Wellcome Co., Research Triangle Park, North Carolina.

their antidepressant activities. The antidepressant actions of imipramine and iproniazid in man, and their effectiveness as antagonists of the sedation produced in animals by reserpine-induced depletion of brain biogenic amines, contributed early to the formulation of the amine hypothesis of affective disorders (Schildkraut, 1965, 1969; Schildkraut and Kety, 1967). As originally stated, this theory suggested that depressive illness is associated with a deficiency of catecholamines, norepinephrine in particular, at adrenergic receptor sites in the brain. The possibility that a deficiency of serotonin (5-HT) may underlie some types of depression has more recently also gained much attention (Coppen, 1967; Lapin and Oxenkrug, 1969; Prange *et al.*, 1974), and there is evidence that an increase in the concentration of 5-HT in central synaptic clefts may underlie the antidepressant effectiveness of tricyclic antidepressants and MAOIs. For an extensive discussion of the amine hypothesis, see Chapter 5.

1.2. Purposes of this Review and a Limitation

The first purpose of this review is to describe the structure–activity relationships among the various chemical classes of MAOIs and, in addition, the structure–activity relationships for the tricyclic antidepressants as inhibitors of the uptake of three important biogenic amines—norepinephrine (NE), dopamine (DA), and 5-HT. The second purpose is to relate these structure–activity relationships to clinical efficacy.

The first purpose is readily accomplished, and in several instances the structure–activity relationships are sufficiently clear to permit hypotheses to be expounded regarding the conformations of drugs when they are attached to their active sites and regarding the nature of the binding involved. Unfortunately, the second purpose is exceedingly difficult to achieve in any firm, factual way. When one attempts to relate relatively precise *in vivo* and *in vitro* biochemical measurements in animals to the amelioration of a complicated array of symptoms which reflect depressed mood and drive in humans, the situation becomes complex. Human depression undoubtedly includes a number of subtypes which respond differently to various therapies and which may be completely unrelated to simple animal models (Klerman, 1971; Berger, 1975; Baldessarini, 1975). Some patients who do not respond well to tricyclic antidepressants show a remarkable improvement when MAOIs are administered, and vice versa, while some depressed patients respond to neither type of drug, and some can be classified as placebo responders (Pare, 1970; Hollister, 1972; Morris and Beck, 1974; Klerman, 1971).

The high placebo response among depressed patients, between 30 and 60% in various studies, has complicated many attempts to evaluate the clinical efficacy of antidepressant drugs. Malitz and Kanzler (1971) have concluded that the inclusion of a placebo group is essential in such studies.

Further difficulties arise from diagnostic inconsistencies among patient groups, lack of adequate dosages in some studies, and individual differences in rates of drug metabolism (Braithwaite and Goulding, 1975). In a recent review, Morris and Beck (1974) have summarized clinical studies accomplished between 1958 and 1972 which could be considered well-controlled—i.e., which were performed on a double-blind basis with either a placebo or a drug control group. These authors concluded that the tricyclic agents amitriptyline and imipramine were generally more effective than the MAOIs phenelzine and isocarboxazid. Tranylcypromine was the most effective MAOI and was judged similar in efficacy to imipramine. As pointed out by the authors, these general conclusions do not take into consideration any specificities of the various drugs with respect to depressive subtypes. Hollister (1972) has recommended that for classic retarded or endogenous depression a tricyclic antidepressant such as amitriptyline should be the drug of first choice. Other workers have reported that the MAOI phenelzine may have a particularly favorable effect in anxious or agitated depressive syndromes (Tyrer *et al.*, 1973; Robinson *et al.*, 1973; Johnson, 1975) and in obsessional neurosis (Jain *et al.*, 1970). Pare (1970) suggested that two specific genetically determined types of depression may be defined, one of which responds favorably to tricyclic antidepressants and the other to MAOIs and that knowledge of the drug response among relatives could be useful in determining the most effective treatment for a particular individual.

Within the obviously tenuous clinical framework described above, we have examined the structure–activity data for the tricyclic antidepressants and the MAOIs for any information which may shed light on antidepressant actions in man. Since the literature to be reviewed is extensive, some selection has necessarily been made among the many contributions in the field. The authors have endeavored, however, to quote all directly pertinent work and hope that they have not inadvertently overlooked any significant contribution.

2. TRICYCLIC AND RELATED COMPOUNDS

2.1. Neuronal Membrane Mechanisms for the Uptake of Biogenic Amines

2.1.1. Norepinephrine and Dopamine

Whitby *et al.* (1961) demonstrated that tissues which contained an adrenergic innervation bound tritiated NE. At the same time, Strömblad and Nickerson (1961) and Hertting *et al.* (1961) reported that following adrenergic denervation there was a drastic reduction in the capacity of tissues to accumulate exogenous NE. Hamberger *et al.* (1964) brought these two observations into focus when they demonstrated by histofluorescence techniques that the adrenergic neuron was able to take up NE and related amines by a mechanism that was localized in the cell membrane. Unlike reserpine, which did not prevent uptake of NE, but prevented its accumulation and retention, cocaine pretreatment blocked the uptake of catecholamines by the adrenergic nerves in the rat iris (Hillarp and Malmfors, 1964). These authors noted that their observations demonstrated, directly, that a very efficient uptake of NE into adrenergic nerves was achieved by a mechanism located in the cell membrane and that this mechanism could be inhibited by a drug. Detailed studies of the characteristics of the uptake system in adrenergic membranes have been carried out. From experiments with the uptake of [^{3}H]NE by heart slices, brain slices, and pineal glands, *in vitro,* the uptake mechanism was shown to exhibit properties consistent with saturation kinetics of the Michaelis–Menten type (Dengler *et al.*, 1961, 1962*a,b*). These investigators suggested that active membrane transport was involved in the uptake. The results of Iversen (1963, 1967) clearly indicated that the uptake of [^{3}H]NE by isolated perfused heart obeyed saturation kinetics. The K_m was 6.7×10^{-7} M and the V_{max} was 1.3 nmol/min per g wet wt. of tissue. It was soon made clear through the work from several laboratories that the uptake system for NE was depressed by cold, heat, cardiac glycosides, and low Na^+ (Lindmar and Muscholl, 1964; Bogdanski and Brodie, 1966; Carlsson, 1966; Giachetti and Shore, 1966; Iversen and Kravitz, 1966; Berti and Shore, 1967). This saturable, energy-dependent, active transport system is commonly known as the *amine pump.*

Study of the uptake of NE by brain tissue was facilitated by the demonstration of its active uptake by purified synaptosomal preparations from whole brains of rats (Colburn *et al.*, 1967, 1968). Colburn *et al.* (1968) reported the K_m for NE uptake to be 5.6×10^{-7} M and the V_{max} to be 0.6 nmol/min per g wet wt. of brain. The kinetics of the uptake of NE and other amines into purified and crude preparations of synaptosomes from several brain regions were subsequently studied. Snyder and Coyle (1969) presented K_m and V_{max} values for NE and DA uptake into six brain regions of the rat (Table 1). Unlike NE, DA was accumulated by two uptake systems in all areas other than the striatum. The high-affinity (neuronal) uptake for DA in these areas appeared to use the NE transport system. It should be noted that in all regions including the striatum, the K_m for the uptake of NE is 5 times greater than the K_m values for the high-affinity uptake of DA. In addition, the K_m values for uptake of both amines in the striatum are 5 times greater than those in the other brain regions. These results suggest that NE and DA utilize the same receptor site in all regions, that the receptor site in striatum differs somehow from all other areas, and that the β OH of NE diminishes the affinity of this amine for striatal receptor sites as well as for receptor sites of other regions by a factor of 5. Ferris and Stocks (1972), however, reported a high- and low-affinity uptake for NE as well as for DA in crude synaptosomal preparations from the hypothalamus and striatum of the rat.

TABLE 1

Kinetic Constants for Catecholamine Uptake by Rat Brain Homogenates[a]

Region	NE constants		DA constants			
	K_m (M)	V_{max}[b]	V_{max_a}[b]	K_{m_a} (M)	K_{m_b} (M)	V_{max_b}[b]
Striatum	2.0×10^{-6}	100	100	4.0×10^{-7}		
Hypothalamus	4.0×10^{-7}	5.0	3.3	0.8×10^{-7}	1.4×10^{-6}	17.0
Cerebral cortex	4.0×10^{-7}	4.0	2.5	0.8×10^{-7}	1.4×10^{-6}	12.5
Midbrain	4.0×10^{-7}	3.7	2.8	0.8×10^{-7}	1.4×10^{-6}	16.6
Medulla oblongata–pons	4.0×10^{-7}	3.3	2.6	0.8×10^{-7}	1.4×10^{-6}	14.0
Cerebellum	4.0×10^{-7}	2.8	1.7	0.8×10^{-7}	1.4×10^{-6}	12.5

[a] From Snyder and Coyle (1969).
[b] V_{max} is expressed as μmol/g pellet per 5 min.

The low-affinity uptakes had K_m values of approximately 2×10^{-6} M for both substrates. Ferris (personal communication) found the K_m values for the high-affinity uptakes in striatum to be 8×10^{-7} M (NE) and 5×10^{-7} M (DA) and in hypothalamus 4×10^{-7} M (NE) and 5×10^{-7} M (DA). These results do not confirm the marked differences observed by Snyder and Coyle (1969) and suggest that the high-affinity (neuronal) uptake for DA and NE is similar, if not identical, in striatum and hypothalamus.

2.1.2. Serotonin

The discovery of a 5-HT pump was stimulated by the description of the NE pump. Ross and Renyi (1967a, 1969) demonstrated that slices of mouse brain stem accumulated 5-[^{3}H]HT when incubated in low concentrations (1×10^{-7} M) of this amine. NE and DA were only weak inhibitors of this uptake, suggesting that accumulation of 5-HT occurred in specific serotonin neurons. Similar conclusions were reached by Alpers and Himwich (1969).

Blackburn et $al.$ (1967) demonstrated that approximately 60% of the 5-HT taken up in 5 min by slices of whole rat brain was recovered in the nerve-ending (synaptosomal) fraction following sucrose-density centrifugation. These authors also showed that the rate of uptake during 5-min exposure at 37°C was not directly proportional to the 5-HT concentration in the medium but approached a maximum at high concentrations. This implied that a saturable carrier mechanism was involved. The kinetic values were 5.7×10^{-7} M for K_m and 0.9 nmol/min per g wet wt. of tissue for V_{max} . DA and NE were weak inhibitors of the uptake from 3×10^{-8} M 5-[^{14}C]HT. Ross and Renyi (1969) found a K_m value of 7×10^{-7} M and a V_{max} of 0.23 nmol/min per g wet wt. of tissue for 5-[^{3}H]HT uptake into brain slices of the rat. Ross and Renyi (1969) commented that their values were close to those found by Blackburn et $al.$ (1967) and to those for the uptake of sympathomimetic amines in slices of mouse brain. Shaskan and Snyder (1970) described two components of 5-HT accumulation, a high-affinity (uptake$_1$) and a low-affinity (uptake$_2$) transport system. In the striatum and the hypothalamus, the high-affinity uptake had a K_m of approximately 2×10^{-7} M and the V_{max} values were approximately 1 nmol/min per g wet wt. of tissue. K_m values for the low-affinity uptake were approximately 60 times greater than for the high-affinity uptake. Shaskan and Snyder (1970) suggested that uptake$_2$ for 5-HT represented its passage into norepinephrine neurons. Wong et $al.$ (1973) confirmed, in rat whole-brain synaptosomes, the dual transport processes described by Shaskan and Snyder (1970). These authors found a K_m value of 1×10^{-7} M and a V_{max} of 1.13 nmol/min per mg synaptosomal protein for the high-affinity uptake (uptake$_1$). The K_m value for the low-affinity uptake was 7.91×10^{-6} M. Kannengiesser et $al.$ (1973) demonstrated that crude preparations from whole rat brain concentrated 5-HT by a process that was saturable, temperature-dependent, and linked to the activity of Na^+K^+-ATPase.

2.1.3. General Comments

As discussed above, the uptake mechanisms for NE and DA in noradre-nergic and dopaminergic nerves and 5-HT in serotonergic nerves exhibit the properties of active transport systems. Unfortunately, as pointed out by several authors, the complexity of the biologic systems has not allowed direct rigorous proof of this point (Mitchell and Oates, 1970; Thoenen *et al.*, 1968). For purposes of this discussion, however, the systems will be considered to be carrier-mediated processes. The terms *amine pump, norepinephrine, dopamine,* or *serotonin uptake process,* and *carrier macromolecule* are used interchangeably to describe the specialized "machinery" in the cell membranes of adrenergic, dopaminergic, and serotonergic neurons which transport the appropriate substrate across the cell membrane. This machinery is considered to be directly comparable to the carrier molecules of other transport systems, or to an enzyme, or to a pharmacologic receptor molecule. The terms *pump receptor site* and *receptor site for norepinephrine, dopamine,* or *serotonin* are used interchangeably to describe the site on the carrier specifically adapted to receive the substrates. This site is comparable to the receptor site in other carrier systems, enzymes, or pharmacologic receptors.

The considerable space allotted below to discussion of the structure–activity relationships for inhibitors of NE and 5-HT pumps is justified on the grounds of the "amine theory of depression" and also on the basis that the therapeutically effective, tricyclic antidepressant drugs are among the most potent inhibitors of the uptake systems both *in vivo* and *in vitro*. Also, since one of the main goals of this review is to define structure–activity relation-ships for inhibitors of the various pumps we have relied heavily on *in vitro* data. Under *in vitro* conditions, variables such as drug concentration, distribution, and metabolism can be much more readily controlled than under *in vivo* conditions. Control of the concentrations of substrates is very important in uptake studies, since passive uptake, independently of active neuronal uptake, is greatly exaggerated at high concentrations. Indeed, concentrations of NE or 5-HT in excess of 3×10^{-7} M should probably not be used for studies concerning active neuronal uptake of these amines. Results from studies, *in vivo*, have been incorporated in Section 2.5, where the relationship between structure and activity for drugs inhibiting amine pumps is examined for the information it might yield regarding the biochemical basis underlying therapeutic effectiveness.

2.2. Inhibition of Norepinephrine Uptake

2.2.1. General Structure–Activity Relationships for Tricyclic Inhibitors in Vitro

Callingham (1967) reported on a systematic study of the structure–activity relationships in a series of tricyclic antidepressant compounds. This author determined the IC_{50} values for these compounds as inhibitors of the 10-min uptake from 6×10^{-8} M [^{3}H]NE into isolated perfused rat hearts. Callingham (1967) concluded that the most potent inhibitors contained a dihydrodibenzazepine ring system (e.g., desmethylimipramine, IC_{50} value 7.1 $\times 10^{-9}$ M). Only a 3- or 4-fold difference in potency existed between the most potent and the least potent ring systems. When the length of the 3-carbon side chain of either imipramine or desmethylimipramine was increased by one methylene group or was reduced by one methylene group, activity was considerably reduced. Branching of the propylamine side chains greatly lowered the potency of the compounds. Potencies also varied with the nature of the substitution on the terminal nitrogen of the side chain: NHMe > NMe$_2$ = N$^+$Me$_3$ > NH$_2$. Maxwell et al. (1969), using rabbit aorta, and Salama et al. (1971), using slices of rat cortex, confirmed many of the observations of Callingham (1967) and extended them to other series of tricyclics. The IC_{50} value of desmethylimipramine in aorta was 1.3×10^{-8} M and in rat cortex was 1.5×10^{-7} M. Interestingly, Salama et al. (1971) found that compounds in the dibenzocycloheptatriene (protriptyline) series which contained NH$_2$, NHMe, and NMe$_2$ were equipotent, unlike their differing efficacies in rat heart and rabbit aorta (Maxwell et al., 1969).

Horn et al. (1971) reported that in the amitriptyline series the NHMe compound (nortriptyline) was approximately 20-fold less potent than the NMe$_2$ compound (amitriptyline) in inhibiting NE uptake into hypothalamic synaptosomes. Ross and Renyi (1975a) found nortriptyline to be 4 times more potent than amitriptyline in inhibiting the uptake of NE into rat midbrain–hypothalamic synaptosomes. These results of Ross and Renyi (1975a) with nortriptyline and amitriptyline agreed with those of Maxwell et al. (1969) and Salama et al. (1971). Ross and Renyi (1975a) suggested that the use of heavily reserpinized rats in the experiments of Horn et al. (1971) might have contributed to their widely discrepant values.

2.2.2. Stereochemical Considerations for Inhibitors of the Uptake of Norepinephrine

a. Tricyclic and Related Compounds. Maxwell et al. (1969, 1970a) and Salama et al. (1971) showed that the uptake of NE into adrenergic nerves of rabbit aorta and into rat cortex slices was competitively inhibited by desmethylimipramine and related substances. Maxwell et al. (1969, 1970b) noted in a series of tricyclic antidepressants and related compounds that if the rings were coplanar the compounds were only poorly active, whereas strong potency was attained if the phenyl rings were held at dihedral angles of greater than 90° and less than 180°. It was suggested that the low potency of the coplanar tricyclic compounds might be due to the projection of the ring system into the binding site for the nitrogen atom.

In confirmation of the observations of Callingham (1967), compounds containing a terminal NHMe were found to be approximately 10 times more potent than derivatives containing NH_2 or NMe_2. However, N-ethyl, N-isopropyl, and N-butyl derivatives were only weakly active.

It was found, additionally, that NH_2, NMe_2, or N^+Me_3 derivatives of desmethylimipramine were nearly equipotent. The pK_a values of the potent, nonquaternary compounds were 8.4 or greater. Therefore, over 90% of the molecules had protonated nitrogen atoms at physiological pH. It was concluded that the positively charged form of the inhibitors was the form which interacted with the receptor site. With respect to this conclusion it was worthy of note that the pK_a for NE, the physiologic substrate of the uptake system, is 9.78 and therefore, like the inhibitors, almost all this amine is protonated at physiologic pH.

Several dicyclic antihistamine compounds had reasonable efficacy with IC_{50} values ranging from 5×10^{-8} to 4×10^{-6} M (Maxwell et al., 1969, 1974). Obviously, a tricyclic ring system was not a *sine qua non* for activity.

Studies were performed with the optical isomers of methylphenidate and deoxypipradrol and with cocaine (Maxwell et al., 1970b). Sharp differences in potency were associated with the isomers, with one isomer containing the preponderance of activity. The $2R : 2'R$-(+)-*threo* enantiomer of methylphenidate, the R-(−) enantiomer of deoxypipradrol and the $2R : 3S$ enantiomer of cocaine were most active with IC_{50} values of 1×10^{-7} M, 6×10^{-8} M, and 5×10^{-7} M, respectively. Models of these active stereoisomers and of desmethylimipramine and phenethylamine were found to have key groups superimposable over one another. When all the structure–activity relationships were taken into consideration, the simplest explanation of the facts was that NE and other phenethylamine derivatives fit the amine pump receptor site while in the planar, *anti* conformation (Fig. 1) and that the inhibitors took the conformations presented in Fig. 2. It was proposed that the phenethylamines (and the inhibitors as well) bind by a single phenyl ring to a hydrophobic surface and that the N^+ binds to a negatively charged area within the same plane as the phenyl ring. Adjacent to the negatively charged area in the receptor site is a hydrophobic area which specifically receives only a methyl substitution on the side chain N.

Maxwell et al. (1970a) calculated ΔF_i° (free energy of binding) values for desmethylimipramine and its primary amine derivative by making use of the

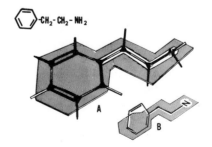

Fig. 1. (A) Molecular model of β-phenethylamine in the planar *anti* conformation. Shaded overlay defines the plane of the phenethylamine. (N) Nitrogen. (B) Drawing on a smaller scale of the model shown in (A), but with the phenyl ring rotated 90° out of the plane of the *anti* ethylamine chain. Also shown is the structural formula for β-phenethylamine. From Maxwell et al. (1974).

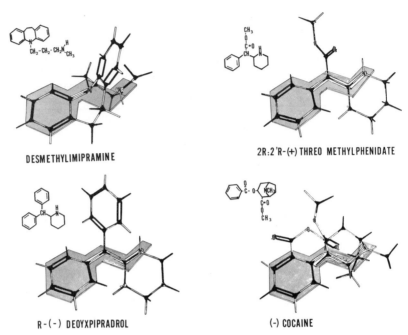

DESMETHYLIMIPRAMINE

2R:2'R-(+) THREO METHYLPHENIDATE

R-(-) DEOYXPIPRADROL

(-) COCAINE

FIG. 2. Molecular models of several inhibitors of NE uptake in conformations in which one phenyl ring and the chain (exocyclic) nitrogen take the same spatial relations as do the phenyl ring and nitrogen of β-phenethylamine in Fig. 1. Shaded overlay defines the "plane of the phenethylamine." Note that the second phenyl ring or a carbomethoxyl group is above the plane of the phenethylamine in all the inhibitors. From Maxwell *et al.* (1970*b*).

well-known equation $\Delta F_i = -RT \ln 1/K_i$. The difference in $\Delta F_i°$ between the primary amine and desmethylimipramine was approximately -1.4 kcal. According to the estimates of Belleau and Lacasse (1964) this difference in binding energy is the amount to be expected if both hydrophobic and van der Waals bonds are formed between a single methyl group and a hydrophobic area. These resutls strongly suggested that the approximate 10-fold difference in potency between desmethylimipramine and its primary amine derivatives occurs because the single methyl on the nitrogen atom forms an intimate "lock-and-key" association with its receptor site.

It was noted by Maxwell *et al.* (1971) that in distinction from what was seen with tricyclic compounds, the secondary methylamine derivatives of phenethylamines, including epinephrine, were only equipotent to, or less potent than, their respective primary amines. This observation had been made earlier by other investigators. The authors pointed out that when a phenethylamine is in the planar *anti* conformation the locus of positions available to the N-methyl group is restricted to an arc of rotation around the α-carbon-to-N bond. It would seem that none of the locations accessible to the N-methyl of phenethylamines under these circumstances approaches close to the *N*-methyl-receiving area in the receptor site. In the tricyclic compounds, the longer alkyl chain not only allows for positioning of one phenyl ring and the chain N such that they superimpose over counterparts in the planar *anti* conformation of phenethylamine, but also simultaneously permits positioning of the *N*-methyl into regions not accessible to the *N*-methyl of phenethylamines, and this presumably is the location of the binding site.

It is of great interest that the secondary methylamine derivatives of the monophenyl and diphenyl analogues of protriptyline and desmethylimipramine are not more potent than their primary amine derivatives (Maxwell *et al.*, 1974), even though, like tricyclic compounds and unlike phenethylamines, they contain propylamine side chains. By way of explanation, Maxwell *et al.* (1974) noted from a study of molecular models that the two-carbon bridge which "fixes" the orientation of the two phenyl rings in tricyclic agents also "fixes" the orientation of the C or N between the two rings and also that of the first C of the propylamine chain. It was concluded that this orientation, which is not present in diphenyl and monophenyl analogues, is necessary to align the whole propylamine side chain so that the *N*-methyl group can make the "lock-and-key" fit with a hydrophobic binding site which was alluded to earlier.

In addition to the tricyclic antidepressants, the active isomers of such potent inhibitors of NE uptake as deoxypipradrol, methylphenidate, and cocaine (Fig. 2) not only bind by a single phenyl ring but also probably bind by a second phenyl ring (or carbomethoxyl group) to a hydrophobic surface "above" the plane of binding of the phenethylamine. In support of this idea, Maxwell *et al.* (1974) showed in two series of monophenyl, diphenyl, and tricyclic compounds that the order of potency was tricyclic > diphenyl > monophenyl ≫ no phenyl. This order of potency was positively correlated with the order of increasing octanol/water partitioning in these compounds. However, it was clear that the correlation was heavily modulated by the three-dimensional display of the phenyl rings. It was reasoned that the great potency of the tricyclic compounds was due in part to the fact that the second phenyl ring (Fig. 2), which participates in binding to the receptor site, is fixed in a relatively optimal position relative to the first phenyl ring by the "two-carbon bridge." This bridge simultaneously forms the tricyclic system, throws the two phenyl rings out of coplanarity, and partially orients the propylamine side chain in a favorable manner. Diphenyl analogues are weaker than the tricyclics because the second phenyl ring is not fixed and may, as a consequence, be in less than an optimal conformation on the receptor site. It was reasoned that deoxypipradrol, a diphenyl compound, was weaker than some tricyclics for probably the same reason. Methylphenidate in turn is weaker than deoxypipradrol because instead of a second phenyl ring it has a carbomethoxyl group available for binding. Cocaine is weaker still, since in addition to having a carbomethoxyl group instead of a second phenyl group, the distance between its phenyl ring and the protonated N is not fixed by a 2-

carbon chain as in deoxypipradrol or methylphenidate, but is dependent on a specific conformational folding for proper spacing to occur.

Horn (1973*a*) presented a theoretical analysis which led him to different conclusions regarding the conformations assumed by NE and tricyclic antidepressants when they occupy the NE pump receptor site. Horn (1973*a*) noted that the preferred conformation of NE in the crystalline state (Bergin and Carlstrom, 1971) has the side chain fully extended and the amino group "above" the plane of the phenyl ring (Fig. 3A). In other words, it is as though one took phenethylamine in the planar *anti* conformation and then rotated the phenyl ring 90° out of planarity (e.g., Fig. 1B). In solution, the side chain has been demonstrated to prefer the extended *anti* conformation (Ison *et al.*, 1973). Horn (1973*a*) proposed the conformation for imipramine at the NE pump receptor site shown in Fig. 3B on the ground "that the imipramine analogue, chlorpromazine, which is a potent inhibitor of noradrenaline uptake (Horn *et al.*, 1971) is known to have a similar structure in the solid state. . . ." As can be seen in Fig. 3C, it is possible to superimpose NE on this conformation of imipramine such that the two most crucial binding sites (one phenyl ring and the chain N) have the same spatial disposition. This rationale of Horn (1973*a*) is reasonable if one accepts the premise that NE and

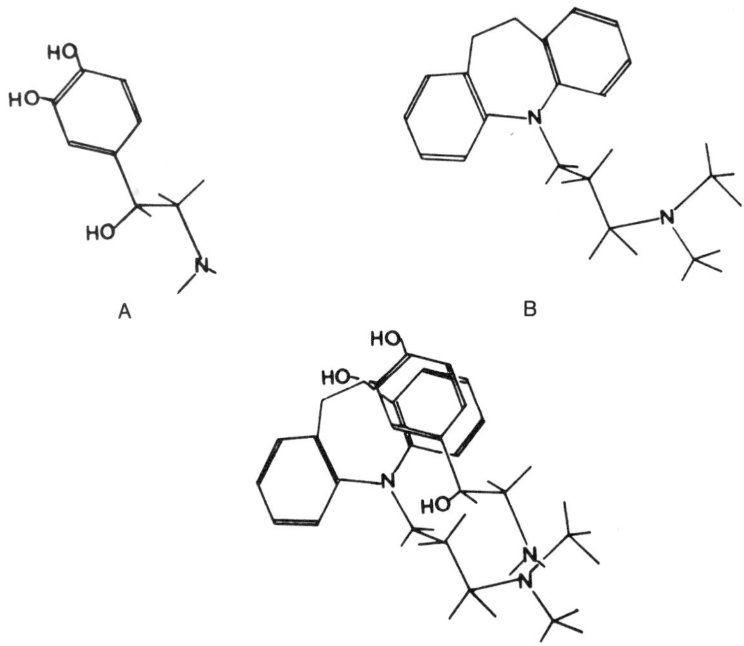

FIG. 3. (A) Conformation of NE as determined by X-ray crystallography. (B) Proposed preferred conformation of imipramine at the uptake site. (C) Superimposition of the two molecules. From Horn (1973*a*).

imipramine fit the receptor site when they hold the conformation which they prefer in crystal or in solution. However, Ison *et al.* (1973) presented evidence from nuclear magnetic resonance studies that the energy differences among rotamers of NE are small (0.83 kcal/mol) and that only 0.2 kcal/mol of this total could be ascribed to steric repulsion between the amino group and the aromatic ring. Hence, the argument for NE assuming the *anti* conformation on the receptor, but necessarily with the phenyl ring out of the plane of the side chain, is not compelling. In addition, X-ray crystallographic studies of imipramine HCl (Post *et al.*, 1975) demonstrated that there are two conformations in the crystalline state. Post *et al.* (1974) observed that "the possibility of conformations other than those found in the crystal, existing in solution cannot be excluded (as a recent NMR study of imipramine and its hydrochloride has shown [Abraham *et al.*, 1974]). . . ." In addition, potential-energy diagrams which were constructed made it apparent that other conformations of the side chain of similar energy to the crystal form could exist and that no *a priori* method of distinguishing which conformation was most likely in the absence of packing constraints was at hand.

b. Spiro Cyclohexyl Compounds. Recently a series of spiro compounds structurally related to tricyclic antidepressants was prepared and studied by Carnmalm *et al.* (1974). In these compounds the structural features of traditional tricyclic antidepressants were preserved, but the flexibility of the side chain was severely limited by incorporating it into a cyclohexene or cyclohexane ring which is quite rigidly attached to the central ring of the tricyclic nucleus. The compounds were studied for their capacity to inhibit the 5-min uptake of [^{3}H]NE from a 10^{-7} M solution into slices of mouse midbrain. The compounds were stated to be competitive inhibitors. The best of these compounds (Fig. 4A) was a tertiary dimethylamine derivative which had an IC_{50} of 3×10^{-7} M. This IC_{50} was approximately equal to that of nortriptyline (Carnmalm *et al.*, 1974). It was also approximately equal to that for imipramine ($IC_{50} = 1.4 \times 10^{-7}$ M) but higher than that for desmethylimi-

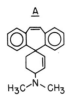

FIG. 4. (A) Structural formula for *N,N*-dimethyl-spiro[5H-dibenzo[a,d]cycloheptene-5,1′-cyclohex-2′-en]-4′-amine. (B) A top view (left) and a side view (right) drawing of a molecular model of the molecule shown in (A) but with a cyclohexane instead of a cyclohexene ring. (a,b,c) Coordinates of the position of the nitrogen atom with respect to the solid line drawn through the central ring of the tricyclic system. From Ross and Renyi (personal communication).

pramine ($IC_{50} = 7 \times 10^{-8}$ M) as reported by Ross and Renyi (1975a). In this series of spiro compounds, in distinction from tricyclic compounds, the order of potency was $NMe_2 > NHMe > NH_2$. These authors remarked that their data indicated that the secondary methylamine group is not necessarily the optimal structural element for tricyclic molecules. However, it must be realized that introducing the spiro ring structure into the flexible tricyclic chain, in addition to markedly reducing the number of positions which can be assumed by the nitrogen atom and its attached methyl group, also introduces two additional carbon atoms and considerable bulk into the chain in the form of a cyclohexene or cyclohexane ring (Fig. 4B). It is possible that some potency is introduced here by binding of these additional hydrophobic groups (or the ring they help form) to heretofore unused sites in the receptor. Additional information is needed. It is possible that within the spiro cyclohexene series the 6-fold increase in potency occurring with the addition of one methyl group to the primary amine derivative may be due to interaction of the methyl group with a different hydrophobic site than that occupied by the N-methyl of desmethylimipramine. Likewise, the 4- to 7-fold increase in potency associated with adding the second methyl group on the nitrogen atom of the spiro cyclohexene compounds may be due to an additional interaction with this hydrophobic area that is not accessible to the second methyl group in the more mobile amitriptyline or imipramine compounds. In short, the spiro compound may be a variant of tricyclics, the "chains" of which have accessibility to a site or sites of binding that are not used by standard tricyclics. Such a possibility may seem more palatable when it is remembered that, as mentioned above, the side chains of tricyclics possess some limited but distinct orientation of their own and are not completely mobile. On a more practical level, Ross and Renyi (1975a) noted that the order of potencies of standard tricyclic inhibitors differed depending on whether brain slices or synaptosome preparations were used for study. With synaptosomes, secondary methylamines were all more active as NE uptake inhibitors than the tertiary derivatives, whereas in brain slices [the same tissue as used in the studies of Carnmalm et al. (1974)] this was not so. In addition, the IC_{50} values of the antidepressant agents were lower in synaptosomal experiments than in slice experiments. Ross and Renyi (1975a) considered that protein and perhaps other constituents in brain tissue bind tricyclic antidepressants, thereby decreasing the free concentrations of compounds. They also suggested that tissue binding was the main reason for the difference in the activities which were observed with the two preparations. It would be of interest to know whether the secondary methylamine in the spiro cyclohexene series had greater nonspecific binding in brain slices than the tertiary dimethylamine compound.

    c. 4-Phenyl-1-aminotetralins. Sarges et al. (1974), on the basis of studies concerned with the capacity of relatively rigid tetralin derivatives and of standard inhibitors to inhibit the uptake of [^{3}H]NE by rat hearts *in vivo*, proposed that the conformation of desmethylimipramine at the NE pump receptor was as shown in Fig. 5C. This conformation is distinctly different from that postulated by Maxwell *et al.* (1969, 1970*b*, 1974) [see Section 2.2.2(a)].

The tetralins can be considered to be tricyclic-like compounds in which the side chains are constrained into a relatively inflexible orientation by inclusion into a ring. In the studies of Sarges *et al.* (1974), rats were pretreated with drug intraperitoneally followed 20 min later by intravenous injection of [³H]NE. Rats were sacrificed 1 hr after [³H]NE. One of the tetralins (shown in Fig. 5A,B) was found to be approximately one-half as potent as desmethylimipramine and forms the basis of the conformation for desmethylimipramine proposed by Sarges *et al.* (1974) and shown in Fig. 5C. Unfortunately, in these studies the concentrations of inhibitors at the amine pump were not known and the effects of variations in tissue distribution or metabolism of the several compounds were not taken into account. Moreover, the competitive nature of the tetralin inhibitors was not established. The work of these authors awaits verification in *in vitro* experiments.

It is clear from an inspection of the spiro cyclohexyl compounds of Carnmalm *et al.* (1974) that the conformation of the "chain" is just as inflexibly fixed within a ring as it is in the tetralins. If the potency data are taken at face value, both groups of compounds were approximately equipotent, being approximately one-fourth to one-half as active as desmethylimipramine. A comparison of the molecular configuration of these two compounds from models built according to Figs. 5B and 4B makes it clear that

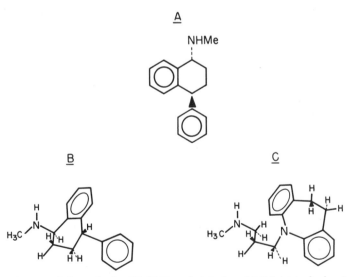

FIG. 5. (A) Structural formula for 1*R*,4*S*-*N*-methyl-4-phenyl-1,2,3,4-tetrahydro-1-naphthylamine. (B) Drawing of molecular model of the molecule in (A). (C) Postulated active conformation of desmethylimipramine. The aminoalkyl side chain is folded toward the aromatic ring system in such a way that both phenyl rings and the aminoalkyl side chain overlap with the corresponding atoms in (B). After Sarges *et al.* (1974).

the conformations of the "chains" dictated by these molecules are markedly different. Further work is needed here to explain how these two distinct conformations for the propylamine chain can both be "the correct" conformation.

   d. *Bicyclic Compounds (Lu 3-010).* Carlsson *et al.* (1969a) concluded on the basis of *in vivo* and *in vitro* histochemical and *in vivo* biochemical studies that the activity of Lu 3-010 (Fig. 6A) on peripheral adrenergic neurons was comparable with that of desmethylimipramine and protriptyline. Maxwell and Ferris (unpublished) have verified this potency *in vitro* in rabbit aorta and hypothalamic synaptosomes, as have other investigators. One of the stereoisomers of Lu 3-010 can readily superimpose over the planar *anti* conformation of phenethylamine in a manner very similar to that of desmethylimipramine (compare Fig. 6B with Fig. 2). Since the phenyl ring is not fixed as in desmethylimipramine, it is perhaps surprising that the compound is as potent as desmethylimipramine. Work in the authors' laboratory indicates that the presence of the two methyl groups on the bicyclic ring adds significantly to the potency of this compound, since removal of either one or both of these groups sharply reduces potency to a level which is consonant with diphenyl compounds. This suggests that additional hydrophobic binding sites which are not utilized by desmethylimipramine or other standard tricyclics are available to the methyl groups of Lu 3-010 and help to account for its high potency.

2.3. Inhibition of Catecholamine Uptake into Dopaminergic Neurons

   Carlsson *et al.* (1966) demonstrated by histofluorescent techniques that desmethylimipramine, protriptyline, and Lu 3-010 (Fig. 6) strongly inhibited the uptake of α-methyl NE into slices of cortex and hypothalamus at

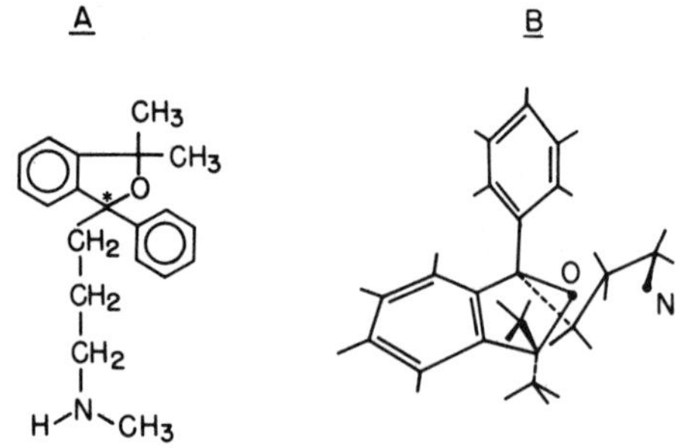

FIG. 6. (A) Structural formula of LU 3-010. (B) LU 3-010 in the conformation in which the horizontal phenyl ring and the nitrogen take the same spatial relations as do the phenyl ring and nitrogen of β-phenethylamine in Fig. 1 and in the inhibitors in Fig. 2. Note the similarities to and differences from desmethylimipramine in Fig. 2. The second (vertical) phenyl is rotatable. Two methyl groups are attached to the five-membered, oxygen-containing ring in such a way that one projects above and one projects below the "plane of the phenethylamine" which is described in Figs. 1 and 2. (- - - -) Projection below the plane; (*) asymmetric carbon atom.

concentrations which did not significantly inhibit the uptake of this amine into the caudate nucleus–putamen. Amphetamine, by way of contrast, was equally effective in inhibiting the accumulation of α-methyl NE by slices from all three brain regions. Glowinski *et al.* (1966) reported results from *in vivo* studies in the rat which indicated a similar differential effect of tricyclic drugs on the uptake of NE and DA in brain. Hamberger (1967) and Fuxe *et al.* (1967) also reported that desmethylimipramine was not an effective inhibitor of the transport mechanism in dopamine neurons.

Ross and Renyi (1967*b*) determined IC_{50} values for tricyclic and related compounds as inhibitors of the uptake of tritiated NE and DA from 10^{-7} M solutions of these amines into slices of mouse cerebral cortex and of rabbit striatum. Lu 3-010 and desmethylimipramine were potent inhibitors of the uptake of NE into slices of cortex but were approximately 1600 and 5000 times less active, respectively, in inhibiting the uptake of DA into slices of striatum. Cocaine was approximately 33 times less potent than desmethylimipramine in inhibiting NE uptake. However, unlike desmethylimipramine and Lu 3-010, cocaine was as effective against DA uptake as it was against NE uptake, and thus was significantly more potent than either desmethylimipramine or Lu 3-010 in this regard.

Horn *et al.* (1971) reported that a series of six tricyclic antidepressants (desmethylimipramine, amitriptyline, nortriptyline, protriptyline, imipramine, and doxepin) were poor inhibitors of the uptake of labeled DA into rat striatal synaptosomes. The drugs were markedly less potent in inhibiting the uptake of DA into striatal synaptosomes than they were in inhibiting the uptake of NE into hypothalamic synaptosomes.

Horn *et al.* (1971) presented evidence that the inhibition of DA uptake into striatum produced by the tricyclic antidepressants was noncompetitive. These authors also commented that the poor affinity of the tricyclic compounds for dopamine neurons might be a reflection of the constraints on the mobility of the phenyl rings and the enforcement of a relatively rigid dihedral angle between these rings in the tricyclic ring system. Presumably, this molecular arrangement is not compatible with a good fit to the catecholamine-uptake receptor site in the striatum. By way of contrast, the phenethylamine derivatives, (+)- and (−)-amphetamine, were noted to inhibit catecholamine uptake competitively in both brain regions.

Ferris *et al.* (1972) commented that the diphenyl compound (−)-deoxypipradrol, in addition to being a potent inhibitor of DA uptake into striatal synaptosomes, exhibited competitive kinetics. This suggested that diphenyl compounds which have relatively mobile phenyl rings as compared with tricyclic compounds could fit the receptor site for catecholamine uptake in striatal tissue.

Birkmayer and Riederer (1975) demonstrated that the DA levels in striatum, nucleus ruber, and raphe were reduced in 4 elderly, depressed patients as compared with values found in 12 control nondepressed subjects.

NE and 5-HT were also lower in some brain regions. The authors speculated that the DA deficiency might be responsible for loss of drive, while NE deficiency might be responsible for the postural changes and 5-HT deficiency for the sleep changes characteristic of depression.

2.4. Inhibition of Serotonin Uptake

2.4.1. General Structure–Activity Relationships for Tricyclic and Related Inhibitors in Vitro

A relatively large number of authors have addressed themselves specifically to the influence of N-substitution on potency. This unusual level of interest stems from a primary concern with the therapeutic utility of these agents (see Section 2.5). In direct contrast to the results found with NE uptake, tertiary dimethylamine tricyclic agents, e.g., imipramine and amitriptyline, were found to be approximately 5–10 times more potent in inhibiting the uptake of 5-HT than were the corresponding secondary methylamines, desmethylimipramine and nortriptyline. These differences in potencies were demonstrated by Blackburn et al. (1967) with slices of whole rat brain, Ross and Renyi (1967a, 1969) with slices of mouse brain stem, Alpers and Himwich (1969) with slices of rabbit brain stem, Carlsson (1970) with slices of mouse brain, Shaskan and Snyder (1970) with rat hypothalamic slices, Kannengiesser et al. (1973) with rat whole-brain synaptosomes, Horn and Trace (1974) with homogenates of rat hypothalamus, and Ross and Renyi (1975a) with slices and crude synaptosomal preparations of rat midbrain–hypothalamus.

Horn and Trace (1974) noted that the primary amine derivative and trimethyl quaternary derivative were approximately equipotent to imipramine. All three agents were 5–10 times more potent than desmethylimipramine in inhibiting 5-HT uptake into homogenates of rat hypothalamus. Ross and Renyi (personal communication) also found the trimethyl quaternary derivative of imipramine to be nearly as potent as imipramine itself.

It should be noted that although imipramine is more potent than desmethylimipramine in blocking 5-HT uptake, direct estimations show that both compounds are more potent in blocking the uptake of NE than the uptake of 5-HT. Thus, Shaskan and Snyder (1970), with slices of rat hypothalamus, reported an IC_{50} for imipramine against NE uptake of $\sim 2 \times 10^{-7}$ M. This was approximately 3- to 4-fold lower than the IC_{50} of imipramine against 5-HT uptake. Likewise, Ross and Renyi (1975a) reported 5- and 21-fold differences in favor of the inhibition of NE uptake into synaptosomes and into slices from rat midbrain–hypothalamus region. Moreover, van der Zee and Hespe (1973) found imipramine to be approximately 20 times more potent against NE uptake than against 5-HT uptake. On the other hand, Lidbrink et al. (1971) reported that imipramine was more potent against 5-HT uptake than against NE uptake into rat whole-brain synaptosomes. However, the IC_{50} values for NE reported by Lidbrink *et al.* (1971) were approximately 100-fold higher than comparable values of Ross and Renyi (1975*a*) and Shaskan and Snyder (1970), and this suggested that some technical problem was distorting the results. Lidbrink *et al.* (1971) suggested that the difference in potency of desmethylimipramine on [^{3}H]NE uptake as reported by Shaskan and Snyder (1970) and by themselves was probably due to the fact that the whole-brain synaptosomal preparations used in their own study contained a large number of dopamine terminals which were very little affected by desmethylimipramine.

Wong *et al.* (1974) reported that the K_I value of imipramine as an inhibitor of 5-HT uptake was 2×10^{-7} M, while its K_I as an inhibitor of NE uptake was 2.4×10^{-5} M. As with the results of Lidbrink *et al.* (1971), this very high K_I value against NE may be due to the fact that whole-brain synaptosomes were used. Also, the high concentration of NE ($0.3-1 \times 10^{-6}$ M) employed in these kinetic studies may have contributed to this discrepancy. It seems reasonably clear that both the secondary methylamine and tertiary dimethylamine compounds have greater affinity for the NE-uptake receptor sites than for 5-HT-uptake receptor sites. The significant difference is that desmethylimipramine has considerably more affinity for the NE site and considerably less affinity for the 5-HT site than imipramine has.

Horn and Trace (1974) carried out a structure–activity study of the capacity of a limited number of tricyclic compounds to inhibit the uptake of 5-HT into homogenates of rat hypothalamus. They noted the following:

1. Reducing or increasing the chain length of imipramine by one methylene group reduced activity by 8 or 7 times, respectively.
2. Substitution of a methyl group on the methylene group adjacent to the chain nitrogen (the α-methyl) or on the methylene group two removed from the chain nitrogen (β-methyl) reduced the potency of imipramine by 17- and 33-fold, respectively.
3. Substitution of a chlorine atom at position 3 on the ring system to produce chlorimipramine (Fig. 7) increased the potency of imipramine by approximately 5-fold. Substitution of a dimethylamino group into the 3 position of the ring system did not significantly affect potency. Carlsson (1970), Shaskan and Snyder (1970), and Ross and Renyi (1975*a*) have all noted that chlorimipramine is 5- to 10-fold more potent than imipramine. Incidentally, Shaskan and Snyder (1970) and Ross and Renyi (1975*a*) noted that chlorimipramine, in distinction from imipramine and desmethylimipramine, is more potent (3- to 10-fold) in inhibiting uptake of 5-HT than of NE.
4. Substitution of a sulfur atom for the two-carbon bridge in imipramine (yielding promazine) and in chlorimipramine (yielding chlorpromazine) reduced potencies by approximately 30- to 50-fold, respectively.

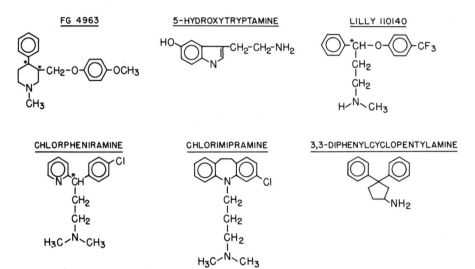

FIG. 7. Structural formulas for 5-HT and several inhibitors of 5-HT uptake. (*) Asymmetric carbon atoms.

Carlsson and Lindqvist (1969) noted in studies *in vivo* that the dicyclic antihistamine chlorpheniramine (Fig. 7) was very potent in inhibiting the uptake mechanism in serotonergic neurons. Lidbrink *et al.* (1971) reported that chlorpheniramine and brompheniramine were potent inhibitors of the uptake of both 5-HT and NE in rat whole-brain synaptosomes. Korduba *et al.* (1973) found that pheniramine was a weak inhibitor of the uptake from 10^{-7} M 5-HT into striatal synaptosomes. Desmethylimipramine had an ID_{50} value of 2.5×10^{-6} M, whereas chlorpheniramine had an ID_{50} value of 9.2×10^{-7} M and 3,4-dichlorpheniramine produced 50% blockade at 8×10^{-8} M. It is clear from these studies that a tricyclic structure is not an absolute requirement for inhibiting the uptake mechanism for 5-HT.

Cocaine inhibited the uptake of 5-HT. Ross and Renyi (1967a) reported an IC_{50} for cocaine of 3×10^{-6} M to inhibit the uptake from 10^{-7} M 5-HT, while Blackburn *et al.* (1967) stated a value of 10^{-5} M for 50% inhibition of the uptake from approximately 5×10^{-8} M 5-HT.

Ross and Renyi (1967a) noted that their IC_{50} for cocaine as an inhibitor of 5-HT uptake was about the same as that found against the uptake of the catecholamines. Thus, cocaine, which has moderate affinity for the NE-uptake receptor site, also has equal affinity for the 5-HT-uptake receptor site.

2.4.2. Stereochemical Considerations for Inhibitors of the Uptake of Serotonin

Many of the publications concerning inhibitors of 5-HT uptake have not defined the nature of the blockade, i.e., whether competitive or noncompetitive (see, for example, Carlsson, 1970; Horn and Trace, 1974; Ross and Renyi, 1969). Wong *et al.* (1974), however, reported that chlorimipramine, imipramine, and nortriptyline were competitive inhibitors of the uptake of 5-HT into synaptosomes from whole rat brain with K_I values of 4×10^{-8}, 2×10^{-7}, and 3.6×10^{-6} M, respectively. Ross and Renyi (1975a) presented evidence that the inhibition by chlorimipramine of the uptake of 5-HT into slices of rat midbrain–hypothalamus region was competitive with a K_I of 2×10^{-7} M. These authors considered that tissue binding of the tricyclic antidepressants was probably the main reason that considerably higher concentrations of these compounds were required to inhibit amine uptake into brain slices as compared with uptake into synaptosomes.

It is necessary to have evidence of competitive inhibition to justify the view that inhibitors and substrates are acting at the same site (the receptor site) in the receptor macromolecule involved in the uptake process. When dealing with competitive inhibition the stereochemical features of the inhibitors can be interpreted in a meaningful way and the principal of complementarity can be employed to permit conclusions to be drawn regarding the nature of the receptor site.

For purposes of this discussion, tryptamine (by analogy to phenethylamine in considerations concerning NE uptake) is taken as the prototype compound for uptake by serotonin neurons. The primary binding is considered to be by the planar indole surface and the terminal nitrogen in its protonated form.

Horn (1973b) studied the structure–activity relations among 5-HT analogues as inhibitors of the uptake of 5-[³H]HT from a 10^{-7} M solution of this amine into hypothalamic synaptosomes (Table 2). It is likely that these analogues of 5-HT are competitive substrates for uptake rather than true inhibitors, whereas the bulky compounds described below, including imipramine, are true inhibitors.

Removal of the hydroxyl group from 5-HT dropped potency (as compared with the K_m for 5-HT) by approximately 10-fold, whereas methylation of the hydroxyl group reduced activity by approximately 100-fold. This indicated that an OH group enhanced, and a methoxyl group interfered with, the binding of the tryptamine molecule. A parallel effect is seen in the NE uptake system with the phenethylamine derivatives, NE and its *O*-methylated metabolite, normetanephrine (Burgen and Iversen, 1965).

N,N-Dimethylation of 5-HT reduced activity by approximately 10-fold. This observation is of interest in that the *N,N*-dimethylated inhibitor, imipramine, is equipotent to its primary amine derivative. A parallel exists here to the observation that *N*-methylation of NE to yield epinephrine decreases its affinity for the NE-uptake receptor site, whereas the secondary methylamine inhibitor, desmethylimipramine, is a significantly more potent inhibitor than its primary amine derivative. It appears that the effects of *N*-substitution on potency can differ depending on whether a substrate or inhibitor is being substituted.

TABLE 2

Effect of Various 5-HT Analogues on the Uptake of 5-HT into Hypothalamic Homogenates[a]

Substitution		IC_{50}
$R_1 = OH$	$R_2 = R_3 = H (5\text{-}HT)$	$K_m 2 \times 10^{-7} M^{b}$
$R_1 = OH$	$R_2 = H$ $R_3 = -\overset{\displaystyle O}{\overset{\displaystyle \|}{C}}-CH_3$	$6.6 \times 10^{-5} M$
$R_1 = OCH_3$	$R_2 = R_3 = H$	$2.5 \times 10^{-5} M$
$R_1 = OH$	$R_2 = R_3 = CH_3$	$1.5 \times 10^{-6} M$
$R_1 = H$	$R_2 = R_3 = H$	$2.8 \times 10^{-6} M$
4-OH	$R_2 = R_3 = H$	$4.5 \times 10^{-6} M$
6,7-di-OH	$R_2 = R_3 = H$	$4.4 \times 10^{-6} M$

[a] From Horn (1973b).
[b] Value for hypothalamic slices from Shaskan and Snyder (1970). (IC_{50}) Concentration of inhibitor required to produce a 50% inhibition of the uptake of 5-[^{3}H]HT. Each drug was tested at three concentrations and a mean value ± SEM was obtained for 3–5 determinations at each concentration. The IC_{50} values were obtained by a graphic method.

Wong *et al.* (1974) described the properties of Lilly 110140 (Fig. 7). It was found to be a competitive inhibitor of 5-HT uptake into whole-brain synaptosomes and to have a K_1 of 5.2×10^{-8} M. It was approximately equipotent to chlorimipramine and 4 times more potent than imipramine. Buus Lassen *et al.* (1975) have reported a new compound, FG 4963 (Fig. 7), to be a selective inhibitor of the uptake of 5-HT. These authors reported an IC_{50} of approximately 2×10^{-7} M for FG 4963 in inhibiting uptake of 5-HT into hippocampal synaptosomes. FG 4963 was approximately one-third as potent as chlorimipramine and 3 times more potent than imipramine. FG 4963 was somewhat less than one-half as potent against NE uptake as it was against 5-HT uptake. As was mentioned earlier, chlorpheniramine (Fig. 7) is also a potent inhibitor of the uptake of 5-HT by brain slices and synaptosomes (Carlsson and Lindqvist, 1969; Lidbrink *et al.*, 1971; Korduba *et al.*, 1973). Carnmalm *et al.* (1975) noted that 3,3-diphenylcyclopentylamine (Fig. 7) was a moderately potent inhibitor (IC_{50}, 6×10^{-7} M) against the uptake of labeled 5-HT.

Since these compounds are aliphatic amines their pK_a values are probably 8.4 or greater, and therefore they are highly protonated at pH 7.4.

In addition, the quaternary derivative of imipramine is approximately as potent as imipramine. It is concluded that it is the charged form of the compounds that fit the 5-HT pump.

It is obvious from a perusal of Fig. 7 that chlorimipramine, chlorpheniramine, 3,3-diphenylcyclopentylamine, Lilly 110140, and FG 4963 are multiringed compounds of considerably more bulk than 5-HT. A similar difference in "bulkiness" exists between the structure of NE and the structures of its potent inhibitors. In addition, all five of the inhibitor compounds pictured in Fig. 7 are structurally dissimilar to each other. One common factor of Lilly 110140 and FG 4963 is that between the *para*-substituted phenyl ring in each compound there is a common O–C–C–C–N. In FG 4963 the segment –C–C–N is built into a piperidine ring, whereas in Lilly 110140 it exists as an ethylamine chain. It should be noted that Lilly 110140, and chlorpheniramine as well, have an asymmetric carbon atom so that they exist as racemic mixtures. FG 4963 has two asymmetric carbon atoms, and therefore has four isomers. The *S* isomer of Lilly 110140, the *S-trans* isomer of FG 4963, and the *S* isomer of chlorpheniramine, as well as chlorimipramine and 3,3-diphenylcyclopentylamine, all exhibit interesting three-dimensional similarities when put into conformations in which they superimpose over a specific conformation of the 5-HT molecule. This can be seen with molecular models if the substituted phenyl ring of each inhibitor is made to overlap with the phenyl segment of the indole ring of 5-HT such that its substituents will also overlap or lie in proximity to the OH in 5-HT (Fig. 8). The use of this particular superimposition as a common starting point is justified on the grounds that the four substituents involved are similar in size and in electrical field effects. The field constants are Cl, 0.41; OMe, 0.26; CF_3, 0.38; OH, 0.29 (Hansch *et al.*, 1973). Part of the indole ring of 5-HT is mimicked, and the amine nitrogen atoms of all the inhibitors overlap the terminal nitrogen atom of 5-HT. Simultaneously, in "superimposing" the inhibitors over the 5-HT conformation shown in Fig. 8, a second phenyl ring (or pyridine ring) of the inhibitors is placed "in front" and below the plane of the indole ring into a fairly circumscribed region. This last observation suggests that a noncoplanar arrangement of two phenyl rings is associated with good potency. Pertinent to this idea, it has been pointed out earlier by Ross *et al.* (1971) that iprindole, which has a tricyclic ring system that is considerably more planar than that of imipramine or chlorimipramine, is only a poor inhibitor of 5-HT uptake into mouse-brain slices. Similar results were obtained with iprindole in synaptosomes prepared from whole rat brains (Rosloff and Davis, 1974). Iprindole is also a very poor inhibitor of NE uptake. Ross and Renyi (personal communication) found that the greater the dihedral angle between phenyl rings of tricyclic antidepressants (more nearly coplanar) the weaker was their capacity to inhibit 5-HT uptake. These authors also noted that in a tricyclic spiro series coplanarity of the rings reduced activity against 5-HT uptake.

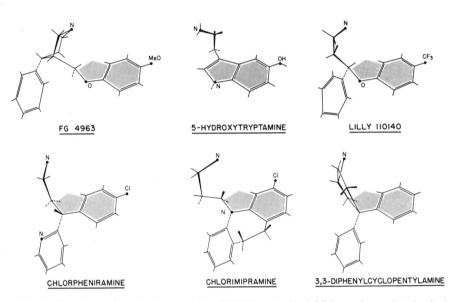

FIG. 8. Drawings of molecular models of 5-HT, and the inhibitors shown in Fig. 7, in conformations in which the phenyl rings and their substituent OH, MeO, CF$_3$, and Cl can superimpose (or nearly so in chlorimipramine). In these conformations, the amine nitrogen atoms of the inhibitors will all superimpose over the nitrogen atom of 5-HT. Note that the segments of the inhibitors adjacent to the phenyl ring form part of a planar surface which is analogous to that of the nitrogen-containing, 5-membered ring of the indole nucleus. All the inhibitors project a phenyl ring (or pyridine ring in chlorpheniramine) to the "front" and "below" the planar surface of the indole. (- - - -) Projection below the indole plane. Methyl substitutions on the nitrogen atoms have been omitted.

These conformational speculations are of interest in that (1) they suggest a conformation of 5-HT at the uptake receptor in serotonin neurons, (2) they put some order into the various structures of the inhibitors where no apparent order existed, and (3) they suggest subsequent compounds to be synthesized. It would be of great interest to know which of the isomers of Lilly 110140, FG 4963, and chlorpheniramine are the most active. It would also be of interest to know whether a *para* OH would improve activity beyond that of the current *para* substituents—trifluromethyl, methoxy, and chloro—or whether indole analogues would be active. If it were found to be true, in a direct comparison, that Lilly 110140 were more potent than FG 4963, it would be of interest to study the FG compound which had the phenyl ring substituted on the methylene adjacent to the oxygen atom rather than on the piperidine ring. It would be of interest to know whether the second phenyl ring (or pyridine ring of chlorpheniramine) is necessary for potency.

2.5. Relationship between Inhibition of the Uptake of Biogenic Amines and Antidepressant Activity *in Vivo*: Influence of Structural Modifications

2.5.1. Amine Substitution in Tricyclic Compounds

Fuxe and Ungerstedt (1967), using histofluorescent techniques, noted that the uptake mechanism for 5-HT in the areas adjacent to the lateral ventricles of rats appeared to be resistant to desipramine (the secondary methylamine derivative). These authors later reported that imipramine (the tertiary dimethylamine derivative) blocked 5-HT uptake (Fuxe and Ungerstedt, 1968). Carlsson *et al.* (1968) subsequently found that 20–30 mg imipramine/kg i.p. produced a partial blockade of the accumulation of intraventricularly administered 5-HT in many serotonergic cell bodies, nonterminal axons and terminals lying close to the cerebral ventricles, and the ventral part of the subarachnoid space in rats. In addition, imipramine (25–50 mg/kg i.p.) virtually completely blocked the reduction in 5-HT levels of mouse brain produced by a α-methyl-*m*-tyramine, presumably by preventing the uptake of this depleting agent into the serotonergic neurons. The α-methyl-*m*-tyramine reduced the content of 5-HT in mouse brain from 0.40 to 0.18 μg/g, while in the imipramine-pretreated animals the level fell to only 0.37 μg/g. Carlsson *et al.* (1968) concluded that their data indicated that imipramine selectively blocked the uptake of 5-HT at the level of the nerve cell membrane. In subsequent papers, Carlsson *et al.* (1969c) demonstrated by histochemical (rats) and biochemical (mice) techniques that the central and peripheral NE-depleting effects of 4,α-dimethyl-*m*-tyramine (H77/77) were largely prevented by protriptyline and desipramine, presumably by their preventing the uptake of this depleting substance into adrenergic neurons. Imipramine showed only slight activity in preventing depletion of central NE. Carlsson *et al.* (1969b) used the related agent 4-methyl-α-ethyl-*m*-tyramine (H75/12), which caused depletion not only of central catecholamine but also of central 5-HT stores. Tertiary amine tricyclic antidepressants, e.g., chlorimipramine, imipramine, and amitriptyline, were more potent in preventing 5-HT depletion than were secondary amines, in contrast to previous observations concerning the effects of these agents on central and peripheral noradrenergic neurons (Table 3) (Carlsson *et al.*, 1969b,c).

Lidbrink *et al.* (1971) determined the effects of antidepressant drugs on the accumulation of intraventricularly administered 5-HT in rats pretreated with reserpine and nialamide. The effects were evaluated histochemically in serotonin terminals and cell bodies lying close to the aqueduct of Sylvius and the fourth ventricle. Chlorimipramine, in the dose range of 5–15 mg/kg i.p., inhibited the appearance of fluorescence. Amitriptyline was less potent, producing only modest inhibition at 15 mg/kg i.p. Chlorimipramine and amitriptyline were observed not to have any effect on the appearance of

TABLE 3

Effect of Thymoleptics on 5-HT Displacement in Brain by H 75/12 and on NE Displacement in Brain by H 77/77[a]

Compound	ED$_{50}$ (mg/kg)	
	Brain 5-HT	Brain NA
Imipramine·HCl	20	>25
Desipramine·HCl	≥50	15
Chlorimipramine·HCl	7	>25
Chlordesipramine	20	—
Amitriptyline·HCl	12	>25
Nortriptyline·HCl	20	>25
N-Methylprotriptyline·HCl	≥25	—
Protriptyline·HCl	>25	4

[a] After Carlsson *et al.* (1969a).

fluorescence in norepinephrine nerve terminals close to the fourth ventricle (especially in the nucleus tractus solitarius).

Carlsson *et al.* (1969b) noted that Kielholz and Poldinger (1968) reported that in man, with respect to psychomotor activity (increase in drive), secondary amines such as desmethylimipramine and nortriptyline appeared more potent than tertiary amines such as imipramine and amitriptyline, while as regards brightening of mood the tertiary amines appeared to be superior. Carlsson *et al.* (1969b) therefore suggested, as a consequence of their results, that norepinephrine neurons were involved in the first instance (psychomotor activation) and serotonin neurons were involved in the second (mood elevation).

Lidbrink *et al.* (1971) concluded that their results supported the view that tertiary amines of the tricyclic compounds such as amitriptyline, imipramine, and chlorimipramine preferentially block 5-HT uptake in the central serotonin neurons, whereas the secondary amines such as desmethylimipramine preferentially block NE uptake in the central adrenergic neurons. The authors felt that the antidepressant action of the frequently used tertiary amine antidepressant drugs might be related to their capacity to block the presynaptic reuptake of 5-HT and thereby elevate its concentration at postsynaptic receptor sites

Ross and Renyi (1975b) determined the inhibition of the simultaneous uptake of 1-[^{3}H]norepinephrine and 5-[^{14}C]HT into slices of the midbrain–hypothalamus region of the rat brain. These slices were prepared from animals 2 hr after they had received oral administration of desipramine, imipramine, nortriptyline, amitriptyline, chlordesipramine, and chlorimipramine. In contrast to Carlsson *et al.* (1969b,c) and Lidbrink *et al.* (1971), these authors found that all the compounds including the tertiary dimethylamine derivatives were more active against NE uptake than against 5-HT uptake. Among the tertiary amine derivatives, chlorimipramine was almost as active on 5-HT uptake as on NE uptake (Table 4). The authors pointed out that absorption from the gastrointestinal tract, and the distribution and metabolism to which the compounds were subjected following oral administration, had undoubtedly influenced the potency estimates, as they also would following oral administration of these drugs to man.

Tuck and Punell (1973) incubated rat cortical slices with plasma from patients taking chlorimipramine, imipramine, or amitriptyline to determine the effect of clinical doses on [^{3}H]NE and 5-[^{3}H]HT uptake. As can be seen in Table 5, only chlorimipramine produced significant blockade of 5-HT uptake. Imipramine and amitriptyline produced little or no blockade of 5-HT uptake. All three groups, however, inhibited NE.

Ross and Renyi (1975b) pointed out that the methods of intraventricular injection employed by Carlsson et al. (1969b,c) and Lidbrink et al. (1971) had the disadvantage that the amines would not penetrate readily to brain regions some distance from the ventricles. In addition these authors felt that with indirect "displacement" methods used by Carlsson et al. (1969a,c), compounds could interfere with the release mechanism and the efflux of the transmitters as well as with the membrane uptake mechanism.

Ross and Renyi (1975b) felt that if absorption from the gastrointestinal tract and distribution and metabolism of tricyclic compounds in rats bore any relationship to the same processes in man, it was clear that the event common to all the tricyclic compounds was inhibition of NE uptake, whereas 5-HT uptake was poorly inhibited by most of the compounds.

2.5.2. Ring Modifications

a. *Maprotoline (Ludiomil®)*. Maprotoline differs from typical tricyclic agents in that it contains a dibenzo-bicyclo-octadiene ring system (see Fig. 9).

TABLE 4

Comparison of the Inhibitory Effects of Amitriptyline, Imipramine, and Chlorimipramine Administered Orally on the Uptake of 1-[^{3}H]NE and 5-[^{14}C]HT in Midbrain–Hypothalamus Slices[a]

Compound	ED$_{50}$ (mg/kg)	
	1-[^{3}H]NE	5-[^{14}C]HT
Amitriptyline	>50	>50
Imipramine	8	50
Chlorimipramine	20	35

[a] The rats were killed after 2 hr and the ED$_{50}$ values were determined from dose–response curves based on at least three doses with four animals in each dose. From Ross and Renyi (1975b).

TABLE 5

Uptake of [³H]NE and 5-[³H]HT by Rat Cerebral Slices Incubated in Plasma from Patients Treated with Tricyclic Antidepressants[a]

Drug	Number of patients[b]	Uptake of 5-[³H]HT (% of control)[c]	Uptake of [³H]NE (% of control)[d]
Chlorimipramine (25–50 mg i.m. twice daily)	9	72 ± 5	43 ± 3
Imipramine (25–50 mg p.o. thrice daily)	10	97 ± 6	33 ± 3
Amitriptyline (25–50 mg p.o. thrice daily)	10	93 ± 5	39 ± 3

[a] From Tuck and Punell (1973).
[b] The same patient's plasma was in separate experiments incubated both with [³H]NE and 5-[³H]HT.
[c] The slices were first incubated in the patient's plasma for 15 min before addition of 5-[³H]HT to a final concentration of 2×10^{-9}M. After incubation for 15 min, the slices were quickly rinsed in drug-free Krebs–Ringer bicarbonate buffer for a few seconds and the radioactivity was determined. The values are calculated as percentages of the 5-[³H]HT uptake in plasma, drawn before treatment. The values are expressed as the mean ± S.E.
[d] The procedure was as for 5-[³H]HT except that final concentration of [³H]NE was 2×10^{-8}M.

Mâitre *et al.* (1971) demonstrated in experiments *in vivo* that maprotoline (34276-Ba) inhibited the uptake of labeled NE by the brain of rats and chicks. Maprotoline was demonstrated by Mâitre *et al.* (1974) to be 20–30 times less effective than imipramine in inhibiting uptake from 1.9×10^{-9} M 5-HT into rat midbrain synaptosomes. Imipramine and maprotoline, on the other hand, were approximately equipotent in inhibiting uptake of NE.

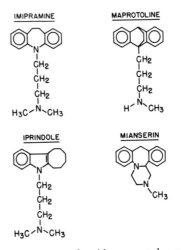

Fig. 9. Structures of antidepressant drugs.

Maprotoline was over 100 times more potent in inhibiting the uptake of NE than of 5-HT. Imipramine was 3 times more potent against NE than against 5-HT. *In vivo*, 300 mg maprotoline/kg p.o. was inactive in inhibiting the depletion of 5-HT from rat brain caused by administration of H75/12, presumably by failing to prevent the uptake of this depleting substance by the 5-HT membrane pump. Imipramine and desmethylimipramine, by way of comparison, were effective in doses of 10–100 mg/kg p.o. in preventing the 5-HT depletion produced by H75/12. Maprotoline appeared to be an active antidepressant with activity that is not distinguishable from standard tricyclic agents (Murphy, 1975*a*).

The evidence with maprotoline suggests that antidepressant activity of the type usually associated with imipramine or amitriptyline is not strictly dependent on its capacity to inhibit 5-HT pumps, but may be associated with inhibition of NE pumps.

b. Iprindole. Gluckman and Baum (1969) reported that iprindole, which differs from imipramine only in the configuration of the ring system (Fig. 9), was an active antidepressant in animal models. Gluckman and Baum (1969) noted that iprindole had no effect on the uptake of [^{3}H]NE by rat heart and brain in doses adequate to produce antidepressant effects in rats. Comparable doses of imipramine effectively reduced the uptake of [^{3}H]NE by rat heart and brain. Like imipramine, iprindole did not inhibit the oxidation of tyramine by brain or liver MAO in concentrations as high as 10^{-3} M.

Ross *et al.* (1971) reported that iprindole was a very weak inhibitor of the uptake of NE ($IC_{50} = 9 \times 10^{-6}$ M) and of 5-HT ($IC_{50} = 5 \times 10^{-5}$ M) in mouse-brain slices, *in vitro*. Imipramine was more than 100 times more potent than iprindole (IC_{50} against NE, 8×10^{-8} M; against 5-HT, 2×10^{-7} M). In additional studies, imipramine and iprindole were administered to mice and rats, their brains were removed, and uptake into slices prepared from the brains was determined. Iprindole inhibited the uptake of NE and 5-HT by less than 50% at 100 mg/kg i.p., whereas imipramine gave 50% inhibition of NE uptake at 10 mg/kg i.p. and 50% inhibition of serotonin uptake at 30 mg/kg i.p.

In a double-blind, 4-week study conducted with 100 depressed and anxious–depressed patients and general practice outpatients, iprindole was found to be similar in efficacy to imipramine (Rickels *et al.*, 1973). Likewise, in a 4-week controlled, double-blind study carried out by Master and Bastani (1972) on 60 outpatients suffering from various types of depression of moderate to severe degree, iprindole and imipramine were comparable in their therapeutic effect.

The evidence from basic and clinical studies with iprindole clearly suggests that antidepressant activity of the type associated with tricyclic antidepressants may not require inhibition of either 5-HT or NE uptake.

c. Mianserin (GB-94). Mianserin, which is a tetracyclic compound, is structurally quite different from a standard tricyclic (see Fig. 9). An ethylamine rather than the usual propylamine side chain is contained within a piperazine ring. This structure orients the "chain" to a considerable degree as compared with its mobility in standard tricyclic agents. Mianserin did not affect the depletion of NE or DA evoked by H77/77 in rat brain (Kafoe and Leonard, 1973; Leonard, 1974). This indicated that mianserin had little capacity to inhibit the NE "pump" in brain. Furthermore, the uptake of 5-[^{14}C]HT into cortex slices prepared from brains of rats pretreated with mianserin (40 mg/kg i.p.) was not diminished as compared with untreated controls. In the same dose range mianserin decreased the turnover of 5-HT in the mouse and increased that of NE and DA in the rat (Kafoe and Leonard, 1973; Leonard, 1974).

Mianserin has been studied in several controlled clinical trials in depressed inpatients (Vogel *et al.*, 1974; Cassano *et al.*, 1974) and in the treatment of depressive disorders in general practice (Murphy, 1975*b*). These studies indicated that mianserin had a therapeutic effect similar to that of amitriptyline and imipramine.

The data accumulated with mianserin, as with those accumulated with iprindole, suggest that clinical antidepressant activity observed with tricyclic agents may not be associated with inhibition of the uptake of either NE or 5-HT by brain tissue. It appears that, as suggested by Kafoe and Leonard (1973), alteration in amine levels in appropriate synapses may be brought about by other means, e.g., effects on turnover, independent of effects on reuptake.

3. MONOAMINE OXIDASE INHIBITORS

Monoamine oxidase (MAO) is an enzyme which catalyzes the oxidative deamination of a wide variety of endogenous substrates. During recent years reports from a number of laboratories have provided evidence that the enzyme is characterized by multiple catalytic sites with differing substrate specificities. Whether these sites occur on different molecular forms of the enzyme, as suggested by electrophoretic separations of sonicated enzyme (Youdim *et al.*, 1969; Collins *et al.*, 1970) and by immunoprecipitation experiments (McCauley and Racker, 1973), or are part of a single molecular complex, as suggested by other experiments (Houslay and Tipton, 1974; White and Glassman, 1977), is still an unsettled question. Nevertheless, there is general agreement that the design of MAOIs which show specificity in preventing the oxidation of selected substrates offers promise as a new approach to the treatment of depression and perhaps other illnesses (Fuller, 1972; Ho, 1972, Biel, 1972; Sandler, 1973; Van Praag, 1974; Martin and Biel, 1974*a*; Neff *et al.*, 1974). Therefore, in this review structure–activity relationships relating to substrate or tissue specificity will be emphasized.

3.1. The Active Site of Monoamine Oxidase

Before discussing the major classifications of potent MAOIs, it is appropriate that we consider what is known about the site to which these inhibitors bind—i.e., the active site of the enzyme.

Extensive studies of the kinetics of the enzymatic reaction of pig brain, rat liver, or beef liver MAO with benzylamine as substrate are consistent with a Ping-Pong mechanism in which the cofactor, flavin adenine dinucleotide (FAD), participates in the oxidation of benzylamine to benzaldehyde in the presence of molecular oxygen (Tipton, 1968; Houslay and Tipton, 1973; Oi et al., 1970). FAD is covalently bound through the 8 α-methyl group of riboflavin to a cysteine moiety of the enzyme (Kearney et al., 1971). One FAD is bound per 10^5 molecular-weight units of MAO. Additional thiol groups have been postulated as being necessary for activity because the enzyme is inhibited by thiol reagents (Singer and Barron, 1945). However, sulfhydryl groups may regulate protein conformation and are not necessarily located in the active-site region. Hiramatsu et al. (1975), using agents which are known to react with histidine, have demonstrated that 2 mol histidine/10^5 g enzyme protein are necessary for activity.

Proteolytic digestions of both pig liver (Oreland et al., 1973) and beef liver MAO (Kearney et al., 1971) have yielded a peptide having the amino acid sequence Ser-Gly-Gly-Cys-(FAD)-Tyr, with an aspartic acid at one end of this chain. The presence of serine, tyrosine, and aspartic acid suggests a rather nucleophilic active-site region. However, it should be remembered that in the native enzyme other parts of the three-dimensional protein structure would also comprise the active site. From studies with a variety of inhibitors of the deamination of phenethylamine and other substrates by solubilized pig liver mitochodrial MAO, Severina (1973) has postulated that at the active center of the enzyme there is a hydrophobic region as well as a nucleophilic polar region, both of which may be involved in substrate or inhibitor binding.

The observed increase in catalytic rate as pH is raised has led to the suggestion that the unprotonated amine may be bound to the enzyme. The rate-determining step in the catalytic sequence may be the removal of a hydrogen from an α-carbon of the amine, with the result that the α–β carbon bond acquires some of the properties of a double bond (Belleau and Moran, 1963). Hellerman and Erwin (1968) have proposed, on the basis of their studies of the interaction of pargyline and other inhibitors with bovine kidney MAO, that a nucleophilic moiety on the enzyme may participate in the abstraction of a proton from the methylene carbon vicinal to the nitrogen of an amine substrate or inhibitor. From plots of pK_m and V_{max} as a function of pH, Oi et al. (1971) have proposed that one amino acid moiety of the enzyme (tyrosine, lysine, or cysteine) having a pK of 10–10.3 may be involved in binding of the amine, while a group with a pK of 7–7.3 (perhaps unprotonated imidazole) may be related to cleavage of the amine. However, their conclusions were based entirely on experiments with solubilized beef liver MAO using benzylamine as the substrate. Huszti (1972), who studied the effect of pH on apparent Michaelis constants obtained with several other MAO substrates and rat brain MAO, concluded that different ionizing groups are probably involved in the binding of different substrates. More extensive studies of the same type may be expected to yield useful information concerning the nature of the multiple substrate-binding sites of MAO.

3.2. Structure–Activity Relationships among Substrates of Monoamine Oxidase

MAO catalyzes the oxidation of many primary amines, N-methyl secondary amines, and to a much lesser extent tertiary amines (Blashko, 1963). In general the best substrates can be characterized as having an aromatic moiety separated by at least one carbon atom from an amine nitrogen. The α-carbon must be unsubstituted, since one α-hydrogen is required for binding, while the other is apparently necessary for catalysis (Zeller, 1960). Compounds with only a single hydrogen on the α-carbon (e.g., amphetamine) are therefore inhibitors rather than substrates.

The finding by Zeller (1963) that m-iodobenzylamine was a good substrate for beef liver MAO, while o-iodobenzylamine was an inhibitor, led to his suggestion that substrates and inhibitors may bind to the active-site region of MAO in more than one way. He postulated that catalysis would occur only if the orientation were such that the amine moiety assumed a proper orientation with its receptor. This hypothesis also supplied a reasonable explanation for the inactivity of mescaline as a substrate.

To consider structure–activity relationships among substrates for the enzyme, apparent K_m values offer the best available approximation of relative binding affinities, although it is important to remember that K_m values are not necessarily enzyme–substrate dissociation constants. They include catalytic rate constants as well as binding constants and may vary with ionic strength, pH, and concentration of other substrates (Webb, 1963). In Table 6 are summarized some values for apparent K_m obtained by several workers. Although various investigators have observed that K_m values for MAO are not significantly influenced by the purity of mitochondrial preparations, from the diversity of data in Table 6, it is obvious that apparent K_m values may vary with species, tissue, method of assay, and undoubtedly other conditions. Nevertheless, it is possible to make some interesting speculations regarding substrate affinity. The two endogenous substrates with lowest K_m values are β-phenethylamine and tryptamine, which are the nonhydroxylated analogues of most of the others. Adding one hydroxyl group to phenethylamine to produce tyramine causes a marked increase in K_m and therefore appears to decrease the affinity of the amine for MAO. With

TABLE 6

Apparent K_m Values Obtained for Mitochondrial MAO with Several Substrates

Source and reference	Method	pH	Apparent K_m (μM)[a]						
			5-HT	Trypt	NE	DA	Tyra	PEA	BA
Pig brain									
Williams (1974)	O$_2$ electrode	7.4					110	11	625
Tipton (1972)	O$_2$ electrode	7.2	28	115	75		120		
Rat brain									
Huszti (1972)	Spectrophotometric	7.6	60	24	370		1300		
Rat liver									
Weetman and Sweetman (1971)	O$_2$ electrode	7.4	57	18	75	171	46		
Robinson et al. (1968)	Radiometric	7.2	40	450			63		
Tipton (1972)	O$_2$ electrode	7.2	70	980	392		870		450
Rat liver mitochondrial outer membrane									
Housley and Tipton (1974)	Spectrophotometric	7.2	187	19	416[b]	405	282	21	245
Bovine brain									
Achee et al. (1974)	Radiometric	7.4	93	11		160	62		
Rabbit brain									
Achee et al. (1974)	Radiometric	7.4	130	16		250	180		
Jain et al. (1973)	Radiometric	7.4	90	30		210	290		
Human brain									
White and Wu (1975b)	Radiometric	7.4	95	16	440	140	85	5	100
Housley et al. (1974)	Spectrophotometric	8.2				111	79		91
Human liver									
White and Wu (unpublished)	Radiometric	7.4	240	34	310	220	260	11	100

[a] (Trypt) tryptamine; (NE) l-NE; (Tyra) tyramine; (PEA) β-phenethylamine; (BA) benzylamine.
[b] O$_2$ electrode method used with NE in this instance.

additional hydroxyl group substitution (DA and NE), the enzyme–substrate affinity appears to decrease further. Likewise, most workers report a much higher K_m value for 5-HT than for tryptamine. Houslay and Tipton (1974) also found that 5-methoxytryptamine exhibits a K_m of 15.9 μM, similar to that of tryptamine, and m-O-methylation of NE reduced the K_m from 416 to 200 μM.

While an increase in K_m may result from an increase in the rate of enzymatic catalysis rather than decreased substrate affinity, an examination of some relative V_{max} data in Table 7 would suggest that this is probably not the reason for K_m differences among the substrates named above. For example, the maximum velocities for oxidation of the hydroxylated substrates, DA and NE are similar to or lower than the V_{max} for phenethylamine. Therefore, one may tentatively conclude that hydroxyl group substitutions on an amine tend to decrease binding affinity to MAO.

Benzylamine, which differs by only one aliphatic carbon from phenethylamine, appears to bind much more weakly to MAO (see Table 6). This emphasizes the desirability of at least a two-carbon side chain connecting the aromatic ring with the amine nitrogen.

3.3. Multiple Substrate-Binding Sites

Mitochondrial MAO from several species and organs has been characterized as having at least two classes of substrate-binding sites (MAO-A and MAO-B), largely on the basis of studies with substrate-selective inhibitors (Johnston, 1968; Squires, 1968; Goridis and Neff, 1971; Fuller, 1972; Yang and Neff, 1973, 1974; Houslay and Tipton, 1974). An understanding of the nature of these different types of MAO sites can help to define the kind of

TABLE 7
Relative V_{max} of Mitochondrial MAO[a]

Substrate	Rat liver (Houslay and Tipton, 1974)	Human brain (White and Wu, 1975b)
Serotonin	1.0	1.0
Tryptamine	0.65	0.55
5-Methoxytryptamine	0.53	—
Norepinephrine	0.57	0.75
m-O-Methylnorepinephrine	0.44	—
Dopamine	0.90	1.4
Tyramine	1.6	2.2
β-Phenethylamine	0.95	1.1
Benzylamine	0.80	—

[a] Maximum velocities were extrapolated from Lineweaver–Burke plots and expressed relative to that for serotonin.

specificity which may be possible in the development of new MAO-inhibiting drugs.

On the basis of plots of percentage inhibition vs. concentration of clorgyline (a 5-HT-selective inhibitor) or deprenyl (a phenethylamine-selective inhibitor), 5-HT has been designated a specific substrate for MAO-A, β-phenethylamine appears to be specific for MAO-B, and tyramine is catalyzed at either type of site (Yang and Neff, 1973). There is, however, considerable disagreement about most of the other common substrates with respect to which enzyme site or sites they favor. Some of these discrepancies may be caused by differences in the stability of A and B sites, since one site may be much more labile during extract preparation or storage than another. With human brain or liver mitochondria, enzyme activity with 5-HT as substrate was more labile than was activity with phenethylamine as substrate (White and Glassman, 1977). During solubilization of the enzyme by detergents, 5-HT activity decreased while phenethylamine activity remained constant. When such preparations were assayed with tyramine as substrate, the percentage inhibition observed at low clorgyline concentrations was much lower than that obtained with extracts in which the ratio of 5-HT/phenethylamine activity was preserved. If 5-HT activity was completely lost, the clorgyline inhibition profile (the curve relating percentage inhibition to log dose of inhibitor) with tyramine closely matched that obtained with β-phenethylamine as substrate. Therefore, when inhibition profiles are used to estimate proportions of a particular substrate which are catalyzed at either A or B sites, one must first ascertain that the ratio of A/B activity in the extract is similar to that in the original mitochondrial preparation.

Figure 10 illustrates clorgyline inhibition profiles obtained with six endogenous substrates using mitochondrial extracts of human brain and liver (White and Wu, 1975a). At the concentrations at which clorgyline showed specificity (10^{-8}–10^{-6} M), oxidations of DA, tyramine, tryptamine, and NE were all partially inhibited, suggesting that these four substrates can be metabolized at multiple enzyme sites. Obviously, an inhibitor with a clorgyline-like specificity can be expected to partially inhibit the oxidation of these four substrates in both brain and liver. This is of particular importance in the case of tyramine, since if peripheral tyramine oxidation is only partially inhibited, it may be possible to avoid some of the well-known side effects of MAOIs, which are attributed largely to inhibition of tyramine oxidation.

Information concerning the nature of multiple enzyme active sites can also be obtained from substrate-competition experiments. If two substrates are metabolized at the same active site on the enzyme, each will be a competitive inhibitor of the other. The competition among six endogenous substrates of human brain mitochondrial MAO was evaluated by White and Wu (1975b). From these experiments it was concluded that 5-HT and β-phenethylamine do not compete with one another as substrates, but appear to be metabolized at independent sites on the enzyme. This is consistent with the concept of A and B sites. Tyramine, as would be expected for a common

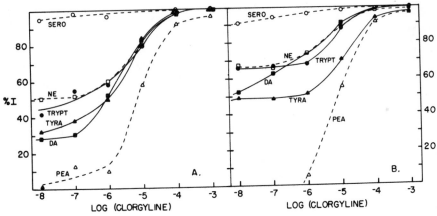

FIG. 10. Inhibition of human MAO by clorgyline in brain mitochondrial extract (A) and liver mitochondrial extract (B). Clorgyline was preincubated with enzyme for 15 min at 37°C prior to addition of radioactive substrates. Incubations in the presence of substrates (at their K_m concentrations) were for 20 min at 37°C. Blank assays contained 2 mM pargyline. Percentage inhibition was calculated from 100 [1 − (dpm$_i$/dpm$_0$)] where dpm$_0$ and dpm$_i$ = radioactivity, in disintegrations per minute, of product formed in the absence and presence, respectively, of clorgyline. (SERO) Serotonin; (NE) 1-norepinephrine; (TRYPT) tryptamine; (TYRA) tyramine; (DA) dopamine; (PEA) β-phenethylamine.

substrate, showed competition with all the other substrates, and, in turn, its oxidation was inhibited by all of them. NE was a competitive inhibitor of 5-HT oxidation, but the oxidation of NE was poorly inhibited by 5-HT. This indicated that NE may be catalyzed at an additional site not shared with 5-HT. That this site may be of the B variety is suggested by the data in Table 8, which show that in the presence of a concentration of harmine (1 μM) sufficient to inhibit all 5-HT (or A-type) activity so that only B-type activity remained, inhibition of NE oxidation by phenethylamine was increased 4-fold. Under the conditions of these experiments, the magnitude of inhibition

TABLE 8

Phenethylamine as a Substrate Inhibitor of 1-[³H]NE Oxidation by Human Brain MAO

Treatment	Product from 1-[³H]NE (nmol)	Inhibition (%)
Control	1.151	—
+ β-Phenethylamine	1.027	10.8
Harmine-treated[a]	0.433	—
+ β-Phenethylamine	0.233	46.2

[a] 1 μM harmine: Activity with 5-HT as substrate was completely inhibited; activity with β-phenethylamine as substrate was unaffected. NE concentration was 0.44 mM, and phenethylamine where present was 10 μM (White and Wu, 1975a).

expected on theoretical grounds for simple competition between the two substrates at the same active site was 50%. These results imply that at least in human brain extracts, the oxidation of NE may be catalyzed by both A and B classes of MAO sites. In rat brain (Yang and Neff, 1973, 1974) and in human liver extracts (White and Wu, 1975a) a larger proportion of NE oxidation was inhibited by low concentrations of clorgyline.

Results of substrate-competition experiments are consistent with patterns of inhibition obtained with known substrate-selective inhibitors. However, it is not certain that A and B sites represent the only classes of MAO sites, and, as emphasized by Neff and Yang (1974), the A and B classifications may each comprise more than one type of site.

3.4. General Structural Requirements for Monoamine Oxidase Inhibition

Almost any aromatic amine which is not a substrate for MAO will inhibit the enzyme *in vitro* at a concentration of 0.1 mM or above. Although it is conceivable that such a weak inhibitor might be specifically accumulated in a particular tissue so that a sufficiently high concentration is achieved *in vivo* to inhibit the enzyme, this review is primarily concerned with potent inhibitors which can be reasonably expected to exhibit *in vivo* effects attributable to MAO inhibition. The major types of classic MAO inhibitors are listed in Table 9, along with examples of representative structures and references to important reviews and other sources which can be consulted for further information.

The general structure which describes most of the known MAO inhibitors is given by formula (1), in which the aryl moiety may be phenyl, indole, or substituted analogues; X is an aliphatic group containing one or more carbons and sometimes an oxygen; N may be an amino, amide, or hydrazine nitrogen; R_1 may be a hydrogen or methyl; and R_2 may be one of a wide variety of different moieties ranging from hydrogen to much larger groups. In the most potent irreversible inhibitors R_2 is a group which binds irreversibly to the enzyme, e.g., a hydrazine, propargyl, or cyclopropyl moiety. A cyclopropyl group may alternatively be introduced

$$\text{Aryl—X—N—R}_2 \qquad (1)$$
$$|$$
$$\text{R}_1$$

into the X portion of (1), as in tranylcypromine, a modification which tends to markedly increase inhibitory potency. β-Carbolines also fit the structural pattern of (1) if they are thought of as cyclized indolealkylamines.

The requirement of an aromatic moiety and a nitrogen suggests that in order to bind to the active center of the enzyme, the inhibitor must bear some resemblance to a substrate. As mentioned before, the best MAO substrates contain an aromatic moiety separated by at least one carbon atom

TABLE 9

Major Classifications of Potent MAOI

Inhibitor type	Examples	References
Hydrazines and hydrazides	(benzene ring)—$CH_2CH_2NHNH_2$ Phenelzine (Nardil)	Biel *et al.* (1964), Ho (1972), Patek and Hellerman (1974)
	(benzene ring)—$CH_2NHNHCC$=N (with O double bond, H_2C, O, CH, CH_3 ring) Isocarboxazid (Marplan)	
Propargylamines	(benzene ring)—CH_2NCH_2C≡CH, CH_3 Pargyline (Eutonyl)	Swett *et al.* (1963), Zirkle and Kaiser (1964), Ho (1972), Martin *et al.* (1975)
Cyclopropylamines	(benzene ring)—CH——CHNH$_2$, CH_2 Tranylcypromine (Parnate)	Zirkle *et al.* (1962), Belleau and Moran (1963), Zirkle and Kaiser (1964)
β-Carbolines	H_3CO (tricyclic ring system) N, H, CH_3 Harmine	Zirkle and Kaiser (1964), McIsaac and Estevez (1966), Ho *et al.* (1968), Ho (1972)

from an amine nitrogen atom. The initial enzyme–inhibitor interaction would therefore be relatively weak and reversible, but if other features of the inhibitor provide favorable binding properties, the affinity can become very strong and perhaps irreversible, especially if the enzyme and inhibitor are preincubated at 37°C before addition of a substrate. This concept is illustrated by analogues of the substrate phenethylamine (Fig. 11). (+)-Amphetamine, a close analogue of phenethylamine, is a weak reversible inhibitor of the oxidation of β-phenethylamine, since it can bind to the enzyme, but the presence of the α-methyl group prevents catalysis (Belleau and Moran, 1963). The other three compounds in Fig. 11, tranylcypromine, pheniprazine, and pargyline, are all similar in structure to phenethylamine, but each of these contains a moiety which causes an irreversible attachment of the inhibitor to the enzyme after the initial reversible binding step.

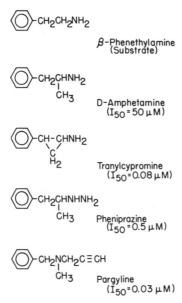

FIG. 11. Structures of the MAO substrate β-phenethylamine and some representative MAOIs. Molar IC_{50} values were determined with [^{14}C]phenethylamine (5 μM) as the substrate for rat brain mitochondrial MAO, as described in footnote c to Table 10.

Fujita (1973) has attempted to analyze the hydrophobic, electronic, and steric effects of substituents on the aromatic ring of various classes of MAOIs using free-energy-related parameters and regression analysis. This study can be questioned because the data used in the analysis were taken from the experiments of many investigators who used different tissue sources, substrates, and techniques in their MAO assays. Also, a number of assumptions were necessary to compensate for a lack of experimental data. Nevertheless, Fujita was able to conclude that the function of the aromatic moiety is probably similar in all MAOIs and that in the enzyme–inhibitor complex this moiety is bound to an electron-rich, noncatalytic region of the enzyme. Changes in MAO inhibitory potency as a result of substitution on the aromatic ring were in general markedly dependent on steric effects of these substituents.

3.5. Structure–Activity Relationships among Inhibitors of Monoamine Oxidase

3.5.1. Hydrazine-Type Inhibitors

The first MAOIs to be used clinically as antidepressants belonged to this category, following the initial discovery by Zeller *et al.* (1952) that iproniazid was a potent MAO inhibitor. Despite the nonspecificity and toxic properties associated with this class of compounds, three of the five MAOIs currently listed in the *Physicians' Desk Reference* (1975) are hydrazines or hydrazides: phenelzine (Nardil), nialamide (Niamid), and isocarboxazid (Marplan). Maximum inhibition with hydrazines is achieved only when the enzyme and inhibitor are incubated in the presence of oxygen. Patek and Hellerman (1974) have shown that phenylhydrazines first bind at the active site of bovine kidney cortex MAO as if they were substrates. The enzyme then catalyzes their oxidation to produce phenyldiazenes, which interact with the flavin moiety of MAO to cause potent irreversible inhibition.

Hydrazides (Fig. 12C,D) apparently require conversion to the corresponding hydrazines, which are the active inhibitors (Ho, 1972). Although a large number of such compounds have been synthesized in efforts to facilitate transport into brain tissues and alleviate side effects of this class of inhibitors (see the earlier reviews of Biel *et al.*, 1964; Ho, 1972), the very simple hydrazine, phenelzine, has emerged as the most acceptable hydrazine-type antidepressant in clinical use at present.

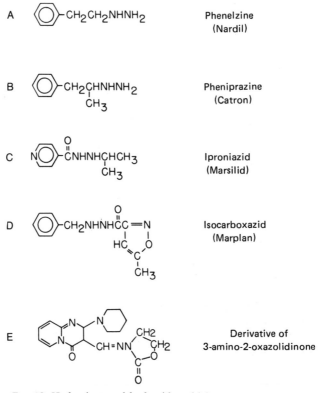

FIG. 12. Hydrazines and hydrazides which are potent MAOIs.

In a recent attempt to facilitate transport of hydrazines to brain, and thereby reduce toxicity in peripheral tissues, Hsu *et al.* (1975) have acylated the hydrazine moiety of benzylhydrazine, phenelzine, and pheniprazine with eleostearic acid. This modification reduced the *in vitro* inhibitory potency of these compounds when they were tested with mouse brain mitochondrial MAO using *m*-iodobenzylamine as substrate. However, their *in vivo* inhibitory potencies and acute toxicities were not diminished.

A number of 3-amino-2-oxazolidinone derivatives (Fig. 12E) have been shown to be more potent than pargyline as MAOIs and antihypertensive agents *in vivo,* but were not MAOIs when tested *in vitro* (Stern *et al.*, 1967; George *et al.*, 1971; Kaul and Grewal, 1972). The critical portion of these structures, 3-amino-2-oxazolidinone (3AO), was also active by both oral and intravenous routes at 1 mg/kg in rats, but was not an inhibitor *in vitro*. Stern *et al.* (1967) and Magyar *et al.* (1974) have suggested that the simple hydrazine 2-hydroxyethylhydrazine, which may be a metabolite of 3-amino-2-oxazolidinone, could be the active metabolite.

The hydrazine class of MAOIs has not in general been noted for marked substrate specificity. However, Popov *et al.* (1970) reported that in brain or liver homogenates of pretreated rats, some unsubstituted analogues of phenelzine in which the length of the acyclic carbon chain was increased exhibited somewhat greater inhibition when DA, tyramine, or 5-HT, rather than benzylamine or tryptamine, was substrate. When several hydrazines and hydrazides, which have been used clinically in depression, were tested *in vitro* using rat brain mitochondrial MAO and in homogenates of brain from pretreated rats, with [^{14}C]phenethylamine and 5-[^{3}H]HT as substrates, the IC_{50} values shown in the top portion of Table 10 were obtained (Howard and White, in prep.). Phenelzine appeared to be about 5 times more potent when 5-HT was the substrate, both *in vitro* and *in vivo*. Nialamide exhibited a similar substrate specificity, although it was less potent. While a 5-fold difference in specificity is probably not sufficient for distinguishing *in vivo* effects of these irreversible inhibitors, especially since the specificity can be expected to diminish at higher doses and with longer exposure times, it is important to note that substrate specificities obtained from *in vitro* experiments do appear to parallel the specificities attained *in vivo*.

3.5.2. Propargylamines

Within the class of acetylenic MAOIs remarkable differences in substrate specificity can be observed, in particular when the MAO-A specificity of clorgyline (Johnston, 1968) is compared with the MAO-B selectivity of deprenyl (Knoll and Magyar, 1972). These differences are illustrated by the data given in Table 10 for propargylamines. In the *in vitro* experiments clorgyline inhibited the deamination of 5-HT in preference to phenethylamine by a concentration factor of 1400, while deprenyl exhibited a similar strong specificity as an inhibitor of phenethylamine deamination. Pargyline

TABLE 10

Substrate-Selective Inhibition by MAOI[a]

Compound	IC_{50}^{b} (in vitro)[c]			ED_{50}^{b} (in vitro)[d]		
	5-HT (μM)	PEA (μM)	S/P	5-HT (mg/kg i.p.)	PEA (mg/kg i.p.)	S/P
Hydrazines and hydrazides						
Phenelzine	0.06	0.33	0.18	2.5	14.5	0.17
Pheniprazine	0.3	0.5	0.60	1	1.5	0.67
Isocarboxazid	0.9	0.5	1.8	2.5	2.1	1.2
Iproniazid	5.0	5.0	1.0	55	25 → 50	1 → 2
Nialamide	1.3	>10	<0.1	15	70	0.21
Propargylamines						
Clorgyline	0.005	7.0	0.0007	1	42	0.024
Pargyline	2.5	0.03	83.3	8.8	0.6	14.7
Deprenyl	30	0.02	1500	50	0.4	125
Others						
Tranylcypromine	0.35	0.08	4.4	0.59	0.24	2.5
Harmine	0.02	50	0.0004	10	>100	<0.1

[a] From Howard and White (in prep.).

[b] IC_{50} is the molar concentration and ED_{50} is the mg/kg dose of inhibitor which resulted in 50% inhibition.

[c] Rat brain mitochondrial MAO was preincubated for 15 min with inhibitor. MAO activity was assayed in double-label experiments using K_m concentrations of $[^{14}C]\beta$-phenethylamine (PEA) and 5-$[^{3}H]HT$ as substrates. Pargyline (2 mM) was included with all other components in blank assays.

[d] Long-Evans rats were treated intraperitoneally 1 hr before sacrifice. Whole brains were homogenized in 5% sucrose–0.1 M potassium phosphate, pH 7.4. A 1:10 ratio of tissue wt./buffer vol. was used with irreversible inhibitors. Harmine samples and corresponding saline controls were homogenized at a 1:1 tissue wt./vol. ratio to minimize dilution of the reversible inhibitor. Homogenates were assayed with 5-$[^{3}H]HT$ and $[^{14}C]\beta$-phenethylamine. Blank assays contained 2 mM pargyline and all other components.

was very similar to deprenyl in its potency as an inhibitor of phenethylamine oxidation, but apparently had a higher affinity than deprenyl for the 5-HT site on the enzyme.

Pargyline and presumably other acetylenic inhibitors, after initially binding to a substrate site on the enzyme, cause a reduction of the flavin moiety of MAO and during this process become covalently bound to the enzyme (Hellerman and Erwin, 1968; Hellerman *et al.*, 1972). When pig liver MAO was reacted with [^{14}C]pargyline and submitted to proteolytic digestion, the small peptide fragment which contained the flavin moiety also included the radioactive pargyline in a 1 : 1 ratio (Oreland *et al.*, 1973). Zeller *et al.* (1972) have described the nonenzymatic formation of covalent addition products from flavins and acetylenic MAOIs.

An examination of the structures of the three compounds in Fig. 13 allows some tentative speculations about their remarkable differences in specificity. The distance between the aromatic ring and the nitrogen is greater in the extended conformation of clorgyline than in the other two structures. The corresponding distance in the substrate, 5-HT, is also longer than in phenethylamine. When one builds space-filling molecular models of the three compounds in Fig. 13, deprenyl, with its two methyl groups, has a bulkier side chain than pargyline, while the aliphatic chain of clorgyline can attain a variety of conformations, including one that is in the same plane as the aromatic ring. Since the potency of propargylamines is known to result from a covalent interaction between the acetylenic moiety and the flavin cofactor on the enzyme, it may be reasonable to postulate that after an initial, nonselective, reversible binding at both MAO-A and MAO-B substrate-binding sites, the development of a strong irreversible inhibition may occur if the acetylenic moiety becomes optimally oriented relative to the flavin. The shorter aromatic ring–nitrogen distance in deprenyl and pargyline may favor

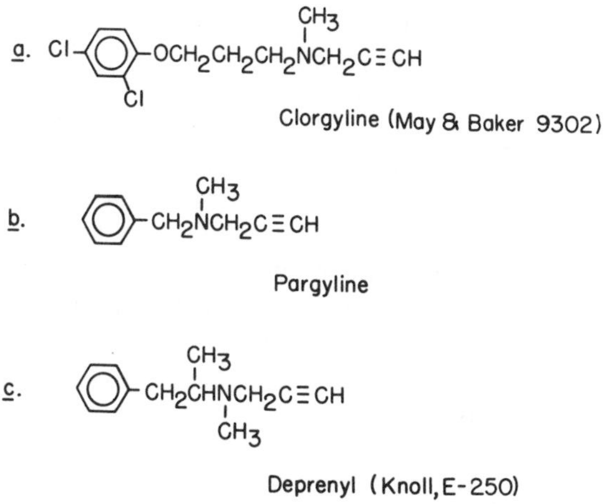

a. $Cl-\langle\bigcirc\rangle-OCH_2CH_2CH_2\overset{\overset{\displaystyle CH_3}{|}}{N}CH_2C\equiv CH$

Clorgyline (May & Baker 9302)

b. $\langle\bigcirc\rangle-CH_2\overset{\overset{\displaystyle CH_3}{|}}{N}CH_2C\equiv CH$

Pargyline

c. $\langle\bigcirc\rangle-CH_2\overset{\overset{\displaystyle CH_3}{|}}{\underset{\underset{\displaystyle CH_3}{|}}{C}}HNCH_2C\equiv CH$

Deprenyl (Knoll, E-250)

FIG. 13. Propargylamines which are potent, substrate-selective MAOIs.

this interaction at MAO-B (phenethylamine) sites, while the longer distance in clorgyline may favor a similar interaction at MAO-A (5-HT) sites. Comparing deprenyl with pargyline, the extra bulkiness of the deprenyl side chain does not appear to affect its affinity for B sites, but does decrease its ability to form a covalent bond at A sites. The chlorine substitution on the ring of clorgyline would increase the lipophilicity of this molecule, suggesting that perhaps the 5-HT-binding site is in a more hydrophobic environment. This would be consistent with recent work (Olivecrona and Oreland, 1971; Tipton et al., 1973; Houslay and Tipton, 1973) which suggests that the integrity of MAO is dependent on mitochondrial phospholipids. These phospholipids may differentially influence the binding of some substrates and inhibitors.

A regression analysis of MAO inhibitory potency with a large number of propynylamines has contributed some new insights relating to structure–activity relationships among this class of inhibitors (Martin and Biel, 1974b; Martin et al., 1975). Unfortunately, these very interesting compounds were tested only with 5-HT as the substrate and with a very crude assay procedure in which the prevention of a color change in 5-HT during a 2.5-hr incubation with rat liver MAO was used as a measure of inhibition. It is to be hoped that data with other substrates, in particular with β-phenethylamine, will eventually be available so that structural parameters which influence substrate selectivity may be analyzed. Martin et al. (1975) concluded that inhibitory potency of pargyline analogues, with 5-HT as substrate, was strongly favored by ortho-substitution on the aromatic ring. The 2-chloro, 2,4-dichloro, and 2-ethoxy analogues were at least 10 times more potent than pargyline, as was also the naphthyl analogue. When the methyl group on the amine nitrogen was replaced by a hydrogen, inhibitory potency decreased by a factor of nearly 10, but if this methyl group was replaced by ethyl or propyl, potency was decreased by a factor of 1000. Lengthening the distance between the aromatic ring and the nitrogen by increasing the number of aliphatic carbons to three or five did not affect potency, while with four carbons the potency was lowered. Adding one methyl group to the α-carbon of pargyline had no effect, but with two methyl groups on this carbon there was a marked decrease in potency with 5-HT as substrate.

Although none of the compounds synthesized for the study cited above were as active as clorgyline, the enhanced potency of the 2,4-dichloro analogue of pargyline suggests that this substitution favors 5-HT-selective inhibition. It would be of considerable interest to know whether some of the structural changes which markedly decreased activity with 5-HT would favor inhibition with phenethylamine as substrate.

Alemany et al. (1975) have synthesized a series of pargyline analogues in which the aromatic ring is replaced by an indole moiety. Their most active compound was slightly less potent than pargyline as an inhibitor of bovine liver MAO using the common substrate, tyramine. If these interesting analogues can be tested with 5-HT and phenethylamine as substrates, they may provide useful information concerning the nature of the multiple binding sites of MAO.

The availability of clorgyline and deprenyl has offered a unique opportunity for studying the pharmacologic and clinical effects of selectively inhibiting either MAO-A or MAO-B forms. Christmas *et al.* (1972) found that clorgyline caused a dose-dependent increase in 5-HT and NE in rat brain, while deprenyl did not. Clorgyline was also much more effective as an antagonist of tetrabenazine-induced sedation in rats, by a factor of about 50 on a milligram per kilogram basis. Neff *et al.* (1974) have shown that clorgyline, but not deprenyl, can prevent the syndrome caused in rats by acute reserpine treatment, which is often used as an animal model of depression. These workers also measured brain amine levels in rats after treatment with the two inhibitors and found that clorgyline at 1 mg/kg 2 hr before sacrifice caused a significant increase in 5-HT, NE, and DA, while deprenyl caused increases in DA, but not the other two amines. They concluded that inhibition of deamination of 5-HT and NE might therefore be responsible for reversal of the reserpine syndrome. Knoll *et al.* (1965) distinguished between acute and chronic effects in animal models as representing psychostimulant and antidepressive properties, respectively. They found that deprenyl at 2 mg/kg reversed the depression caused by chronic treatment with repeated small doses of reserpine.

In preliminary clinical studies (Varga, 1965), deprenyl, presumably the racemic mixture, was administered at a dose of 50–200 mg/day to 10 patients with endogenous depression. All the patients exhibited cardiovascular side effects, including a drop in blood pressure. However, in half of these patients symptoms of depression disappeared within a few days, and with 3 others a favorable response was achieved. In the same study the drug appeared to be ineffective in 9 schizophrenic patients. Tringer *et al.* (1967) administered 20 mg/kg of the (−) isomer of deprenyl, which was a more effective MAOI than the (+) isomer (Knoll and Magyar, 1972), to 30 endogenous depressives. These workers also reported a rapid improvement during the first week of therapy. After 10–14 days, 9 patients were free of symptoms, 12 showed partial recovery, and 9 were not improved. The conclusions reached in these uncontrolled clinical studies were that deprenyl may be useful in treating endogenous depression, but that it should not be prescribed for patients who suffer from anxiety or somatic complaints, since these symptoms became worse during treatment. An interpretation of the clinical responses to this compound must include a consideration of its effects on uptake (Section 4.1) as well as its unique MAO inhibitory properties. More extensive clinical studies in which either a placebo or another antidepressant is used for comparison would be desirable.

Clinical trials with clorgyline have been more extensive. In an uncontrolled pilot study (Herd, 1969) with 116 depressed patients, clorgyline at 15–30 mg/day generally resulted in noticeable improvement within 1 week. Complete recovery occurred in 57% of these cases, while partial improvement was observed in an additional 19%. A further double-blind controlled study with 31 depressed patients was then carried out by the same workers (Herd, 1969). The response to clorgyline at doses of 20–30 mg/day was compared with amitriptyline at 100–150 mg/day for a period of 4–6 weeks. A tranquilizer, pericyazine, was also prescribed for patients receiving clorgyline, since the pilot study had indicated that this drug did not influence the results. Of 16 patients treated with clorgyline, 87.5% recovered or were significantly improved, while only 46.7% of the patients receiving amitripty-line were benefited. It was noted that clorgyline appeared more successful in reactive and neurotic depression than in endogenous depression, but was superior to amitriptyline in all three types.

Another trial (Wheatley, 1970) in which clorgyline at 30 mg/day was compared with imipramine at 150 mg/day in a total of 92 depressed patients resulted in 72% recovery or improvement for patients receiving either drug. Although the investigator concluded that the therapeutic value of clorgyline was similar to that of imipramine, it is worth noting that in this study the percentage of complete recoveries was higher with clorgyline than with imipramine (39 vs. 27%).

In both the clinical trials cited above, side effects observed with clorgyline were minimal, and no hypertensive crises occurred. However, all patients had received and apparently obeyed instructions concerning dietary restrictions, and therefore it was not possible to determine whether clorgyline is intrinsically safer than other MAOIs as regards interactions with tyramine.

3.5.3. Cyclopropylamines

The most familiar member of this series is tranylcypromine (Fig. 14), which may be thought of as an analogue of amphetamine or phenethylamine in which the two carbons which separate the phenyl and amine moieties are retained in a *trans* or *anti* configuration by inclusion in a cyclopropyl ring. This structural modification is apparently responsible for the marked po-tency of this compound in comparison with the weak inhibition observed with amphetamine and with the cyclobutyl analogue of tranylcypromine (Zirkle *et al.*, 1962).

Belleau and Moran (1963) have suggested that tranylcypromine, because of the polarizability of the cyclopropane bonds, may induce a conformational change in MAO which mimics a transition state of the enzyme–substrate complex. However, Zirkle *et al.* (1962), who measured the effect of many cyclopropylphenylamines on the potentiation of tryptamine-induced convul-sions in rats, proposed that stereochemical factors are largely responsible for the potent inhibition by this type of compound. In any case, steric or electronic properties, or both, of the tranylcypromine molecule favor a very tight, essentially irreversible, binding to the enzyme.

Although tranylcypromine is recognized as a clinically effective antide-pressant, the occurrence of serious side effects, in particular hypertensive

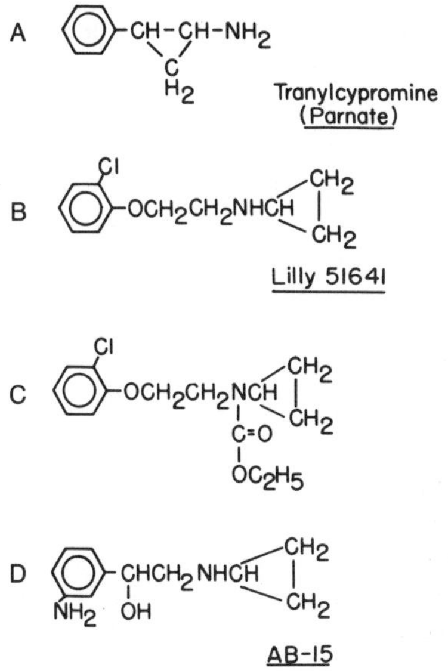

FIG. 14. Examples of cyclopropylamines which inhibit MAO.

crises after ingestion of pressor-amine-containing foods, has limited its use and has stimulated attempts to improve the safety factor, while retaining the antidepressant properties. Some cyclopropylamines have been shown to exhibit different potencies as MAOIs depending on the substrate employed. The *in vitro* IC_{50} values obtained for tranylcypromine inhibition of rat brain MAO showed a 4-fold greater inhibition of the B form of MAO, and a similar specificity was indicated by the *in vivo* data (Table 10). This is approximately the reverse of the specificity seen with phenelzine and may bear some relevance to the observations that tranylcypromine appears to be less effective than tricyclics or neuroleptics in agitated or atypical depressions (Náhunek and Švestka, 1972), while phenelzine may be especially helpful in such conditions (Robinson *et al.*, 1973; Tyrer *et al.*, 1973). However, in making such a comparison one should also consider the effect of tranylcypromine on uptake mechanisms (Section 4.1).

Fuller (1968, 1972) has described some interesting analogues in which the cyclopropyl moiety is in the R_2 position of the general inhibitor formula. Lilly 51641 (Fig. 14B), which bears a structural resemblance to clorgyline (Fig. 13A), was 400–600 times more potent in inhibiting rat brain or liver MAO when 5-HT was used as the substrate than when phenethylamine was used (Fuller, 1968). This compound was at least 10-fold more potent than tranylcypromine as an inhibitor of 5-HT deamination in isolated rat brain mitochondria (Fuller, 1968; Fuller *et al.*, 1970; Christmas *et al.*, 1972), and its substrate selectivity was retained when MAO in brain homogenates of pretreated rats was assayed (Christmas *et al.*, 1972). As a measure of its potential antidepressant activity, Lilly 51641 was active at oral doses of 10–100 mg/kg as an antagonist of tetrabenazine-induced sedation in rats. Fuller's observation that 2-chloro substitution appears to increase selective inhibition of tryptamine deamination relative to that of phenethylamine suggests that *ortho*-substitution may increase binding to MAO-A in this series as well as in the propargylamine compounds discussed earlier. One analogue of Lilly 51641 (Fig. 14C) exhibited a unique tissue specificity. It was not an inhibitor *in vitro*, but apparently was metabolized *in vivo* to an active inhibitor, presumably the parent compound. When tested at 10 mg/kg i.p. in mice, MAO activity, assayed with tryptamine in liver homogenates, was essentially unchanged, while activity in brain homogenates was about 40% of control values (Fuller, 1972).

Another substrate-selective cyclopropylamine is shown in Fig. 14D. This compound, designated AB-15, inhibited 5-HT oxidation in rat brain extracts with an IC_{50} of 4 μM when 5-HT was the substrate and was 2- and 10-fold less potent with NE and tyramine, respectively. This compound also showed activity *in vivo* as an MAOI and as an antagonist of reserpine (Huszti *et al.*, 1969).

3.5.4. β-Carbolines

The β-carbolines differ from the other major classes of potent MAO inhibitors discussed thus far in that these compounds do not become covalently bound to the enzyme, but can be removed by dialysis. Belleau and Moran (1963) have proposed that these planar compounds may interact with MAO by forming charge–transfer complexes with the flavin cofactor at the active site. Because β-carbolines compete with substrates, IC_{50} values depend on the concentration of substrate employed. For this reason IC_{50} values reported for many β-carbolines and other competitive MAOIs are misleading, and large discrepancies are encountered when one attempts to compare the data of different workers. An appropriate measure of inhibitory potency among competitive inhibitors can be obtained if one employs substrates at their K_m concentrations. In this situation the I_{50} concentration of a simple competitive inhibitor will be equal to twice its binding constant or K_I value. Probably the most reliable procedure is a direct determination of K_I from a reciprocal plot of data obtained by varying substrate concentration (Webb, 1963).

Among the β-carbolines, harmine (Fig. 15A) is the most potent MAOI which has been studied to any extent. At low concentrations it shows a marked specificity for inhibition of 5-HT oxidation (Long, 1962; Fuller, 1968). With K_m concentrations of the MAO-A- and MAO-B-specific substrates, 5-HT and phenethylamine, IC_{50} values for harmine differed by a factor of 2500 (Table 10).

Other workers have employed common MAO substrates, tyramine and tryptamine, in evaluating β-carboline analogues. Reduction of the pyridine

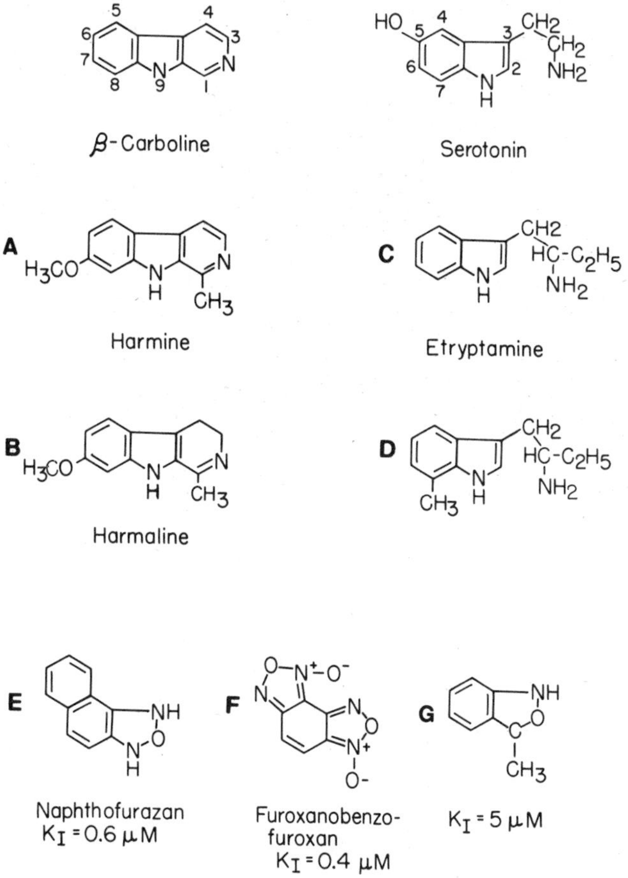

FIG. 15. β-Carbolines, indolealkylamines, and other indoleamine analogues. K_I values are from Bolt *et al.* (1974).

ring to give dihydro- (Fig. 15B) or tetrahydro-β-carbolines, in which the ring structure would no longer be coplanar, resulted in progressively decreased inhibitory potencies, while removal of or acetylation of the pyridine nitrogen completely destroyed inhibitory activity (McIsaac and Estevez, 1966). A variety of methyl or methoxy substitutions on the aromatic ring did not markedly affect potency, but a hydroxyl substituent in the 6 position substantially reduced activity (McIsaac and Estevez, 1966). A methyl group on the N-9 nitrogen of tetrahydro-β-carboline gave a 35-fold increase in potency over the parent compound, while a similar substitution on the completely aromatic β-carboline produced a 3-fold increase in potency. The inhibitions obtained with these two N-9 methyl analogues were therefore very similar, when both were tested with sonicated beef liver mitochondria using tryptamine as substrate (Ho *et al.*, 1968), even though the potencies of the parent compounds differed by a factor of 10. Methyl substitution in the C-8 position of tetrahydro-β-carboline did not influence activity, but a chlorine in the same position gave a 3-fold increase in potency (Ho et al., 1969). Replacement of the indolic nitrogen with a sulfur to produce a benzo[b]thiophene analogue of harmaline (S-harmaline) resulted in a 50-fold increase in potency in vitro with rat liver MAO and tryptamine as substrate (Bosin et al., 1972). A similar analogue of harmine did not show increased potency. Partition coefficients of harmaline and S-harmaline indicated that the lipid solubility of the latter compound was 200 times that of the former. Obviously, it would be of interest to know the effects of the modifications discussed above on inhibitions obtained with the substrates 5-HT and phenethylamine.

Ho et al. (1973) synthesized β-carbolinium analogues in an effort to obtain a tissue-specific inhibitor which, because of the charge on the quaternary nitrogen, would not penetrate the blood–brain barrier. They reasoned that such compounds would have a potential use either in angina pectoris or, in combination with irreversible MAOIs, to protect peripheral MAO during antidepressant therapy with irreversible MAOIs. The 2,9-dimethyl-substituted β-carbolinium iodide appeared to be the most potent inhibitor found in this study, with K_I values ranging from 0.8 and 0.9 μM with human liver and heart MAO to 67 μM with human brain enzyme. The very different procedures used for the solubilization of MAO from different tissues may have influenced this apparent in vitro tissue specificity. In vivo data were not reported.

3.5.5. Indolealkylamines

The β-carboline structure may be regarded as a cyclized derivative of the structure of 5-HT or tryptamine. Noncyclized analogues of these two substrates appear to be much weaker MAOIs. Vane (1959) first noted the MAO inhibitory properties of α-methyltryptamine. Both α-methyl (Indopan) and α-ethyl tryptamine (etryptamine or Monase, Fig. 15C) were found to preferentially inhibit 5-HT oxidation by MAO from guinea pig liver, while 5-hydroxy-α-methyltryptamine was inactive against 5-HT oxidation (Greig et al., 1959). The selective inhibition of 5-HT oxidation by α-methyl tryptamine was confirmed by Gorkin et al. (1967), who used rat liver and brain MAO. Following a number of clinical trials during 1961–1962, Monase was reported to be beneficial in both agitated and withdrawn depression (review of Zirkle and Kaiser, 1964). However, the prevalence of undesirable side effects caused it to fall into disuse. Several analogues of etryptamine were synthesized by Hester et al. (1964) in an attempt to find a similar compound which would not interfere with 5-HT synthesis as etryptamine apparently did (Greig et al., 1959; Hester et al., 1964). The 7-methylindole derivative (Fig. 15D) was more potent than etryptamine as an MAOI with guinea pig liver MAO. However, these workers reported IC_{50} values obtained only at a relatively high concentration of 5-HT, and since these compounds would be expected to compete with 5-HT, their K_I values would be much more informative.

3.5.6. Oxazoles, Oxadiazoles, and Benzooxadiazoles

Bolt *et al.* (1974) have reported K_I values, obtained with [^{14}C]tryptamine and rat liver mitochondria, for an interesting series of heterocyclic 5-membered ring structures and their benzo derivatives. Thiazoles and isothiazoles were less active than their oxygen analogues. Fusion of the heterocyclic ring with an aromatic ring enhanced inhibitory potency at least 100-fold (Fig. 15E–G). N-Oxide formation and a combination of two oxadiazole rings with an aromatic nucleus were also favorable for inhibition, as illustrated by furoxanobenzofuroxan (Fig. 15F), the most potent inhibitor found in this study. This compound, which bears a resemblance to the planar structure of harmine, was a reversible inhibitor *in vitro*, and since it selectively increased brain 5-HT levels in rats at the relatively low dose of 15 mg/kg, Bolt and Sleigh (1974) suggested that it was specific in inhibiting oxidation of indoleamines. These authors did not perform *in vitro* assays with 5-HT as the MAO substrate. However, their plot of percentage inhibition of tryptamine deamination vs. inhibitor concentration began to level off at about 60% inhibition, suggestive of a preferential inhibition of a portion of MAO sites, presumably those shared by both 5-HT and tryptamine. *In vitro* assays with 5-HT and other substrates would allow a more definitive conclusion about the specificity of this compound.

3.5.7. Some Miscellaneous Inhibitors of Particular Interest

a. NSD-2023. NSD-2023 (γ-morpholinobutyrophenone, Fig. 16A). was reported by Squires and Buus Lassen (1968) to be much more potent as an inhibitor of mouse brain MAO *in vivo* than *in vitro*, and therefore a metabolic conversion to a more active irreversible inhibitor was suspected. In addition, only a partial block of tryptamine or kynuramine deamination was achieved in either *in vitro* or *in vivo* assays of brain homogenates from pretreated rats. Mouse brain MAO was inhibited 50–60% 1 hr after a single oral dose of 2 mg/kg. At 100 times this dose, the percentage inhibition reached only 70%. Christmas *et al.* (1972) observed that NSD-2023 produced only a partial inhibition of 5-HT or tyramine deamination. When brain homogenates of rats were assayed with 5-HT, tyramine, and benzylamine 1 hr after oral administration of NSD-2023, the compound inhibited 5-HT deamination most strongly (About 70%) and benzylamine very weakly. Therefore, NSD-2023 is a substrate-selective MAOI which appears unique in that it inhibits only a portion of MAO-A sites. Because of the apparent requirement for metabolic conversion of NSD-2023, this specificity was

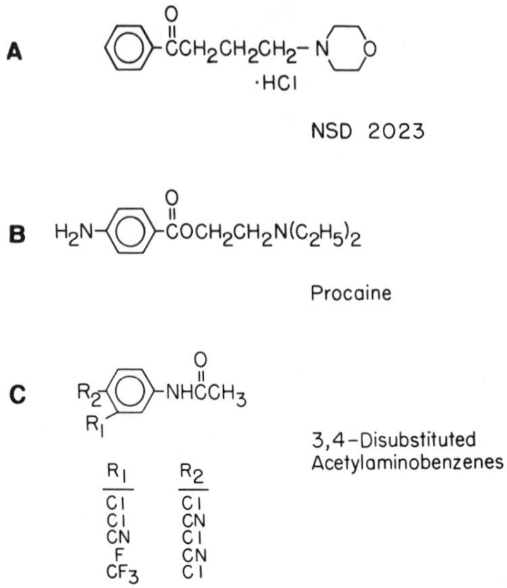

A

NSD 2023

B   Procaine

C   3,4–Disubstituted Acetylaminobenzenes

R_1	R_2
Cl	Cl
Cl	CN
CN	Cl
F	CN
CF$_3$	Cl

FIG. 16. Miscellaneous MAOIs.

observed only *in vivo* and may represent selective metabolism or distribution of the compound within brain tissue.

b. Procaine. Procaine (Fig. 16B) has been employed for over 20 years in Europe as an antidepressant and mild euphoriant in geriatric patients (Aslan, 1956). The pharmaceutical preparation, Gerovital, is a 2% solution of procaine, which also contains benzoic acid, *p*-aminobenzoic acid, and inorganic buffer ions. Sakalis *et al.* (1974), in an uncontrolled clinical study using intramuscular treatment with 300–600 mg Gerovital H3/week in 10 senile–depressed individuals, reported only a transient mild euphoriant effect of this drug. However, Zung *et al.* (1974), in a double-blind controlled study in which Gerovital H3 was administered orally for 4 weeks to elderly depressed patients, found that this drug was superior to either imipramine or placebo.

The MAO inhibitory properties of procaine (Philpot, 1940), procaine-amide, and the *N*-dimethyl analogue of procaine (Ozaki *et al.*, 1960) have long been recognized. MacFarlane and Besbris (1974) have suggested that the antidepressant action of Gerovital H3 may result from the weak, competitive inhibition of MAO by procaine. These authors obtained a K_I value of 89 μM with kynuramine as the substrate for rat brain MAO. However, procaine is much more potent as an inhibitor of 5-HT oxidation. The K_I was 1.9 μM with 5-HT as the substrate for human brain MAO, while no inhibition of phenethylamine oxidation occurred at concentrations of procaine up to 100 μM (White and Wu, 1975a). Therefore, this compound may be classed as a substrate-selective MAOI, similar in specificity to harmine, although much weaker. Its marked substrate selectivity, as well as the reversible and competitive nature of the inhibition, may account for the absence of side effects at therapeutic doses.

c. 3,4-Disubstituted Acetylaminobenzenes. These compounds (Fig. 16C) were reported to be potent inhibitors of rat brain MAO, a property which correlated well with their antagonism of tetrabenazine-induced sedation in mice (Grivsky and Hitchings, 1974). An amino or formamido moiety in place of the acetylamino group caused a drop in potency, as did substitution of *N*-acyl groups with more than two carbons. One compound in this series, 2-chloro-4-acetylamino benzonitrile, was a competitive and reversible inhibitor of rat brain MAO with K_I values of 0.4 and 0.6 μM with the substrates tryptamine and tyramine, respectively. This compound also inhibited 5-HT and phenethylamine oxidation at similar concentrations, and therefore was not substrate-selective (White, unpublished).

4. MAOIs AS INHIBITORS OF THE UPTAKE OF BIOGENIC AMINES AND TRICYCLIC COMPOUNDS AS INHIBITORS OF MONOAMINE OXIDASE

4.1. MAOIs as Inhibitors of Amine Uptake

Hendley and Snyder (1968) noted that six potent MAOIs had significantly differing capacities to inhibit the uptake of tritiated metaraminol from a 10^{-7} M solution of this amine into chopped rat cerebral cortex (Table 11). Tranylcypromine was the most potent inhibitor of uptake. Phenelzine and pargyline were considerably less potent, and nialamide, isocarboxazid, and iproniazid produced no inhibition of uptake at 10^{-4} M. The order of activity of these compounds as MAOIs was different from their order of activity as uptake inhibitors (Table 11). Hendley and Snyder (1968) pointed out that there was a positive relationship between the relative potency of the drugs as

TABLE 11
Differential Potencies of MAOIs[a]

Drug	Inhibition of metaraminol uptake (ID_{50}) (M)	Inhibition of monoamine oxidase (ID_{50}) (M)
Tranylcypromine	0.5×10^{-5}	0.85×10^{-7}
Phenelzine	6.2×10^{-5}	0.37×10^{-7}
Pargyline	1.2×10^{-4}	1.5×10^{-7}
Iproniazid	Ineffective	1.6×10^{-6}
Nialamide	Ineffective	3.0×10^{-7}
Isocarboxazid	Ineffective	1.0×10^{-7}

[a] From Hendley and Snyder (1968). Tyramine was the MAO substrate.

inhibitors of metaraminol uptake and a ranking for clinical efficacy as derived by the authors from the psychiatric literature. This suggested that the antidepressant action of the clinically effective MAOIs might be related to inhibition of NE reuptake mechanisms, rather than to MAO inhibition *per se,* and thus might provide a unitary explanation for the antidepressant efficacy of MAOIs and tricyclic drugs.

Ferris *et al.* (1975) measured uptake and release of labeled NE and 5-HT in hypothalamic synaptosomes, DA uptake and release in striatal synaptosomes, and MAO inhibition in rat brain mitochondrial extracts using 5-HT and phenethylamine as substrates. Correlations were made between these measurements and a ranking of the clinical efficacy of these compounds which the authors compiled from the literature. Significant correlations occurred between clinical efficacy and inhibition of NE uptake ($r = +0.96$) and DA uptake ($r = +0.83$), and stimulation of DA release ($r = +0.92$). Ferris *et al.* (1975 and personal communication) found essentially the same rank order for the MAOIs as inhibitors of the uptake of NE (and DA) as did Hendley and Snyder (1968) for metaraminol. In addition, pheniprazine was found to be slightly more potent than phenelzine. These findings supported the idea of Hendley and Snyder (1968) that the clinical efficacy of MAOIs might be related to their effects on uptake of amines.

Horn and Snyder (1972) pointed out that of the two isomeric forms of tranylcypromine, ($-$)-tranylcypromine was approximately 3–4 times more potent than ($+$)-tranylcypromine in inhibiting the uptake of tritiated NE and DA from 10^{-7} M solutions of these amines into synaptosomal preparations from rat hypothalamus and striatum. Zirkle *et al.* (1962) noted that the ($+$) isomer was approximately 4-fold more potent than the ($-$) isomer as an MAO inhibitor in brain homogenates of pretreated rats. Horn and Snyder "suggested that a determination of the antidepressant efficacy of ($+$)- and ($-$)-tranylcypromine may help to elucidate the extent to which inhibition of either catecholamine uptake or monoamine oxidase activity is responsible for the drugs' clinical effects."

Escobar *et al.* (1974) tested ($+$)- and ($-$)-tranylcypromine under double-blind conditions in a total of 11 depressed patients. Placebo-treated patients were not included. These authors reported that ($-$)-tranylcypromine was a more effective antidepressant and produced fewer side effects than did ($+$)-tranylcypromine. These findings should be subjected to wider study, and additional comparisons should be made with ($\pm$)-tranylcypromine and placebo. One wonders if the 3- to 4-fold differences between the two isomers that are seen in *in vitro* uptake experiments are great enough to be carried over to the *in vivo* situation. Also, since ($-$)-tranylcypromine is not devoid of MAO inhibitory activity and is irreversible in its action, it might be expected that MAO inhibition would become significant over a 3- to 4-week period. Also, it would seem that administration of ($\pm$)-tranylcypromine would combine two effects—MAO inhibition and inhibition of NE uptake—and might therefore be the best drug.

Like tranylcypromine, deprenyl is a racemic mixture. The (−) isomer of deprenyl is more potent as an MAOI but less potent as an inhibitor of amine uptake than is the (+) isomer (Knoll and Magyar, 1972). Unlike other irreversible MAOIs, deprenyl (racemic mixture) does not potentiate the effects of tyramine on blood pressure (Knoll *et al.*, 1968). The lack of tyramine potentiation caused by deprenyl is apparently not attributable to a specificity of its inhibitory effect on MAO, but to its capacity to inhibit uptake of tyramine by adrenergic nerve endings.

From a structural point of view, the MAOIs which are the most potent inhibitors of metaraminol, NE, or DA uptake are those which most closely resemble the phenethylamine structure. Compare the structures of tranylcypromine, pheniprazine, phenelzine, and pargyline with that of phenethylamine (Figs. 11 and 12). Contrast these with the structures of iproniazid and isocarboxazid (Fig. 12). Nialamide also bears little resemblance to phenethylamine.

These comparisons strongly suggest that the more potent inhibitors of uptake fit the active site of the amine pumps better than the less potent agents. It is possible that the active agents are substrates for the uptake sites and thereby compete with NE for uptake. They are not necessarily very good substrates, since none of these MAOIs is a very potent uptake inhibitor. All the compounds are considerably more potent MAOIs than they are uptake inhibitors.

At present, it is probably best to consider the hypothesis of Hendley and Snyder (1968) as interesting but unproved. Correlations between *in vitro* biochemical measurements and psychiatric measurements in man run a very high risk of being merely fortuitous. Considering the variable dosages of the drugs given to humans, the differences in distribution and metabolism of the compounds, plus the relatively crude psychiatric measurement techniques that are employed to diagnose the various types of depression and to measure therapeutic effects, one must be cautious in accepting these correlations as proof of anything.

4.2. Tricyclic Compounds as MAOIs

Because several tricyclic and related compounds which are clinically effective as antidepressants, e.g., iprindole and mianserin (Org GB-94), are not potent inhibitors of the uptake of NE or 5-HT, some questions have been raised regarding the validity of amine uptake inhibition as an explanation for the antidepressant actions of tricyclic antidepressants as a group.

As pointed out in Section 3.4, any compound having an aromatic moiety separated by a carbon chain from an aliphatic amine can be expected to serve as either a substrate or inhibitor of MAO at sufficiently high concentrations. Roth and Gillis (1974*a,b*, 1975) and Roth (1975) have proposed that the antidepressant activities of imipramine, desmethylimipramine, amitriptyline, mianserin (Org GB-94), doxepin, and related tricyclics may be attributed to the ability to these compounds to selectively inhibit the B form of MAO. In most of their experiments with rabbit brain or lung mitochondria these authors employed a very low substrate concentration (1.8 μM) well below the K_m concentration, a condition which would tend to exaggerate the observed percentage inhibitions of these competitive inhibitors. However, for three tricyclics they reported K_I values, which were obtained using either 5-HT or phenethylamine as the MAO substrate. These data, shown in Table 12, indicate a preferential inhibition of the B form of MAO. Roth and Gillis (1975) concluded that tricyclic compounds having a double bond between the ring system and the aliphatic side chain were the more potent inhibitors of the B form. Thus, the antidepressant amitriptyline and the neuroleptic chlorprothixene (Table 12) were 7- or 8-fold more potent than imipramine and chlorpromazine, which have saturated side chains. On the other hand, Edwards and Burns (1974) did not observe this effect of the exocyclic double bond in their studies with MAO of sonicated human platelets. These workers, who used a phenethylamine concentration of 4.9 μM, found that IC_{50} values for amitriptyline, nortriptyline, and imipramine all ranged from 4 to 6 μM.

It has been suggested (Mosnaim et al., 1973; Sabelli et al., 1974) that reduced levels of endogenous phenethylamine may represent a biochemical lesion in depression. In addition, tricyclic antidepressants and MAOIs were shown to elevate phenethylamine concentrations in human urine and rat brain (Fischer et al., 1972). Despite these observations, the significance of the results of Roth and Gillis (1974a,b) is somewhat clouded by the fact that the 8- to 40-fold ratios of K_I values (Table 12) for inhibition of A and B sites of MAO do not reveal a very high degree of specificity for these compounds as inhibitors of phenethylamine deamination when one considers that the ratio of IC_{50} values obtained in vitro with the more potent selective inhibitor of the B form, deprenyl, was 1500 (see Table 10). In addition, the tricyclic compounds are weak MAOIs in comparison with the standard inhibitors

TABLE 12

Binding Constants for Several Tricyclic Psychoactive Drugs to Type A and B MAO[a]

	K_I	
Inhibitor	Type A (M)	Type B (M)
Imipramine	3×10^{-4}	4×10^{-5}
Amitriptyline	2×10^{-4}	5×10^{-6}
Chlorprothixene	8×10^{-5}	6×10^{-6}

[a] From Roth and Gillis (1975).

(Table 10). Although MAO inhibition cannot at present be excluded as a contributing factor in the antidepressant activity of the tricyclics, especially in tissues where a preferential accumulation of these compounds may occur, the relatively low potencies of tricyclic antidepressants as MAOIs compared with their much greater effectiveness as inhibitors of the uptake of biogenic amines, plus the fact that neuroleptics also exhibit similar weak MAO inhibition, suggest that MAO inhibition is not a likely specific basis for the antidepresssant action of tricyclics.

5. SUMMARY AND PERSPECTIVE

The authors intend to take the liberty of synthesizing in a speculative, and we hope a stimulating, way many of the observations covered in this review. The following information has been run through the filter of our own biases and judgments for the intended purpose of projecting a coherent picture out of occasionally contradictory information. The reader is therefore urged to read the body of this review and draw his own conclusions if the ones presented here are unpalatable.

At present, the amine hypothesis of affective disorders is under question. There is evidence, based largely on drug effects, which favors norepinephrine as the important mediator in depression and other evidence which puts serotonin into a key position. There is additional evidence favoring a role for both agents, while other evidence suggests that neither mediator may be important. Simultaneously, the biochemical basis for the clinical effectiveness of tricyclic antidepressants is being questioned. Several tricyclic and related drugs, which have little effect on the uptake of biogenic amines, have been described as effective in the treatment of depression. Indeed, some workers suggest that tricyclic agents work not by inhibiting the uptake of biogenic amines but because they are MAOIs which selectively inhibit the catabolism of endogenous phenethylamine. At the other extreme, several laboratories present data to show that potent MAOIs may not elicit their antidepressant effects by inhibiting MAO, but by inhibiting the uptake of biogenic amines in a manner similar to the tricyclic agents. At the same time potent irreversible MAOIs have been developed which selectively inhibit phenethylamine or serotonin oxidation, and their clinical effectiveness is a point of argument for a role of these mediators in depression. Needless to say, considerable clarification is needed. At present, it seems reasonable to consider that the properties of inhibition of uptake of biogenic amines and inhibition of MAO, if they are present in a single compound, are probably both involved in determining therapeutic efficacy.

If one considers in detail the structure–activity relationships among substrates and inhibitors of the pumps processing biogenic amines, as has been done in this review, some interesting lines of speculation arise.

Norepinephrine, dopamine, and serotonin are three molecules with much in common structurally but with some differences. All three are ethylamine derivatives. The ethylamine chain is connected to a phenyl ring in norepinephrine and dopamine and to an indole ring in serotonin. All three bear a hydroxyl in the 3 position of the phenyl ring or an analogous position in the indole ring. Phenyl rings and indole rings are planar structures. The distance between the nitrogen atom and the phenyl ring of norepinephrine and dopamine is shorter by one C–C bond than is the distance between the nitrogen atom and phenyl segment of the indole ring. Indeed, serotonin can be considered to be a phenylpropylamine in which the two carbon atoms closest to the phenyl ring are fixed in their orientation. When molecular models of these three compounds are compared and the phenyl moieties of the indole and of the catecholamines are superimposed with their 3-OH groups aligned, this partially fixed orientation of serotonin precludes close overlap of the nitrogen atoms if dopamine and norepinephrine are in a planar *anti* conformation. Perhaps this is why serotonin is not a good substrate for catecholamine pumps, since these pumps may require a substrate to assume a planar *anti* conformation. On the other hand, the proclivity of the serotonin receptor site for the partially fixed orientation of serotonin and for the larger planar indole surface may explain why the shorter, more flexible catecholamines, with smaller planar surfaces available for binding, are not good substrates for the serotonin-uptake site.

At present, the authors favor the view that the uptake receptor sites in striatum do not differ markedly from similar sites in other brain regions in their capacity to recognize norepinephrine and dopamine. The β-hydroxyl group of norepinephrine may reduce affinity for the uptake sites, but it does this to the same extent in all regions (e.g., striatum as well as hypothalamus). Thus, one can conceive of essentially similar restricted regions in the center of striatal and hypothalamic receptor sites to which norepinephrine and dopamine bind reversibly and as a consequence of which they are passed through the membrane. Surrounding this "substrate receptor site" is an array of molecular species, presumably functional groups on the amino acids of proteins, phospholipid constituents, and other compounds. This surrounding "foliage," as it were, provides potential ancillary sites for binding of potent inhibitors. This view is consonant with the fact that potent true inhibitors are "bulkier" molecules than are substrates. The array of potential ancillary binding sites is greater than is used by any one class of inhibitors, e.g., tricyclic antidepressants, and may be the reason other classes of compounds, e.g., Lu 3-010, and spiro cyclohexyl compounds, can be equipotent to desmethylimipramine or imipramine as inhibitors of norepinephrine uptake despite obvious structural and conformational differences from these potent agents. They may simply bind to groups which are not utilized by the tricyclic agents.

Interestingly, the array of molecular species around catecholamine-uptake receptor sites in the striatum is probably very distinct from the array surrounding the other catecholamine or serotonergic regions of the brain or of the periphery. This would explain why the tricyclic ring systems will bind to the uptake site in noradrenergic neurons or in serotonergic nerves but not in striatal neurons. To account for the high potency of the diphenyl compound, (−)-deoxypipradrol, as a competitive inhibitor in the striatum, the receptor in the striatum, in common with the receptors in the other pumps studied, may be capable of receiving two phenyl rings, but the position of the two receptive areas for these rings, with respect to each other, may be different in the striatum than it is in other areas.

Differences in the molecular "foliage" surrounding substrate-receptor sites may also be the basis for why it is that molecules which are potent competitive blockers of the uptake-receptor sites for norepinephrine are quite different structurally from those which are potent competitive blockers of α- or β-adrenergic receptor sites.

Since, as stated earlier, serotonin and the catecholamines have structural similarities, it would seem likely that some inhibitor(s) should exist which would fit both the catecholamine- and the serotonin-receptor sites equally well. Since the compound would have to fit two different "substrate-receptor sites" as well as three differing surrounding "foliages," such an inhibitor molecule would have to be flexible and not locked into a more rigid structure designed to markedly increase its affinity for one site. Such a molecular commitment would surely reduce its affinity for the other sites. According to the work of Ross and Renyi (1967a,b), cocaine appears to be equipotent against norepinephrine uptake into hypothalamus, dopamine uptake into striatum, and serotonin uptake into hypothalamus. As demonstrated in Fig. 2, a model of cocaine can be readily folded into a conformation in which it bears some resemblance to the more potent inhibitors of norepinephrine uptake such as desmethylimipramine, but it is considerably weaker than this agent. Cocaine can also be folded to mimic the conformations of the inhibitors of serotonin uptake shown in Fig. 8, especially that of FG 4963, to which it bears structural similarities (compare Fig. 2 with Fig. 7). In this conformation, cocaine projects a carbomethoxyl group into the region occupied by the unsubstituted phenyl ring of FG 4963. As would be expected, cocaine is only a moderately potent inhibitor of the uptake of norepinephrine, dopamine, and serotonin.

It is worthy of note that mono- or dimethylation of the nitrogen atom in the substrates, norepinephrine and serotonin, either does not affect the affinity for the uptake system or reduces it. It is surmised that in the catecholamine-uptake sites the substrates cannot project their N-methyl groups into an available hydrophobic binding area, while in the serotonin-uptake sites the presence of N-methyl groups on substrates actively interferes with the binding of their nitrogen atoms.

Monomethylation of the primary amine group of tricyclic inhibitors increases affinity for the norepinephrine-uptake site, but reduces affinity for the serotonin site. The two methyl groups of the tertiary amine derivatives appear not to be perceived by either receptor site, since these compounds are approximately equipotent with the primary amine derivatives. Thus, with the tricyclic inhibitors, the single methyl group on the nitrogen atom reaches a specific receptive site in noradrenergic nerves which is inaccessible to the monomethylated phenethylamines. This site can be reached because folding of the longer chain in the tricyclic compounds permits the *N*-methyl to reach a site that cannot be reached by the *N*-methyl in the phenethylamines. A second methyl group attached to the nitrogen atom, as in imipramine, negates the binding of the first methyl group, presumably by steric interference. In serotonergic nerves it appears that there is no receptive site for methyl substituents on the nitrogen atom of the tricyclic agents, since the primary amine, tertiary dimethylamine, and quaternary trimethylamine derivatives are approximately equipotent. The presence of a single methyl group in the secondary methylamine derivatives sharply reduced affinity and probably interferes with the binding of the nitrogen atom.

From the theoretical discussion just presented we would expect that new classes of compounds will be discovered which will be potent inhibitors of catecholamine or serotonin uptake. These compounds at a minimum will have a planar hydrophobic group separated by at least two carbons from an amine nitrogen. The molecules will have additional hydrophobic planar, aliphatic, or carbomethoxyl groups which will not necessarily be sterically analogous to similar groups in the potent compounds available at present.

Since it is uncertain at present whether inhibition of catecholamine and/ or serotonergic pumps is the basis for the clinical effects of tricyclic antidepressant drugs, the practical importance of newly developed inhibitors of uptake is difficult to predict. If inhibition of uptake is important to therapeutic efficacy, perhaps the most effective drugs will inhibit norepinephrine uptake and serotonin uptake in some special ratio which will be optimal treatment for a specific subclass of depression. Development of such drugs is certainly feasible.

With reference to MAOIs, the possibilities for selective inhibitions of the oxidation of one or more substrates should also be emphasized. In fact, if MAOIs are to be widely used as antidepressants in the future, it will probably be necessary to develop safer substrate- or tissue-specific agents which are designed for particular depression subtypes. The information available concerning MAO-A and -B sites (Section 3.3) allows some rational speculations regarding the kind of selectivity which may be possible in the development of new MAOIs. If a specific inhibition of serotonin oxidation is desired, it is unlikely that this can be accomplished without a simultaneous partial inhibition of the oxidation of norepinephrine, tryptamine, tyramine, and to a lesser extent, dopamine. Likewise, a selective inhibitor of phenethylamine oxidation may also be expected to partially affect norepinephrine, dopamine, and tyramine oxidation. However, with either kind of specificity one may predict only a partial inhibition of tyramine oxidation in peripheral tissues and therefore a safer therapeutic agent. This would be especially true if the inhibition were reversible and competitive.

Since norepinephrine may be oxidized at both A and B sites of MAO in human brain, a selective inhibition of norepinephrine oxidation does not appear to be a likely possibility. However, if A and B sites each represent more than one type of site, perhaps differing in substrate affinities or in tissue distribution, it is conceivable that some degree of selectivity may be attained. If a preferential inhibition of dopamine oxidation is desired, this might be accomplished with a B-site inhibitor, since the largest proportion of dopamine is metabolized at MAO-B sites.

From the experiments and conclusions of several workers reviewed in Section 3.1, the substrate sites of MAO may be envisioned as containing an electrophilic (i.e., electron-deficient) binding region for an unprotonated amine nitrogen, a nucleophilic (i.e., electron-rich) region for a hydrogen atom on the carbon vicinal to the nitrogen, and a hydrophobic region for an aromatic moiety. According to the "induced-fit" hypothesis of enzyme–substrate interactions (summarized by Koshland and Neet, 1968), the binding of a substrate may induce a conformational change in the enzyme so that the nitrogen becomes favorably oriented with respect to the flavin cofactor at the active site. This would represent a transition state of the enzyme–substrate complex, and, following the arguments of Belleau and Moran (1963), one may assume that in this state the bond between the nitrogen and the α-carbon of the substrate acquires some double-bond character. Subsequent steps in the redox catalytic mechanism depend on the participation of the flavin and can occur only if the proper positioning of the interacting moieties is achieved.

Any compound which binds reversibly at a substrate site but does not participate effectively in the subsequent series of catalytic reactions would be a competitive inhibitor. A wide variety of aralkyl amines, including amphetamine and some of the tricyclic uptake inhibitors, fall into this category of rather weak inhibitors, with binding constants similar to those of the known substrates ($5 \rightarrow 500$ μM). However, if the compound also contains a group which interacts covalently with the enzyme following the initial relatively weak binding, then a much more potent and irreversible inhibition may occur. Such is the case with the hydrazines and propargylamines, which have been shown to interact with the flavin moiety.

The most potent reversible inhibitors of MAO are compounds such as harmine ($K_I = 0.01$ μM) and furoxanobenzofuroxan (see Fig. 15), which are tricyclic coplanar compounds having very restricted conformations. Interestingly, these compounds are selective inhibitors at MAO-A sites. Planar structures such as these may participate in charge–transfer complexes (Baker, 1967), and as suggested by Belleau and Moran (1963), such a complex between harmine and the flavin moiety of MAO may reinforce the inhibition. One may also expect that these coplanar inhibitors would fit into a relatively narrow crevice or restricted region on the enzyme surface and that the binding affinity might be strengthened by such a fit. To explain the selectivity of inhibition at MAO-A sites, one might speculate that the flavin moiety at A sites is situated so that as soon as harmine binds to the substrate-binding region, a reinforcement of this binding can occur, perhaps by charge–transfer interaction with the flavin. Harmine can also bind to the substrate-binding region of MAO-B sites, since inhibition of phenethylamine oxidation can be demonstrated at higher concentrations (see Table 10). However, at B sites the inhibition is not potentiated and the affinity of harmine is similar to that of a typical substrate. This might imply that the flavin moiety at B sites has a different orientation relative to the substrate-binding region and therefore does not interact with harmine.

Harmine is not used as a therapeutic agent because of its toxic properties. However, the potent inhibition observed with this compound, both *in vitro* and *in vivo*, is a good indication that a reversible MAOI lacking the undesirable properties of harmine might be developed as a potential therapeutic agent. The reversibility and the competitive nature of the inhibition, as well as the marked substrate selectivity of such a compound, would tend to minimize side effects caused by inhibition of MAO in peripheral tissues.

An attempt can be made to apply the speculations relating to selective inhibition by the restricted structure of harmine to the more flexible MAO-A inhibitors such as clorgyline, Lilly 51641, NSD 2023, and procaine (see Figs. 13, 14, and 16). In all these compounds the aliphatic chain between the aromatic moiety and the nitrogen is relatively long compared with that in selective MAO-B inhibitors such as deprenyl or pargyline (Fig. 13). However, simply increasing the aliphatic chain length in pargyline analogues did not enhance inhibition of serotonin oxidation (Martin *et al.*, 1975). *Ortho*-substitution on the aromatic ring of pargyline did potentiate the inhibition of serotonin oxidation by pargyline. *Ortho*-substitution might influence the conformation of the aliphatic portion of the molecule so that it can more easily interact with the flavin at A sites. The ether linkage between the aromatic ring and the aliphatic chain of clorgyline and Lilly 51641 may have a similar effect. It is possible that MAO-A inhibitors may mimic the planar conformation of harmine in order to fit the binding site.

The aliphatic groups of the B-selective inhibitors, deprenyl and pargyline, are shorter and bulkier, and the bulkiest of these is deprenyl, which is the most potent inhibitor at MAO-B sites and the poorest inhibitor at MAO-A sites in Table 10. These structures cannot assume a flat, extended conformation. They may fit optimally into a less extensive substrate-binding region with the flavin moiety oriented quite differently from that at A sites.

These speculations are necessarily very tentative and incomplete since, as pointed out in Section 3.4, much structure–activity work remains to be done. Many interesting analogues of substrate-selective inhibitors have not been tested under appropriate conditions with the substrates serotonin and phenethylamine.

Predictions of the clinical advantages of such selective inhibitions will require a better understanding, on a biochemical level, of which particular biogenic amines may be deficient in various categories of depressive illness. What is really needed is a biochemical classification of depression, as suggested by van Praag (1974), so that diagnostic tests may be developed which, together with information about the symptomatology and etiology, would allow a prediction of the most useful drug for each patient. The availability of new amine-uptake inhibitors and MAOIs which exhibit selectivity with respect to a given substrate, in addition to their therapeutic potential, may become very useful in studies of biochemical mechanisms underlying depressive subtypes.

ACKNOWLEDGMENTS

The authors thank Dr. M. Harfenist for advice concerning conformational analysis of MAOIs, Mrs. Lacala Hall for her patient retyping of the several drafts of the manuscript, and Mrs. Linda Byrd for preparing the figures.

6. REFERENCES

ABRAHAM, R. J., KRICKA, L. J., and LEDWITH, A., 1974, The nuclear magnetic resonance spectra and conformations of cyclic compounds. Part X. Conformational equilibria in 5-substituted 10,11-dihydrodibenz[b,f]azepines, *J. Chem. Soc. Perkin Trans. 2:*1648–1654.

ACHEE, F. M., TOGULGA, G., and GABAY, S., 1974, Studies of monoamine oxidases: Properties of the enzyme in bovine and rabbit brain mitochondria, *J. Neurochem.* **22:**651–661.

ALEMANY, A., FERNÁNDEX ALVAREZ, E., AND MARTINEZ LÓPEZ, J. M., 1975, Inhibiteurs d'énzymes. XV. Préparation de (propargylamino méthyl)-3 indoles, *Bull. Soc. Chim. France*, No. 5–6, pp. 1223–1227.

ALPERS, H. S., and HIMWICH, H. E., 1969, An *in vitro* study of the effects of tricyclic antidepressant drugs on the accumulation of C^{14}-serotonin by rabbit brain, *Biol. Psychiatry* **1:**81–85.

ASLAN, A., 1956, A new method for prophylaxis and treatment of aging with Novocain—eutrophic and rejuvenating effects, *Therapiewoche* **7:**14–22.

BAKER, B. R., 1967, *Design of Active-Site-Directed Irreversible Enzyme Inhibitors*, pp. 28–38, Wiley, New York.

BALDESSARINI, R. J., 1975, The basis for amine hypotheses in affective disorders, *Arch. Gen. Psychiatry* **32:**1087–1093.

BELLEAU, B., and LACASSE, G., 1964, Aspects of the chemical mechanism of complex formation between acetylcholinesterase and acetylcholine-related compounds, *J. Med. Chem.* **7**:768–775.

BELLEAU, B., and MORAN, J., 1963, Deuterium isotope effects in relation to the chemical mechanism of monoamine oxidase, *Ann. N. Y. Acad. Sci.* **107**:822–839.

BERGER, F. M., 1975, Depression and antidepressant drugs, *Clin. Pharmacol. Ther.* **18**:241–248.

BERGIN, R., and CARLSTROM, D., 1971, The crystal and molecular structure of amphetamine sulphate, *Acta Crystallogr. Sect. B:* **27**:2146–2152.

BERTI, F., and SHORE, P. A., 1967, A kinetic analysis of drugs that inhibit the adrenergic neuronal membrane amine pump, *Biochem. Pharmacol.* **16**:2091–2094.

BIEL, J. H., 1972, Summary of Section IV: Pharmacology of monoamine oxidase inhibitors, *Adv. Biochem. Psychopharmacol.* **5**:445–446.

BIEL, J. H., HORITA, A., and DRUKKER, A. E., 1964, Monoamine oxidase inhibitors (hydrazines), in: *Psychopharmacological Agents,* Vol. 1 (M. Gordon, ed.), pp. 359–443, Academic Press, New York.

BIRKMAYER, W., and RIEDERER, P., 1975, Biochemical post-mortem findings in depressed patients, *J. Neural Transm.* **37**:95–109.

BLACKBURN, K. J., FRENCH, P. C., and MERRILLS, R. J., 1967, 5-Hydroxytryptamine uptake by rat brain *in vitro,* *Life Sci.* **6**:1653–1663.

BLASHKO, H., 1963, Amine oxidase, in: *The Enzymes,* Vol. 8, 2nd ed. (P. D. Boyer, H. Lardy, and K. Myrbäck, eds.), pp. 337–351, Academic Press, New York.

BOGDANSKI, D. F., and BRODIE, B. B., 1966, Role of sodium and potassium ions in storage of norepinephrine by sympathetic nerve endings, *Life Sci.* **5**:1563–1569.

BOLT, A. G., and SLEIGH, M. J., 1974, Furoxanobenzofuroxan, a selective monoamine oxidase inhibitor, *Biochem. Pharmacol.* **23**:1969–1977.

BOLT, A. G., GHOSH, P. B., and SLEIGH, M. J., 1974, Benzo-2,1,5-oxadiazoles—a novel class of heterocyclic monoamine oxidase inhibitors, *Biochem. Pharmacol.* **23**:1963–1968.

BOSIN, T. R., CAMPAIGNE, E., and MAICKEL, R. P., 1972, Biochemical pharmacology of benzo[b]thiophene analogs of harmaline and harmine, *Life Sci.* **11**:685–691.

BRAITHWAITE, R., and GOULDING, R., 1975, Effective dosage of tricyclic antidepressants, *Br. Med. J.* **Jan. 1975**:206.

BURGEN, A. S. V., and IVERSEN, L. L., 1965, The inhibition of noradrenaline uptake by sympathetic amines in the rat isolated heart, *Br. J. Pharmacol.* **25**:34–49.

BUUS LASSEN, J., SQUIRES, R. F., CHRISTENSEN, J. A., and MOLANDER, L., 1975, Neurochemical and pharmacological studies on a new 5HT-uptake inhibitor, FG4963, with potential antidepressant properties, *Psychopharmacologia* **42**:21–26.

CALLINGHAM, B. A., 1967, The effects of imipramine and related compounds on the uptake of noradrenaline into sympathetic nerve endings, in: *Proceedings of the First International Symposium on Antidepressant Drugs* (S. Garattini and M. N. G. Dukes, eds.), pp. 35–43. Excerpta Medica, Amsterdam.

CARLSSON, A., 1966, Pharmacological depletion of catecholamine stores, *Pharmacol. Rev.* **18**:541–549.

CARLSSON, A., 1970, Structural specificity for inhibition of [^{14}C]-5-hydroxytryptamine uptake by cerebral slices, *J. Pharm. Pharmacol.* **22**:729–732.

CARLSSON, A., and LINDQVIST, M., 1969, Central and peripheral monoaminergic membrane-pump blockade by some addictive analgesics and antihistamines, *J. Pharm. Pharmacol.* **21**:460–464.

CARLSSON, A., FUXE, K., HAMBERGER, B., and LINDQVIST, M., 1966, Biochemical and histochemical studies on the effects of imipramine-like drugs and (+)-amphetamine on central and peripheral catecholamine neurons, *Acta Physiol. Scand.* **67**:481–497.

CARLSSON, A., FUXE, K., and UNGERSTEDT, U., 1968, The effect of imipramine on central 5-hydroxytryptamine neurons, *J. Pharm. Pharmacol.* **20**:150–151.

CARLSSON, A., FUXE, K., HAMBERGER, B., and MALMFORS, T., 1969*a*, Effect of a new series of bicyclic compounds with potential thymoleptic properties on the reserpine-resistant uptake mechanism of central and peripheral monoamine neurones *in vivo* and *in vitro*, *Br. J. Pharmacol.* **36:**18–28.

CARLSSON, A., CORRODI, H., FUXE, K., and HÖKFELT, T., 1969*b*, Effect of antidepressant drugs on the depletion of intraneuronal brain 5-hydroxytryptamine stores caused by 4-methyl-α-ethyl-*meta*-tyramine, *Eur. J. Pharmacol.* **5:**357–366.

CARLSSON, A., CORRODI, H., FUXE, K., and HÖKFELT, T., 1969*c*, Effects of some antidepressant drugs on the depletion of intraneuronal brain catecholamine stores caused by 4,α-dimethyl-*meta*-tyramine, *Eur. J. Pharmacol.* **5:**367–373.

CARNMALM, B., JACUPOVIC, E., JOHANSSON, L., DE PAULIS, T., RÁMSBY, S., STJERNSTRÖM, N. E., RENYI, A. L., ROSS, S. B., and ÖGREN, S. O., 1974, Antidepressant agents. 1. Chemistry and pharmacology of amino-substituted spiro[5H-dibenz(a,d)cycloheptene-5,1'-cycloalkanes], *J. Med. Chem.* **17:**65–72.

CARNMALM, B., DE PAULIS, T., JACUPOVIC, E., JOHANSSON, L., LINDBERG, V. H., ULFF, B., STJERNSTRÖM, N. D., RENYI, A. L., ROSS, S. B., and ÖGREN, S.-O., 1975, Antidepressant agents. IV. Phenylcycloalkylamines, *Acta Pharm. Suec.* **12:**149–172.

CASSANO, G. B., CASTROGIOVANNI, P., CONTI, L., SARTESCHI, P., 1974, Clinical experiences with GB 94. A new tetracyclic antidepressant compound, *J. Pharmacol.* **5**(2):17.

CHRISTMAS, A. J., COULSON, C. J., MAXWELL, D. R., and RIDDELL, D., 1972, A comparison of the pharmacological and biochemical properties of substrate-selective monoamine oxidase inhibitors, *Br. J. Pharmacol.* **45:**490–503.

COLBURN, R. W., GOODWIN, F. K., BUNNEY, W. E., JR., and DAVIS, J. M., 1967, Effect of lithium on the uptake of noradrenaline by synaptosomes, *Nature (London)* **215:**1395–1397.

COLBURN, R. W., GOODWIN, F. K., MURPHY, D. L., BUNNEY, W. E., JR., and DAVIS, J. M., 1968, Quantitative studies of norepinephrine uptake by synaptosomes, *Biochem. Pharmacol.* **17:**957–964.

COLLINS, G. G. S., SANDLER, M., WILLIAMS, E. D., and YOUDIN, M. B. H., 1970, Multiple forms of human brain mitochondrial monoamine oxidase, *Nature (London)* **225:**817–820.

COPPEN, A., 1967, The biochemistry of affective disorders, *Br. J. Psychiatry* **113:**1237–1264.

CRANE, G. E., 1957, Iproniazid (Marsilid) phosphate, a therapeutic agent for mental disorders and debilitating diseases, *Psychiatr. Res. Rep.* **8:**142–152.

DENGLER, H. J., SPIEGEL, H. E., and TITUS, E. O., 1961, Uptake of tritium-labelled norepinephrine in brain and other tissues of cat *in vitro*, *Science* **133:**1072–1073.

DENGLER, H. J., MICHAELSON, I. A., SPIEGEL, H. E., and TITUS, E. O., 1962*a*, The uptake of labeled norepinephrine by isolated brain and other tissues of the cat, *Int. J. Neuropharmacol.* **1:**23–38.

DENGLER, H. J., WILSON, C. W. M., SPIEGEL, H. E., and TITUS, E., 1962*b*, Uptake of norepinephrine by isolated pineal bodies, *Biochem. Pharmacol.* **11:**795–801.

EDWARDS, D. J., and BURNS, M. O., 1974, Effect of tricyclic antidepressants upon human platelet monoamine oxidase, *Life Sci.* **15:**2045–2058.

ESCOBAR, J. I., SCHIELE, B. C., and ZIMMERMANN, R., 1974, The tranylcypromine isomers: A controlled clinical trial, *Am. J. Psychiatry* **131:**1025–1026.

FERRIS, R. M., and STOCKS, B. D., 1972, Kinetic analysis of ³H-*dl*-norepinephrine and ³H-dopamine uptake into homogenates of rat striatum and hypothalamus and purified synaptosomes of rat whole brain, *Abstracts, Fifth International Congress on Pharmacology*, San Francisco, p. 68.

FERRIS, R. M., TANG, F. L. M., and MAXWELL, R. A., 1972, A comparison of the capacities of isomers of amphetamine, deoxypipradol and methylphenidate to inhibit the uptake of tritiated catecholamines in rat cerebral cortex slices, synaptosomal preparations of rat cerebral cortex, hypothalamus and striatum and into adrenergic nerves of rabbit aorta, *J. Pharmacol. Exp. Ther.* **181:**407–416.

FERRIS, R. M., HOWARD, J. L., and WHITE, H. L., 1975, A relationship between clinical efficacy and various biochemical parameters of monoamine oxidase inhibitors, *Pharmacologist* **17:**257.

FISCHER, E., SPATZ, H., HELLER, B., and REGGIANI, H., 1972, Phenethylamine content of human urine and rat brain, its alterations in pathological conditions and after drug administration, *Experientia* **28:**307–308.

FUJITA, T., 1973, Structure–activity relationships of monoamine oxidase inhibitors, *J. Med. Chem.* **16:**923–930.

FULLER, R. W., 1968, Influence of substrate in the inhibition of rat liver and brain monoamine oxidase, *Arch. Int. Pharmacodyn. Ther.* **174:**32–36.

FULLER, R. W., 1972, Selective inhibition of monoamine oxidase, *Adv. Biochem. Psychopharmacol.* **5:**339–354.

FULLER, R. W., WARREN, B. J., and MOLLOY, B. B., 1970, Selective inhibition of monoamine oxidase in rat brain mitochondria, *Biochem. Pharmacol.* **19:**2934–2936.

FUXE, K., and UNGERSTEDT, V., 1967, Localization of 5-hydroxytryptamine uptake in rat brain after intraventricular injection, *J. Pharm. Pharmacol.* **19:**335–337.

FUXE, K., and UNGERSTEDT, U., 1968, Histochemical studies on the effect of (+)-amphetamine, drugs of the imipramine group and tyramine on central catecholamine and 5-hydroxytryptamine neurons after intraventricular injection of catecholamines and 5-hydroxytryptamine, *Eur. J. Pharmacol.* **4:**135–144.

FUXE, K., HAMBERGER, B., and MALMFORS, T., 1967, The effect of drugs on accumulation of monoamines in tubero-infundibular dopamine neurons, *Eur. J. Pharmacol.* **1:**334–341.

GEORGE, T., KAUL, C. L., GREWAL, R. S., and TAHILRAMANI, R., 1971, Antihypertensive and monoamine oxidase inhibitory activity of some derivatives of 3-formyl-4-oxo-4H-pyrido[1,2-a]pyrimidine, *J. Med. Chem.* **14:**913–915.

GIACHETTI, A., and SHORE, P. A., 1966, Studies *in vitro* of amine uptake mechanisms in heart, *Biochem. Pharmacol.* **15:**607–614.

GLOWINSKI, J., AXELROD, J., and IVERSEN, L. L., 1966, Regional studies of catecholamines in the rat brain. IV. Effects of drugs on the disposition and metabolism of H^3-norepinephrine and H^3-dopamine, *J. Pharmacol. Exp. Ther.* **153:**30–41.

GLUCKMAN, M. I., and BAUM, T., 1969, The pharmacology of iprindole, a new antidepressant, *Psychopharmacology* **15:**169–185.

GORIDIS, C., and NEFF, N. H., 1971, Evidence for a specific monoamine oxidase associated with sympathetic nerves, *Neuropharmacology* **10:**557–564.

GORKIN, V. Z., TAT'IANENKO, L. V., SUVOROV, N. N., and NEKLUDOV, A. D., 1967, On selective inhibition by α-substituted tryptamine derivatives of enzymatic deamination of serotonin, *Biokhimija* **32:**1036–1046.

GREIG, M. E., WALK, R. A., and GIBBONS, A. J., 1959, The effect of three tryptamine derivatives on serotonin metabolism *in vitro* and *in vivo*, *J. Pharmacol. Exp. Ther.* **127:**110–115.

GRIVSKY, E. M., and HITCHINGS, G. H., 1974, Syntheses of 2-chloro-4-acetylaminobenzonitrile isomers and structurally related compounds with biological activities, *Ind. Chim. Belg.* **39:**490–500.

HAMBERGER, B., 1967, Reserpine-resistant uptake of catecholamines in isolated tissues of the rat, *Acta Physiol. Scand. Suppl.* **295:**1–56.

HAMBERGER, B., MALMFORS, T., NORBERG, K.-A., and SACHS, CH., 1964, Uptake and accumulation of catecholamines in peripheral adrenergic neurons of reserpinized animals, studied with a histochemical method, *Biochem. Pharmacol.* **13:**841–844.

HANSCH, C., LEO, A., UNGER, S. H., KIM, K. H., NIKAITIS, D., and LIEN, E. J., 1973, "Aromatic" substituent constants for structure–activity correlations, *J. Med. Chem.* **16:**1207–1216.

HELLERMAN, L., and ERWIN, V. G., 1968, Mitochondrial monoamine oxidase. II. Action of various inhibitors for the bovine kidney enzyme, catalytic mechanism, *J. Biol. Chem.* **243:**5234–5243.

HELLERMAN, L., CHUANG, H. Y. K., and DE LUCA, D., 1972, Approaches to the catalytic mechanism of mitochondrial monoamine oxidase, *Adv. Biochem. Pharmacol.* **5:**327–337.

HENDLEY, E. D., and SNYDER, S. H., 1968, Relationship between the action of monoamine oxidase inhibitors on the noradrenaline uptake system and their antidepressant efficacy, *Nature (London)* **220:**1330–1331.

HERD, J. A., 1969, A new antidepressant—M&B 9302, a pilot study and a double-blind controlled trial, *Clin. Trials J.,* pp. 219–225.

HERTTING, G., AXELROD, J., KOPIN, I. J., and WHITBY, L. G., 1961, Lack of uptake of catecholamines after chronic denervation of sympathetic nerves, *Nature (London)* **189:**66.

HESTER, J., GREIG, M., ANTHONY, W., HEINZELMAN, R., and SZMUSZKOVICZ, J., 1964, Enzyme inhibitory activity of 3-(2-aminobutyl)indole derivatives, *J. Med. Chem.* **7:**274–279.

HILLARP, N.-A., and MALMFORS, T., 1964, Reserpine and cocaine blocking of the uptake and storage mechanisms in adrenergic nerves, *Life Sci.* **3:**703–708.

HIRAMATSU, A., TSURUSHIIN, S., and YASUNOBU, K. T., 1975, Evidence for essential histidine residues in bovine liver mitochondrial monoamine oxidase, *Eur. J. Biochem.* **57:**587–593.

Ho, B. T., 1972, Monoamine oxidase inhibitors, *J. Pharm. Sci.* **61:**821–837.

Ho, B. T., MCISAAC, W. M., WALKER, K. E., and ESTEVEZ, V., 1968, Inhibitors of monoamine oxidase: Influence of methyl substitution on the inhibitory activity of β-carbolines, *J. Pharm. Sci.* **57:**269–274.

Ho, B. T., MCISAAC, W. M., and TANSEY, L. W., 1969, Inhibitors of monoamine oxidase IV: 6(or 8)-Substituted tetrahydro-β-carbolines and their 9-methyl analogs, *J. Pharm. Sci.* **58:**998–1001.

Ho, B. T., GARDNER, P. M., and WALKER, K. E., 1973, Inhibition of MAO by β-carbolinium halides, *J. Pharm. Sci.* **62:**36–39.

HOLLISTER, L. E., 1972, Clinical use of psychotherapeutic drugs. II. Antidepressant and antianxiety drugs and special problems in the use of psychotherapeutic drugs, *Drugs* **4:**361–410.

HORN, A., 1973a, Conformational aspects of the inhibition of neuronal uptake of noradrenaline by tricyclic antidepressants, in: *Frontiers in Catecholamine Research* (E. Usdin and S. Snyder, eds.), pp. 411–413, Pergamon Press, New York.

HORN, A. S., 1973b, Structure–activity relations for the inhibition of 5-HT uptake into rat hypothalamic homogenates by serotonin and tryptamine analogues, *J. Neurochem.* **21:**883–888.

HORN, A. S., and SNYDER, S. H., 1972, Steric requirements for catecholamine uptake by rat brain synaptosomes: Studies with rigid analogs of amphetamine, *J. Pharmacol. Exp. Ther.* **180:**523–530.

HORN, A. S., and TRACE, R. C. A. M., 1974, Structure–activity relations for the inhibition of 5-hydroxytryptamine uptake by tricyclic antidepressants into synaptosomes from serotoninergic neurones in rat brain homogenates, *Br. J. Pharmacol.* **51:**399–403.

HORN, A. S., COYLE, J. T., and SNYDER, S. H., 1971, Catecholamine uptake by synaptosomes from rat brain: Structure–activity relationships of drugs with differential effects in dopamine and norepinephrine neurons, *Mol. Pharmacol.* **7:**66–80.

HOUSLAY, M. D., and TIPTON, K. F., 1973, The nature of the electrophoretically separable multiple forms of rat liver monoamine oxidase, *Biochem. J.* **135:**173–186.

HOUSLAY, M. D., and TIPTON, K. F., 1974, A kinetic evaluation of monoamine oxidase activity in rat liver mitochondrial outer membranes, *Biochem. J.* **139:**645–652.

HOUSLAY, M. D., GARRETT, N. J., and TIPTON, K. F., 1974, Mixed substrate experiments with human brain monoamine oxidase, *Biochem. Pharmacol.* **23:**1937–1944.

HSU, S. Y., HUANG, C. L., and WATERS, I. W., 1975, Effect of acylation with eleostearic acids on the monoamine oxidase inhibitory potency of some hydrazine antidepressants in mice, *J. Med. Chem.* **18:**20–23.

HUSZTI, Z., 1972, Kinetic studies on rat brain monoamine oxidase, *Mol. Pharmacol.* **8:**385–397.

HUSZTI, Z., FEKETE, M., and HAJÓS, A., 1969, Monoamine oxidase inhibiting properties of AB-15—comparison with tranylcypromine, nialamide and pargyline, *Biochem. Pharmacol.* **18:**2293–2301.

Ison, R. R., Partington, P., and Roberts, G. C. K., 1973, The conformation of catecholamines and related compounds in solution, *Mol. Pharmacol.* **9**:756–765.

Iversen, L. L., 1963, The uptake of noradrenalin by the isolated perfused rat heart, *Br. J. Pharmacol.* **21**:523–537.

Iversen, L. L., 1967, *The Uptake and Storage of Noradrenaline in Sympathetic Nerves*, University Press, Cambridge.

Iversen, L. L., and Kravitz, E. A., 1966, Sodium dependence of transmitter uptake at adrenergic nerve terminals, *Mol. Pharmacol.* **2**:360–362.

Jain, V. K., Swinson, R. P., and Thomas, J. G., 1970, Phenelzine in obsessional neurosis, *Br. J. Psychiatry* **117**:237–238.

Jain, M., Sands, F., and Von Korff, R. W., 1973, Monoamine oxidase activity measurements using radioactive substrates, *Anal. Biochem.* **52**:542–554.

Johnson, W. C., 1975, A neglected modality in psychiatric treatment—the monoamine oxidase inhibitors, *Dis. Nerv. Syst.* **36**:521–525.

Johnston, J. P., 1968, Some observations upon a new inhibitor of monoamine oxidase in brain tissue, *Biochem. Pharmacol.* **17**:1285–1297.

Kafoe, W. F., and Leonard, B. E., 1973, The effect of a new tetracyclic anti-depressant compound, Org GB 94, on the turnover of dopamine, noradrenalin and serotonin in the rat brain, *Arch Int. Pharmacodyn. Ther.* **206**:389–391.

Kannengiesser, M. H., Hunt, P., and Raynaud, J.-P., 1973, An *in vitro* model for the study of psychotropic drugs and as a criterion of antidepressant activity, *Biochem. Pharmacol.* **22**:73–84.

Kaul, C. L., and Grewal, R. S., 1972, Antihypertensive and monoamine oxidase inhibitory activity of 3-amino-2-oxazolidinone (3AO) and its condensation product with 2-substituted-3-formyl-4-oxo(4H)pyrido(1,2-a)pyrimidines, *Biochem. Pharmacol.* **21**:303–316.

Kearney, E. B., Salach, J. I., Walker, W. H., Seng, R., and Singer, T. P., 1971, Structure of the covalently bound flavin of monoamine oxidase, *Biochem. Biophys. Res. Commun.* **42**:490–496.

Kielholz, P., and Poldinger, W., 1968, Die Behandlung endogener Depressionen mit Psychopharmaka, *Deutsch. Med. Wochenschr.* **93**:701–704.

Klerman, G. L., 1971, Chemotherapy of depression, in: *Brain Chemistry and Mental Disease Proceedings* (B. T. Ho and W. M. McIsaac, eds.), pp. 379–402, Plenum Press, New York.

Knoll, J., and Magyar, K., 1972, Some puzzling pharmacological effects of monoamine oxidase inhibitors, *Adv. Biochem. Psychopharmacol.* **5**:393–408.

Knoll, J., Ecseri, Z., Kelemen, K., Nievel, J., and Knoll, B., 1965, Phenylisopropylmethylpropinylamine (E-250), a new spectrum psychic energizer, *Arch. Int. Pharmacodyn. Ther.* **155**:154–164.

Knoll, J., Vizi, E. S., and Somogyi, G., 1968, Phenylisopropylmethylpropynylamine (E-250), a monoaminooxidase inhibitor antagonising the effects of tyramine, *Arzneim.-Forsch.* **18**:109–112.

Korduba, C. A., Veals, J., and Symchowicz, S., 1973, The effect of pheniramine and its structural analogues on 5-hydroxytryptamine in rat and mouse brain, *Life Sci.* **13**:1557–1564.

Koshland, D. E., and Neet, K. E., 1968, The catalytic and regulatory properties of enzymes, *Annu. Rev. Biochem.* **37**:359–410.

Kuhn, R., 1958, The treatment of depressive states with G22355 (imipramine hydrochloride), *Am. J. Psychiatry* **115**:459–464.

Lapin, I. P., and Oxenkrug, G. F., 1969, Intensification of the central serotoninergic processes as a possible determinant of the thymoleptic effect, *Lancet* **1**:132–136.

Leonard, B. E., 1974, Some effects of a new tetracyclic anti-depressant compound, Org GB 94, on the metabolism of monoamines in the rat brain, *Psychopharmacology* **36**:221–236.

Lidbrink, P., Jonsson, G., and Fuxe, K., 1971, The effect of imipramine-like drugs and antihistamine drugs on uptake mechanisms in the central noradrenaline and 5-hydroxytryptamine neurons, *Neuropharmacology* **10**:521–536.

LINDMAR, R., and MUSCHOLL, E., 1964, Die Wirkung von Pharmaka auf die Elimination von Noradrenalin aus der Perfusionsflüssigkeit und die Noradrenalinaufnahm in das isolierte Herz, *Naunyn-Schmiedebergs Arch. Exp. Pathol. Pharmakol.* **247**:469–492.

LONG, R. F., 1962, Reversible inhibition of brain monoamine oxidase *in vitro* and *in vivo*, *Acta Neurol. Scand.* **35**(S1):27–28.

LOOMER, H. P., SAUNDERS, J. C., and KLINE, N. S., 1957, A clinical and pharmacodynamic evaluation of iproniazid as a psychic energizer, *Psychiatr. Res. Rep.* **8**:129–141.

MACFARLANE, M. D., and BESBRIS, H., 1974, Procaine (Gerovital H3) therapy: Mechanism of inhibition of monoamine oxidase, *J. Am. Geriatr. Soc.* **22**:365–371.

MAGYAR, K., SÁTORY, E., MÉSZÁROS, Z., and KNOLL, J., 1974, The monoamine oxidase inhibitory effect of new homopyrimidazole derivatives, *Med. Biol.* **52**:384–389.

MÂITRE, L., STAEHELIN, M., and BEIN, H. J., 1971, Blockade of noradrenaline uptake by 34276-Ba, a new antidepressant drug, *Biochem. Pharmacol.* **20**:2169–2186.

MÂITRE, L., WALDMEIER, P. C., BAUMANN, P. A., and STAEHELIN, M., 1974, Effect of maprotoline, a new antidepressant drug, on serotonin uptake, *Adv. Biochem. Psychopharmacol.* **10**:297–304.

MALITZ, S., and KANZLER, M., 1971, Are antidepressants better than placebo?, *Am. J. Psychiatry* **127**:1605–1611.

MARTIN, Y. C., and BIEL, J. H., 1974a, Proceedings: Some considerations in the design of substrate and tissue specific inhibitors of MAO, *Psychopharmacol. Bull.* **10**:8–9.

MARTIN, Y. C., and BIEL, J. H., 1974b, Some considerations in the design of substrate and tissue-specific inhibitors of monoamine oxidase, *Adv. Biochem. Psychopharmacol.* **12**:37–48.

MARTIN, Y. C., MARTIN, W. B., and TAYLOR, J. D., 1975, Regression analysis of the relationship between physical properties and the *in vitro* inhibition of monoamine oxidase by propynylamines, *J. Med. Chem.* **18**:883–888.

MASTER, R. S., and BASTANI, J. B., 1972, Iprindole in depressive states: A controlled, double-blind study, *Curr. Med. Res. Opin.* **1**:3–9.

MAXWELL, R. A., KEENAN, P. D., CHAPLIN, E., ROTH, B., and ECKHARDT, S. B., 1969, Molecular features affecting the potency of tricyclic antidepressants and structurally related compounds as inhibitors of the uptake of tritiated norepinephrine by rabbit aortic strips, *J. Pharmacol. Exp. Ther.* **166**:320–329.

MAXWELL, R. A., ECKHARDT, S. B., and HITE, G., 1970a, Kinetic and thermodynamic considerations regarding the inhibition by tricyclic antidepressants of the uptake of tritiated norepinephrine by the adrenergic nerves in rabbit aortic strips, *J. Pharmacol. Exp. Ther.* **171**:62–69.

MAXWELL, R. A., CHAPLIN, E., ECKHARDT, S. B., SOARES, J. R., and HITE, G., 1970b, Conformational similarities between molecular models of phenethylamine and of potent inhibitors of the uptake of tritiated norepinephrine by adrenergic nerves in rabbit aorta, *J. Pharmacol. Exp. Ther.* **173**:158–165.

MAXWELL, R. A., ECKHARDT, S. B., CHAPLIN, E., and BURCSU, J., 1971, Inhibitors of the uptake of norepinephrine by the adrenergic nerves in rabbit aorta, in: *Proceedings of the Symposium on the Physiology and Pharmacology of Vascular Neuroeffector Systems* (J. Bevan, R. F. Furchgott, R. A. Maxwell and A. P. Somlyo, eds.), pp. 98–110, Karger, Basel.

MAXWELL, R. A., FERRIS, R. M., BURCSU, J., WOODWARD, E. C., TANG, D., and WILLIARD, K., 1974, The phenyl rings of tricyclic antidepressants and related compounds as determinants of the potency of inhibition of the amine pumps in adrenergic neurons of the rabbit aorta and in rat cortical synaptosomes, *J. Pharmacol. Exp. Ther.* **191**:418–430.

MCCAULEY, R., and RACKER, E., 1973, Separation of two monoamine oxidases from bovine brain, *Mol. Cell. Biochem.* **1**:73–81.

MCISAAC, W. M., and ESTEVEZ, V., 1966, Structure–action relationship of β-carbolines as monoamine oxidase inhibitors, *Biochem. Pharmacol.* **15**:1625–1627.

MITCHELL, J. R., and OATES, J. A., 1970, Guanethidine and related agents. I. Mechanism of the selective blockade of adrenergic neurons and its antagonism by drugs, *J. Pharmacol. Exp. Ther.* **172**:100–107.

MORRIS, J. B., and BECK, A. T., 1974, The efficacy of antidepressant drugs, *Arch. Gen. Psychiatry* **30**:667–674.

MOSNAIM, A. D., INWANG, E. E., SUGERMAN, J. H., DE MARTINI, W. J., and SABELLI, H. C., 1973, Ultraviolet spectrophotometric determination of 2-phenylethylamine in biological samples and its possible correlation with depression, *Biol. Psychiatry* **6**:235–257.

MURPHY, J. E. (ed.), 1975a, Ludiomil symposium, *J. Int. Med. Res.* **3**(Suppl. 2).

MURPHY, J. E., 1975b, A comparative clinical trial of Org GB 94 and imipramine in the treatment of depression in general practice, *J. Int. Med. Res.* **3**:251–260.

NÁHUNEK, K., and ŠVESTKA, J., 1972, Therapeutic effect of tranylcypromine in endogenous depressions. Comparison with other antidepressant drugs, *Cesk. Psychiatrie* **68**:3–11.

NEFF, N. H., and YANG, H.-Y. T., 1974, Another look at the monoamine oxidases and the monoamine oxidase inhibitor drugs, *Life Sci.* **14**:2061–2074.

NEFF, N. H., YANG, H.-Y., and FUENTES, J. A., 1974, The use of selective monoamine oxidase inhibitor drugs to modify amine metabolism in brain, *Adv. Biochem. Psychopharmacol.* **12**:49–57.

OI, S., SHIMADA, K., INAMASU, M., and YASUNOBU, K. T., 1970, Mechanistic studies of beef liver mitochondrial amine oxidase, *Arch. Biochem. Biophys.* **139**:28–37.

OI, S., YASUNOBU, K. T., and WESTLEY, J., 1971, The effect of pH on the kinetic parameters and mechanism of beef liver monoamine oxidase, *Arch. Biochem. Biophys.* **145**:557–564.

OLIVECRONA, T., and ORELAND, L., 1971, Reassociation of soluble monoamine oxidase with lipid-depleted mitochondria in the presence of phospholipids, *Biochemistry* **10**:332–340.

ORELAND, L., KINEMUCHI, H., and YOO, B. Y., 1973, The mechanism of action of the monoamine oxidase inhibitor pargyline, *Life Sci.* **13**:1533–1541.

OZAKI, M., WEISSBACH, H., OZAKI, A., WITKOP, B., and UDENFRIEND, S., 1960, Monoamine oxidase inhibitors and procedures for their evaluation *in vivo* and *in vitro*, *J. Med. Pharm. Chem.* **2**:591–607.

PARE, C. M., 1970, Differentiation of two genetically specific types of depression by the response to antidepressant drugs, *Humangenetik* **9**:199–201.

PATEK, D. R., and HELLERMAN, L., 1974, Mitochondrial monoamine oxidase, mechanism of inhibition by phenylhydrazine and by aralkylhydrazines. Role of enzymatic oxidation, *J. Biol. Chem.* **249**:2373–2380.

PHILPOT, F. J., 1940, The inhibition of adrenaline oxidation by local anaesthetics, *J. Physiol.* **97**:301–307.

Physicians' Desk Reference, 1975, Medical Economics Co., Oradell, New Jersey.

POPOV, N., MATTHIES, H., LIETZ, W., THIEMANN, CHR., and JASSMANN, E., 1970, The effect of different substrates on the inhibition of rat brain and liver monoamine oxidase by arylalkylhydrazines, *Biochem. Pharmacol.* **19**:2413–2418.

POST, M. L., KENNARD, O., and HORN, A. S., 1974, Possible pharmacological and theoretical implications of X-ray structure of the tricyclic antidepressant imipramine, *Nature (London)* **252**:493–495.

POST, M. L., KENNARD, O., and HORN, A. S., 1975, The tricyclic antidepressants: Imipramine hydrochloride. The crystal and molecular structure of 5-(3-dimethylaminopropyl)-10,11-dihydro-5H-dibenz[b,f]azepine hydrochloride, *Acta Crystallogr. Sect. 3:* **31**:1008–1013.

PRANGE, A. J., WILSON, I. C., LYNN, C. W., ALLTOP, L. B., and STRIKELEATHER, R. A., 1974, L-Tryptophan in mania, contribution to a permissive hypothesis of affective disorders, *Arch. Gen. Psychiatry* **30**:56–62.

RICKELS, K., CHUNG, H. R., CSANALOSI, I., SABLOSKY, L., and SIMON, J. H., 1973, Iprindole and imipramine in non-psychotic depressed out-patients, *Br. J. Psychiatry* **123**:329–339.

ROBINSON, D. S., LOVENBERG, W., KEISER, H., and SJOERDSMA, A., 1968, Effects of drugs on human blood platelet and plasma amine oxidase activity *in vitro* and *in vivo*, *Biochem. Pharmacol.* **17**:109–119.

ROBINSON, D. S., NIES, A., RAVARIS, C. L., and LAMBORN, K. R., 1973, The monoamine oxidase inhibitor, phenelzine, in the treatment of depressive–anxiety states, *Arch. Gen. Psychiatry* **29**:407–413.

ROSLOFF, B. N., and DAVIS, J. M., 1974, Effect of iprindole on norepinephrine turnover and transport, *Psychopharmacology* **40**:53–64.

ROSS, S. B., and RENYI, A. L., 1967a, Accumulation of tritiated 5-hydroxytryptamine in brain slices, *Life Sci.* **6**:1407–1415.

ROSS, S. B., and RENYI, A. L., 1967b, Inhibition of the uptake of tritiated catecholamines by antidepressant and related agents, *Eur. J. Pharmacol.* **2**:181–186.

ROSS, S. B., and RENYI, A. L., 1969, Inhibition of the uptake of tritiated 5-hydroxytryptamine in brain tissue, *Eur. J. Pharmacol.* **7**:270–277.

ROSS, S. B., and RENYI, A. L., 1975a, Tricyclic antidepressant agents. I. Comparison of the inhibition of the uptake of ^{3}H-noradrenaline and ^{14}C-5-hydroxytryptamine in slices and crude synaptosome preparations of the midbrain–hypothalamus region of the rat brain, *Acta Pharmacol. Toxicol.* **36**:382–394.

ROSS, S. B., and RENYI, A. L., 1975b, Tricyclic antidepressant agents. II. Effect of oral administration on the uptake of ^{3}H-noradrenaline and ^{14}C-5-hydroxytryptamine in slices of the midbrain–hypothalamus region of the rat, *Acta Pharmacol. Toxicol.* **36**:395–408.

ROSS, S. B., RENYI, A. L., and OGREN, S.-O., 1971, A comparison of the inhibitory activities of iprindole and imipramine on the uptake of 5-hydroxytryptamine and noradrenaline in brain slices, *Life Sci.* **10**:1267–1277.

ROTH, J. A., 1975, Inhibition of rabbit monoamine oxidase by doxepin and related drugs, *Life Sci.* **16**:1309–1320.

ROTH, J. A., and GILLIS, C. N., 1974a, Inhibition of lung, liver and brain monoamine oxidase by imipramine and desipramine, *Biochem. Pharmacol.* **23**:1138–1140.

ROTH, J. A., and GILLIS, C. N., 1974b, Deamination of β-phenylethylamine by monoamine oxidase-inhibition by imipramine, *Biochem. Pharmacol.* **23**:2537–2545.

ROTH, J. A., and GILLIS, C. N., 1975, Some structural requirements for inhibition of type A and B forms of rabbit monoamine oxidase by tricyclic psychoactive drugs, *Mol. Pharmacol.* **11**:28–35.

SABELLI, H. C., MOSNAIM, A. D., and VAZQUEZ, A. J., 1974, Phenethylamine: Possible role in depression and antidepressive drug action, in: *Neurohumoral Coding of Brain Function* (R. R. Drucker-Colin and R. D. Meyer, eds.), pp. 331–357, Plenum Press, New York.

SAKALIS, G., OH, D., GERSHON, S., and SHOPSIN, B., 1974, A trial of Gerovital H3 in depression during senility, *Curr. Ther. Res.* **16**:59–63.

SALAMA, A. I., INSALACO, J. R., and MAXWELL, R. A., 1971, Concerning the molecular requirements for the inhibition of the uptake of racemic ^{3}H-norepinephrine into rat cerebral cortex slices by tricyclic antidepressants and related compounds, *J. Pharmacol. Exp. Ther.* **178**:474–481.

SANDLER, M., 1973, New look at monoamine oxidase inhibitors; the new biochemical background, *Proc. R. Soc. Med.* **66**:946–947.

SARGES, R., KOE, B. K., WEISSMAN, A., and SCHAEFER, J. P., 1974, Blockade of heart ^{3}H-norepinephrine uptake by 4-phenyl-1-aminotetralines: Implications for the active conformation of imipramine-like drugs, *J. Pharmacol. Exp. Ther.* **191**:393–402.

SCHILDKRAUT, J. J., 1965, The catecholamine hypothesis of affective disorders: Review of supporting evidence, *Am. J. Psychiatry* **123**:509–522.

SCHILDKRAUT, J. J., 1969, *Neuropsychopharmacology and the Affective Disorders*, Little, Brown, Boston.

SCHILDKRAUT, J. J., and KETY, S. S., 1967, Biogenic amines and emotion, *Science* **156**:21–30.

SEVERINA, I. S., 1973, On the substrate-binding sites of the active centre of mitochondrial monoamine oxidase, *Eur. J. Biochem.* **38**:239–246.

SHASKAN, E. G., and SNYDER, S. H., 1970, Kinetics of serotonin accumulation into slices from rat brain: Relationship to catecholamine uptake, *J. Pharmacol. Exp. Ther.* **175**:404–418.

SINGER, T. P., and BARRON, E. S. G., 1945, Studies on biological oxidations. XX. Sulfhydryl enzymes in fat and protein metabolism, *J. Biol. Chem.* **157**:241–253.

SNYDER, S. H., and COYLE, J. T., 1969, Regional differences in H^3-norepinephrine and H^3-dopamine uptake into rat brain homogenates, *J. Pharmacol. Exp. Ther.* **165**:78–86.

SQUIRES, R. F., 1968, Additional evidence for the existence of several forms of mitochondrial monoamine oxidase in the mouse, *Biochem. Pharmacol.* **17**:1401–1409.

SQUIRES, R. F., and BUUS LASSEN, J., 1968, Some pharmacological and biochemical properties of γ-morpholino-butyrophenone (NSD 2023), a new monoamine oxidase inhibitor, *Biochem. Pharmacol.* **17**:369–384.

STERN, I. J., HOLLIFIELD, R. D., WILK, S., and BUZARD, J. A., 1967, The antimonoamine oxidase effects of furazolidone, *J. Pharmacol. Exp. Ther.* **156**:492–499.

STRÖMBLAD, B. C. R., and NICKERSON, M., 1961, Accumulation of epinephrine and norepinephrine by some rat tissues, *J. Pharmacol. Exp. Ther.* **134**:154–159.

SWETT, L. R., MARTIN, W. B., TAYLOR, J. D., EVERETT, G. M., WYKES, A. A., and GLADISH, Y. C., 1963, Structure–activity relationships in the pargyline series, *Ann. N. Y. Acad. Sci.* **107**:891–898.

THONEN, H., HURLIMANN, A., and HAEFELY, W., 1968, Mechanism of amphetamine accumulation in the isolated perfused heart of the rat, *J. Pharm. Pharmacol.* **20**:1–11.

TIPTON, K. F., 1968, The reaction pathway of pig brain mitochondrial monoamine oxidase, *Eur. J. Biochem.* **5**:316–320.

TIPTON, K. F., 1972, Some properties of monoamine oxidase, *Adv. Biochem. Psychopharmacol.* **5**:11–24.

TIPTON, K. F., HOUSLAY, M. D., and GARRETT, N. J., 1973, Allotopic properties of human brain monoamine oxidase, *Nature (London)* **246**:213–214.

TRINGER, L., HAITS, G., and VARGA, E., 1967, The effect of L-E-250 (L-phenyl-isopropyl-methyl-propinyl-amine HCl) in depressions, *Conferentia Hungarica pro Therapia et Investigatione in Pharmacologia V*, Budapest, pp. 111–113.

TUCK, J. R., and PUNELL, G., 1973, Uptake of [^{3}H]5-hydroxytryptamine and [^{3}H]noradrenaline by slices of rat brain incubated in plasma from patients treated with chlorimipramine, imipramine or amitriptyline, *J. Pharm. Pharmacol.* **25**:573–574.

TYRER, P., CANDY, J., and KELLY, D., 1973, Phenelzine in phobic anxiety: A clinical trial, *Physiol. Med.* **3**:120–124.

VAN DER ZEE, P., and HESPE, W., 1973, Influence of orphenadrine hydrochloride and its N-demethylated derivatives on the *in vitro* uptake of noradrenaline and 5-hydroxytryptamine by rat brain slices, *Neuropharmacology* **12**:843–851.

VANE, J. R., 1959, The relative activities of some tryptamine analogues on the isolated rat stomach strip preparation, *Br. J. Pharmacol.* **14**:87–98.

VAN PRAAG, H. M., 1974, Toward a biochemical classification of depression, *Adv. Biochem. Psychopharmacol.* **11**:357–368.

VARGA, E., 1965, Vorläufiger Bericht über die Wirkung des Präparates E-250 (phenyl-isopropyl-methyl-propinylamin-chlorhydrat), *Conferentia Hungarica pro Therapia et Investigatione in Pharmacologia III*, Budapest, pp. 197–201.

VOGEL, H. P., BENTE, D., and HELMCHEN, H., 1974, Mianserin vs. amitriptyline—a double-blind study evaluated by the AMP-system, *J. Pharmacol.* **5**(2):103.

WEBB, J. L., 1963, *Enzyme and Metabolic Inhibitors*, Academic Press, New York.

WEETMAN, D. F., and SWEETMAN, A. J., 1971, Realistic estimations of kinetic constants for the oxidation of naturally occurring monoamines by monoamine oxidase, *Anal. Biochem.* **41**:517–521.

WHEATLEY, D., 1970, A comparative trial of a new monoamine oxidase inhibitor in depression, *Br. J. Psychiatry* **117**:573–574.

WHITBY, L. G., AXELROD, J., and WEIL-MALHERBE, H., 1961, The fate of H^3-norepinephrine in animals, *J. Pharmacol. Exp. Ther.* **132**:193–201.

WHITE, H. L., and WU, J. C., 1975a, Substrate-selective binding sites of human brain monoamine oxidase, *Fed. Proc.* **34**:283.

WHITE, H. L., and WU, J. C., 1975b, Multiple binding sites of human brain monoamine oxidase as indicated by substrate competition, *J. Neurochem.* **25**:21–26.

WHITE, H. L., and GLASSMAN, A. T., 1977, Multiple binding sites of human brain and liver monoamine oxidase: Substrate specificities, selective inhibitions, and attempts to separate enzyme forms, *J. Neurochem.* (in press).

WILLIAMS, C. H., 1974, Monoamine oxidase. I. Specificity of some substrates and inhibitors, *Biochem. Pharmacol.* **23**:615–628.

WONG, D. T., HORNG, J.-S., and FULLER, R. W., 1973, Kinetics of serotonin accumulation into synaptosomes of rat brain—effects of amphetamine and chloroamphetamines, *Biochem. Pharmacol.* **22**:311–322.

WONG, D. T., HORNG, J. S., BYMASTER, F. P., HAUSER, K. L., and MOLLOY, B. B., 1974, A selective inhibitor of serotonin uptake: Lilly 110140, 3-(p-trifluoromethylphenoxy)-N-methyl-3-phenylpropylamine, *Life Sci.* **15**:471–479.

YANG, H.-Y. T., and NEFF, N. H., 1973, β-Phenylethylamine: A specific substrate for type B monoamine oxidase of brain, *J. Pharmacol. Exp. Ther.* **187**:365–371.

YANG, H.-Y. T., and NEFF, N. H., 1974, The monoamine oxidases of brain: Selective inhibition with drugs and the consequences for the metabolism of the biogenic amines, *J. Pharmacol. Exp. Ther.* **189**:733–740.

YOUDIM, M. B. H., COLLINS, G. G. S., and SANDLER, M., 1969, Multiple forms of rat brain monoamine oxidase, *Nature (London)* **223**:626–628.

ZELLER, E. A., 1960, Studies on the active center of monoamine oxidase, *Experientia* **16**:399–402.

ZELLER, E. A., 1963, A new approach to the analysis of the interaction between monoamine oxidase and its substrates and inhibitors, *Ann. N. Y. Acad. Sci.* **107**:811–820.

ZELLER, E. A., BARSKY, J., FOUTS, J. R., KIRCHHEIMER, W. F., and VAN ORDEN, L. S., 1952, Influence of isonicotinic acid hydrazide (INH) and 1-isonicotinoyl-2-isopropylhydrazine (IIH) on bacterial and mammalian enzymes, *Experientia* **8**:349–350.

ZELLER, E. A., GÄRTNER, B., and HEMMERICH, P., 1972, 4a,5-Cycloaddition reactions of acetylenic compounds at the flavoquinone nucleus as mechanisms of flavoprotein inhibitions, *Z. Naturforsch.* **27**:1050–1052.

ZIRKLE, C. L., and KAISER, C., 1964, Monoamine oxidase inhibitors (nonhydrazines), in: *Psychopharmacological Agents*, Vol. 1 (M. Gordon, ed.), pp. 445–554, Academic Press, New York.

ZIRKLE, C. L., KAISER, C., TEDESCHI, D. H., TEDESCHI, R. E., and BURGER, A., 1962, Substituted cyclopropylamines. II. Effect of structure upon monoamine oxidase-inhibitory activity as measured *in vivo* by potentiation of tryptamine convulsions, *J. Med. Pharm. Chem.* **5**:1265–1284.

ZUNG, W. W. K., GIANTURCO, D., PFEIFFER, E., WANG, H. S., WHANGER, A., BRIDGE, T. P., and POTKIN, S. G., 1974, Pharmacology of depression in the aged: Evaluation of Gerovital H3 as an antidepressant drug, *Psychosomatics* **15**:127–131.

4

TRICYCLIC ANTIDEPRESSANTS: ANIMAL PHARMACOLOGY (BIOCHEMICAL AND METABOLIC ASPECTS)

Fridolin Sulser

1. INTRODUCTION

The prototype of tricyclic antidepressants, imipramine, was developed through molecular modification of the phenothiazine nucleus in promazine, i.e., by replacement of the sulfur with an ethylene group. In contrast to promazine, which is a symmetrical molecule, the molecule of imipramine is asymmetrical, the two benzene rings being twisted against each other (Häfliger, 1959). This molecular modification is obviously responsible for the change in the clinical activity from antipsychotic to antidepressant. It is noteworthy that the antidepressant activity of imipramine was discovered by Kuhn (1957, 1958) while he was evaluating the drug as a potential antipsychotic agent; it could not have been predicted from pharmacologic studies conducted at that time.

The discovery that N-demethylation of the tertiary amine imipramine to the secondary amine desmethylimipramine (desipramine) yields a drug with increased "antidepressant" activity in animal tests (Sulser *et al.*, 1962) triggered the synthesis of a number of secondary amines, e.g., nortriptyline and protriptyline. At present, all tricyclic antidepressants available for the

Fridolin Sulser • Vanderbilt University School of Medicine and Tennessee Neuropsychiatric Institute, Nashville, Tennessee.

treatment of depression or for experimental studies are either tertiary or secondary amines (Table 1), the latter of which can be formed *in vivo* by oxidative *N*-demethylation. Table 2 includes a number of drugs (iprindole, maproptiline, nisoxetine, nomifensine, and fluoxetine) with pharmacologic and biochemical properties which are pertinent for the discussion of the mode of action of tricyclic antidepressants and for a critical evaluation of current hypotheses of affective disorders.

The chemistry, general pharmacology, and clinical applications of tricyclic antidepressants have been extensively reviewed (Häfliger and Burckhard, 1964; Klerman and Cole, 1965; Bickel, 1968; Sigg, 1968; Kupfer, this volume). It is the aim of this chapter to discuss pertinent data on the mode of action of tricyclic antidepressants from both the biochemical and the metabolic points of view.

2. PHARMACOLOGIC TEST PROCEDURES PREDICTING CLINICAL ANTIDEPRESSANT ACTIVITY

Since Kuhn (1957) first described the antidepressant activity of imipramine 20 years ago, no fundamental new advances have been made in the field of tricyclic antidepressants with the exception of some structural modifications (e.g., replacement of the ring nitrogen by carbon, synthesis of secondary amines, and other changes in the side chain) that led to the introduction of a number of similar drugs. This slow process is partly due to the fact that reliable animal models of human depression are lacking and pharmacologic test procedures have been devised on the basis of pharmacologic or biochemical properties of preexisting drugs with proven clinical efficacy, thus making it unlikely that antidepressants with a novel profile will emerge.

The tricyclic antidepressants share with phenothiazine-like antipsychotic drugs anticholinergic and antihistaminic properties, particularly when given in high doses (Domenjoz and Theobald, 1959; Sulser and Watts, 1960; Vernier, 1961; Vernier *et al.*, 1962; Theobald *et al.*, 1964). While the former properties can explain many of the side effects observed following the administration of tricyclic antidepressants (e.g., dry mouth, difficulty in accommodation), the contribution of both pharmacologic actions to the clinical antidepressant activity of this class of drugs in unclear. Neurophysiologic studies also reveal that the tricyclic antidepressants behave like weak phenothiazines (Benesova *et al.*, 1962; Bradley and Key, 1959; Himwich *et al.*, 1964; Monnier and Krupp, 1959; Sigg, 1959; Steiner and Himwich, 1963).

Generally, however, the following pharmacologic properties involving noradrenergic or serotonergic mechanisms or both can distinguish imipramine-like drugs from structurally similar substances lacking antidepressant

TABLE 1
Prototypes of Tricyclic Antidepressants

Structure	Tertiary amine R=CH₃	Secondary amine R=H
I. Iminodibenzyl derivatives		
	Imipramine (Tolfranil®) Chlorimipramine (Anafranil®)	Desipramine (Pertofrane,® Norpramine®) Desmethylchlor-imipramine
II. Dibenzocycloheptadiene derivatives		
	Amitriptyline (Elavil,® Laroxyl®)	Nortriptyline (Aventyl®)
III. Dibenzocycloheptatriene derivatives		
	Ro 4-1577	Ro 4-6011
		Protriptyline (Vivactil®)
IV. Dibenzothiepin derivatives		
	Prothiadene	Northiadene
V. Dibenzoxepin derivatives		
	Doxepin (Sinequan,® Adapin®)	Desmethyldoxepin

TABLE 2
Miscellaneous Drugs with Potential Antidepressant Properties

---

1. Selective blockers of norepinephrine uptake
   Maproptiline (Ludiomil®)   1-(3-Methylaminopropyl)-dibenzo-
                                 [b,e]bicyclo-[2.2.2.]octadiene
   Nisoxetine   3-(o-Methoxyphenoxy)-3-phenyl-
                                 N-methylpropylamine
2. Selective blockers of 5-hydroxytryptamine uptake
   Fluoxetine   3-(p-Trifluoromethylphenoxy)-3-phenyl-
                                 N-methylpropylamine
   Desmethylfluoxetine
3. Blockers of norepinephrine and dopamine uptake
   Nomifensine   8-Amino-2-methyl-4-phenyl-1,2,3,4-
                                 tetrahydroisoquinoline
4. Antidepressants which do not block neuronal uptake
   Iprindole   5-(3-Dimethylaminopropyl)-6,7,8,9,10,11-
                                 hexahydro-5H-cyclooct[6]indole

---

activity: (1) potentiation of exogenous and endogenous catecholamines at peripheral adrenergic receptor sites; (2) potentiation of various central effects elicited by amphetamine-like drugs; (3) antagonism of guanethidine-induced catecholamine depletion and adrenergic neuron blockade; (4) antagonism of the reserpine-like syndrome in rodents; (5) blockade by tricyclic antidepressants of the uptake of catecholamines or 5-HT or both.

2.1. Potentiation of Exogenous and Endogenous Catecholamines at Peripheral Adrenergic Receptor Sites

Sigg (1959) first observed that imipramine enhanced and prolonged pharmacologic responses to injected norepinephrine both at the cardiovascular system and on the nictitating membrane of the cat. The norepinephrine-potentiating properties of imipramine-like drugs on the peripheral sympathetic system have since been demonstrated in many organs and for many species, including man (Schaeppi, 1960; Meduna *et al.*, 1961; Vernier *et al.*, 1962; Izquierdo *et al.*, 1962; Halliwell *et al.*, 1964; Loew, 1964; Häefeli *et al.*, 1964; Cairncross, 1965; Theobald *et al.*, 1965; Fischbach *et al.*, 1966; Schmitt and Schmitt, 1966). Osborne and Sigg (1960) showed that imipramine potentiated noradrenergic responses at low doses, while it blocked them at high doses. The difference between tertiary amines of tricyclic antidepressants and phenothiazines is in this respect only quantitative. Sensitization to exogenous norepinephrine is not a specific property of the tricyclic antidepressants, as it is shared by diverse pharmacologic agents such as cocaine, reserpine, ganglionic blocking drugs, adrenergic neuron blocking drugs, and veratrum alkaloids. Under certain circumstances, even chlorpromazine can potentiate the effect of exogenous norepinephrine (Martin *et al.*, 1960).

Imipramine-like drugs enhance and prolong over a wide dose range noradrenergic responses elicited by pre- or postganglionic sympathic nerve stimulation, e.g., on the nictitating membrane (Sigg *et al.*, 1963; Häefely *et al.*, 1964) and on contraction height of the isolated perfused spleen (Thoenen *et al.*, 1964). Again, while low concentrations of tricyclic antidepressants increase the response elicited by nerve stimulation, higher concentrations of the drugs reduce the intensity of the effects while still prolonging them. Generally, secondary amines of tricyclic antidepressants are more potent than their corresponding tertiary amines in enhancing responses to endogenous or exogenous norepinephrine, and tertiary amines can exert phenothiazine-like sympatholytic properties (Sigg *et al.*, 1963; Häefely *et al.*, 1964; Halliwell *et al.*, 1964; Theobald *et al.*, 1964, 1965; Jori and Garattini, 1965). For example, Häefely *et al.* (1964) have shown that the tertiary amine of a dibenzocycloheptatriene derivative (Ro 4-1577) decreases the effect of sympathetic nerve stimulation, while the corresponding secondary amine (Ro 4-6011) enhances the action of endogenously released norepinephrine. Moreover, Stone *et al.* (1964) demonstrated that the secondary amines protriptyline, desipramine, and nortriptyline antagonize the adrenergic neuron blockade elicited by guanethidine, while the corresponding tertiary amines imipramine and amitriptyline behave like chlorpromazine and fail to exhibit this antagonism.

2.2. Potentiation of Various Central Effects Elicited by Amphetamine-like Drugs

Since amphetamine-like drugs exert many of their central actions through catecholaminergic mechanisms (Glowinski and Axelrod, 1965; Costa and Garattini, 1970; Sulser and Sanders-Bush, 1971; Snyder *et al.*, 1972; Costa, 1973; Stein and Wise, 1973), it is of interest that tricyclic antidepressants enhance and prolong many behavioral effects of amphetamine (Carlton, 1961; Stein and Seifter, 1961; Scheckel and Boff, 1964; Sulser *et al.*, 1964; Halliwell *et al.*, 1964). These amphetamine-enhancing properties of imipramine-like drugs have been used to formulate or support various hypotheses on the central mode of action of tricyclic antidepressants and have provided widely employed methods of screening for potential antidepressants which are devoid of stimulatory activity in normal animals. A number of recent investigations have convincingly demonstrated, however, that the potentiation and prolongation by tricyclic antidepressants of central actions of amphetamine in the rat result from an inhibition in the metabolism of amphetamine (Sulser *et al.*, 1966; Valzelli *et al.*, 1967; Consolo *et al.*, 1967; Lewander, 1969). Although it could be argued that tricyclic antidepressants cause a potentiation of amphetamine by blocking the reuptake of catecholamines released by amphetamine, this cannot be the major mode of action, as tricyclic antidepressants do not potentiate and prolong the action of amphetamine in the mouse, a species in which *para*-hydroxylation is a minor pathway (Dolfini *et al.*, 1969; Lew and Iversen, 1971). Moreover, the new antidepressant iprindole shares with imipramine-like tricyclic antidepressants the ability to enhance and prolong many central effects caused by amphetamine (Gluckman and Baum, 1969; Miller *et al.*, 1970) but does not block the neuronal uptake of norepinephrine while markedly inhibiting the *para*-hydroxylation of amphetamine and thus prolonging the biological half-life of the drug (Freeman and Sulser, 1972). Small doses of chlorpromazine, although they usually reduce the intensity of the psychomotor stimulation caused by amphetamine, have also been shown to prolong many effects of amphetamine (Stein, 1962; Halliwell *et al.*, 1964; Babbini *et al.*, 1961; Spengler and Waser, 1969). Sulser and Dingell (1968) first provided evidence that the potentiating and prolonging effect of chlorpromazine is also associated with an inhibition of the metabolism of amphetamine by chlorpromazine. These results have since been confirmed and expanded by Borella *et al.* (1969*a,b*) and by Lewander (1969). These studies emphasize the importance of metabolic considerations in the proper interpretation of drug interaction studies and reveal that amphetamine potentiation by tricyclic antidepressants is not a reliable model to detect antidepressant drugs, as it can measure drug interactions at a metabolic rather than at a relevant neurochemical level.

2.3. Antagonism of Guanethidine-Induced Catecholamine Depletion and Adrenergic Neuron Blockade

Tricyclic antidepressants can block the peripheral depletion of catecholamines and the "sympatholytic" effects elicited by adrenergic-neuron-blocking drugs such as guanethidine (Stone *et al.*, 1964). Since the guanethidine-induced postganglionic blockade of noradrenergic neurons is prevented by the prior administration of tricyclic antidepressants but cannot be reversed, once established, it is likely that tricyclic antidepressants interfere with the uptake of guanethidine into the noradrenergic neuron. Carlsson and Waldeck (1965*a,b*) have indeed demonstrated that tricyclic antidepressants interfere with the uptake of guanethidine by blocking the transport mechanism located in the neuronal membrane. A similar mechanism may also explain the antagonism by tricyclic antidepressants of the action of indirectly acting sympathomimetic amines such as tyramine, phenylethylamine, and amphetamine in the peripheral sympathetic nervous system (Sigg, 1959; Ryall, 1961; Osborne, 1962; Vernier *et al.*, 1962; Stone *et al.*, 1964). The interference by tricyclic antidepressants with the adrenergic amine transport system is not an exclusive attribute of tricyclic antidepressants. Phenothiazine derivatives, sympathomimetic amines, and antihistaminic drugs can also interfere with this amine transport system, at least in peripheral adrenergic neurons.

2.4. Antagonism of the Reserpine-like Syndrome in Rodents

The reserpine-like syndrome elicited by reserpine and synthetic benzo-quinolizines such as tetrabenazine and Ro 4-1284 has been widely and successfully used as a "model depression" for the screening of antidepressants which are devoid of stimulatory activity in normal animals. Both tricyclic antidepressants and MAO inhibitors with antidepressant activity display antagonistic properties of various degrees. This "model depression" is of particular interest from the clinical point of view, as reserpine is known to precipitate occasionally severe depressive reactions in man (Müller et al., 1955; Bunney and Davis, 1965).

The reserpine-like syndrome is characterized by tranquilization, decreased sympathetic activity, increased central parasympathetic activity, and extrapyramidal symptoms (Sulser and Bass, 1968). Tricyclic antidepressants antagonize or prevent various autonomic effects elicited by reserpine such as ptosis, miosis, hypothermia, stomach ulcers, diarrhea, bradycardia, parasympathetic salivation, and, under certain circumstances, potentiation of anesthetics (Domenjoz and Theobald, 1959; Costa et al., 1960; Sulser and Watts, 1960; Garattini et al., 1962; Halliwell et al., 1964). Moreover, behavioral changes such as decreased exploratory activity elicited by reserpine-like drugs (particularly synthetic benzoquinolizines) are modified or "reversed" (Figs. 1 and 2) by tricyclic antidepressants (Sulser and Brodie, 1961; Sulser et al., 1962, 1964; Vernier et al., 1962).

The antagonism by tricyclic antidepressants of peripheral autonomic symptoms elicited by reserpine-like drugs is, however, not specific for this group of drugs, but is shared by a large number of diverse pharmacologic agents including sympathomimetics, antihistamines, and ganglion-blocking and adrenergic-neuron-blocking drugs. The antagonism of the behavioral changes elicited by reserpine-like drugs (particularly synthetic benzoquinolines such as tetrabenazine and Ro 4-1284) appears to offer a more discriminating test for the detection of antidepressants displaying imipramine-like properties.

Depending on the particular test procedure, tricyclic antidepressants can block both peripheral and central symptoms of the reserpine-like syndrome in rats and mice. Thus, rodents display exophthalmus instead of blepharospasm, mydriasis instead of miosis, and increased exploratory activity and "compulsive" motor activity instead of lack of locomotor and exploratory activity, and a blockade of conditioned avoidance and other behaviors has been reported (Sulser et al., 1962, 1964, 1968; Besendorf et al., 1962; Watts and Reilly, 1966; Matussek and Rüther, 1965; D'Encarnacaco and Anderson, 1970; Scheckel and Boff, 1964; Vernier et al., 1962; Vernier, 1966; Kulkarni

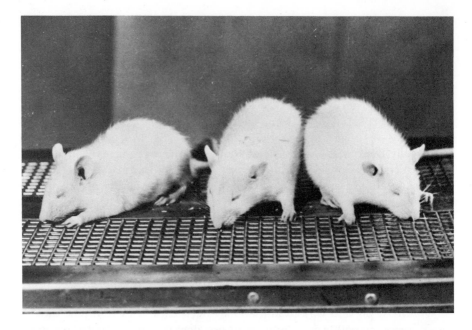

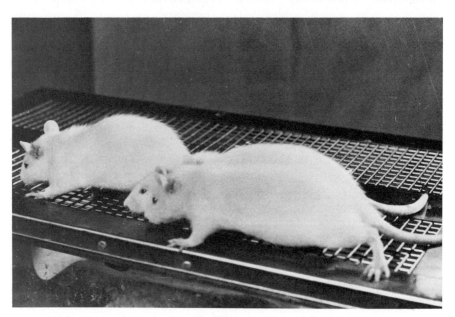

FIG. 1. Effect of desipramine on the reserpine-like syndrome. *Top:* Effect of the reserpine-like drug Ro 4-1284 (10 mg/kg) 60 min after its intraperitoneal administration: blepharospasm, sedation, decreased locomotor and exploratory activity. *Bottom:* Antagonism of the reserpine-like syndrome by desipramine (15 mg/kg i.p.) administered 15 min before Ro 4-1284: exophthalmus, alertness, increased "compulsive" motor activity. From Sulser *et al.* (1962).

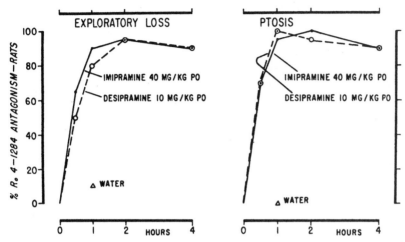

FIG. 2. Time effect curve of imipramine and desipramine for antagonism of Ro 4-1284-induced sedation (loss of exploratory activity) and ptosis in rats. Ro 4-1284 (8 mg/kg i.p.) was administered 30 min prior to observation From Vernier, (1966).

and Bocknik, 1973). These antagonistic effects are chiefly the result of the potentiation of norepinephrine by the tricyclic antidepressants at postsynaptic noradrenergic receptor sites (see Section 3). The degree of reserpine antagonism by tricyclic antidepressants appears to depend on the rate of release of catecholamines (Sulser and Soroko, 1965), which in turn depends on species, strain, dose, and type of reserpine-like drug. Additional evidence for this view is provided by studies which demonstrated that tricyclic antidepressants fail to counteract many effects elicited by reserpine-like drugs (Fig. 3) in rats the brains of which had been selectively depleted of catecholamines (Sulser and Bickel, 1962; Sulser *et al.*, 1964; Scheckel and Boff, 1964).

2.5. Blockade by Tricyclic Antidepressants of the Uptake of Catecholamines and/or 5-HT

Since inhibition of the reuptake of biogenic amines into the nerve terminal is believed to be a major mechanism of action of tricyclic antidepressants (see Section 3), a number of *in vitro* and *in vivo* tests have been utilized to characterize existing tricyclic antidepressants and to detect new drugs with potential antidepressant activity. In Chapter 3, Maxwell and White discuss in detail structure–activity relationships between tricyclic antidepressants and their effects on *in vitro* and *in vivo* uptake systems of biogenic amines. Kinetically, the inhibition of the uptake of norepinephrine by tricyclic antidepressants is competitive in nature, and, generally, secondary amines have been found to be more potent than the corresponding tertiary amines

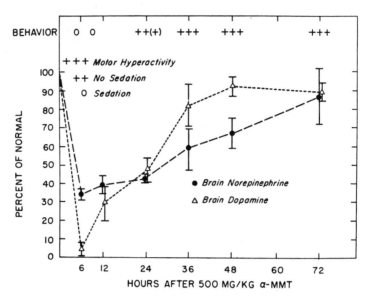

Fig. 3. Relationship between Ro 4-1284 antagonism by desipramine and the levels of brain catecholamines in rats. Catecholamines in brain of rats were depleted by α-methyl-*m*-tyrosine (α-MMT). Desipramine (20 mg/kg i.p.) and Ro 4-1284 (15 mg/kg i.p.) were administered at various times thereafter. Vertical bars represent standard deviations. Normal amine values in μg/g brain ± S.E. are: norepinephrine, 0.63 ± 0.03 (N = 19); dopamine, 0.78 ± 0.05 (N = 9). From Sulser *et al.* (1964).

in blocking the uptake of norepinephrine through the neuronal membrane (Carlsson *et al.*, 1966; Ross and Renyi, 1967; Maxwell *et al.*, 1969; Salama *et al.*, 1971). The correlation among blockade of uptake of norepinephrine, potentiation of norepinephrine, and clinical efficacy is, however, less than ideal. For example, Lahti and Maickel (1971), who measured the inhibition of the *in vivo* uptake of tritiated norepinephrine by the mouse heart, found that a number of antipsychotic drugs exert blocking properties equal to those of tricyclic antidepressants, whereas clinically effective tricyclic antidepressants such as opipramol and iprindole were without effect on this system (Tables 3 and 4).

In recent years, it became clear that tricyclic antidepressants also inhibit the amine uptake mechanism for 5-HT in serotoninergic neurons and in platelets. Using various *in vitro* systems (brain slices, platelets, synaptosomal preparations) as well as *in vivo* studies (depletion of 5-HT in brain with 4-methyl-α-ethyl-*m*-tyramine according to Carlsson *et al.*, 1969a), structure–activity relationships revealed that tertiary amines of tricyclic antidepressants are more potent inhibitors of 5-HT uptake than the corresponding secondary amines (Carlsson *et al.*, 1969a,b; Ross and Renyi, 1969; Todrick and Tait, 1969; Ahtee and Saarnivaara, 1971). Interestingly, this order of potency is the reverse of that found for the inhibition of the uptake of norepinephrine

TABLE 3

Effect of Various Tricyclic Antidepressants on the Uptake of [³H]Norepinephrine by the Mouse Heart[a]

Drug name	Structure	ED_{50} (mg/kg)
Amitriptyline		6.0
Imipramine		5.0
Melitracen		16.0
Desmethylmelitracen		6.0
Protriptyline		1.0
Opipramol		Inactive at 30 mg/kg
Iprindole		Inactive at 200 mg/kg

Amitriptyline: CH—CH₂—CH₂—N(CH₃)₂

Imipramine: CH₂—CH₂—CH₂—N(CH₃)₂

Melitracen: CH₃ CH₃ ; CH—CH₂—CH₂—N(CH₃)₂

Desmethylmelitracen: CH₃ CH₃ ; CH—CH₂—CH₂—NH—CH₃

Protriptyline: CH₂—CH₂—CH₂—NH—CH₃

Opipramol: CH₂—CH₂—CH₂—N⟨⟩N—CH—CH₂—OH

Iprindole: CH₂—CH₂—CH₂—N(CH₃)₂

[a] Drugs were administered intraperitoneally 1 hr prior to intravenous administration of [³H]NE. Mice were sacrificed 3 hr after injection of the labeled drug. Two hearts were used per determination and 3 determinations were made per dosage. Thee doses were used to obtain the dose producing a 50% inhibition of uptake. From Lahti and Maickel (1971).

TABLE 4

Effect of Phenothiazines and Related Drugs on the Uptake of [³H]Norepinephrine by the Mouse Heart[a]

Drug name	Structure	ED_{50}
Promazine		8.0
Desmethylpromazine		5.0
Methdilazine	$R_1 = -CH_2-$ (ring with $-N-CH_3$); $R_2 = -H$	11.0
Chlorpromazine		3.0
Perphenazine	$R_1 = -CH_2-CH_2-CH_2-N$ (piperazine) $N-CH_2-CH-OH$; $R_2 = -Cl$	Inactive at 60 mg/kg
Triflupromazine		6.0
Trifluoperazine	$R_1 = -CH_2-CH_2-CH_2-N$ (piperazine) $N-CH_3$; $R_2 = -CF_3$	Inactive at 25 mg/kg
Thiothixene	$(CH_3)_2NSO_2$ ... $CH_2-CH_2-CH_2-N$ (piperazine) $N-CH_3$	Inactive at 200 mg/kg

[a] Drugs were administered intraperitoneally 1 hr prior to the intravenous administration of [³H]NE. Mice were sacrificed 3 hr after injection of the labeled drug. Two hearts were used per determination and 3 determinations were made per dosage. Three doses were used to obtain the dose producing 50% inhibition of uptake. From Lahti and Maickel (1971).

(Table 5). The blockade of the reuptake of 5-HT, particularly by tertiary amines of tricyclic antidepressants, may result in an accumulation of 5-HT at the synapse analogous to the increased availability of catecholamines at catecholaminergic receptors following blockade of the reuptake of norepinephrine or dopamine. Negative feedback mechanisms might then be activated, resulting in a decreased turnover of cerebral 5-HT (Corrodi and Fuxe, 1969; Meek and Werdinius, 1970; Schildkraut et al., 1969; Schubert et al., 1970). It is noteworthy in this regard that the tertiary amines chlorimipramine, imipramine, and amitriptyline depress the firing rate of raphe neurons, whereas the secondary amines desipramine and protriptyline have been reported to have either minimal or no depressant effect in equivalent doses (Sheard et al., 1972). The effect of the tertiary amines on the physiology of serotoninergic neurons thus parallels their effect on the blockade of uptake of 5-HT. The data obtained with tricyclic antidepressants on flexor and extensor reflex activity in the rat also support the view that the tertiary amines of tricyclic antidepressants preferentially inhibit the uptake of 5-HT, whereas the secondary amines preferentially inhibit the reuptake of norepinephrine. Thus, chlorimipramine, imipramine, and amitriptyline potentiate the effect of tryptophan and 5-hydroxytryptophan plus nialamide on the hindlimb extensor reflex, while the secondary amines desipramine and protriptyline are weak potentiators of this response but cause a marked potentiation of the effect of L-dopa on the hindlimb flexor reflex (Lidbrink et al., 1971; Meek et al., 1970).

Tuomisto (1974) has provided evidence that the molecular requirements for the 5-HT (but not the catecholamine) uptake mechanism in platelets and brain are very close to one another, supporting the conclusion that platelets may be used as a model for studies on serotonergic but not on catecholaminergic mechanisms. Ross et al. (1972) have devised a convenient double-labeling technique for determining the simultaneous uptake or inhibition of

TABLE 5

Effect of Thymoleptics on 5-HT Displacement in Brain by H 75/12 and on NA Displacement in Brain and Heart by H 77/77: ED_{50} (mg/kg)[a]

Drug	Brain 5-HT	Brain NA	Heart NA
Imipramine·HCl	20	>25	12
Desipramine·HCl	>50	15	6
Chlorimipramine·HCl	7	>25	20
Chlordesipramine	20	—	—
Amitriptyline·HCl	12	>25	14
Nortriptyline·HCl	20	>25	15
N-Methylprotriptyline·HCl	>25	—	—
Protriptyline·HCl	>25	4	4

[a] From Carlsson et al. (1969a).

uptake of 5-HT and norepinephrine in brain slices. While the uptake mechanism appears to be rather specific at low concentrations of amines, at high concentrations, considerable uptake of 5-HT into noradrenergic neurons and of norepinephrine into serotonergic neurons may, however, occur (Shaskan and Snyder, 1970). The study of norepinephrine uptake by brain slices or synaptosomes is further complicated by the existence of a highly active catecholamine transport system in dopaminergic neurons (Snyder and Coyle, 1969; Coyle and Snyder, 1969). The tricyclic antidepressants and other currently available antidepressants do not, however, inhibit the uptake of dopamine (Horn et al., 1971; Fuxe and Ungerstedt, 1968) with the exception of the new tetrahydroisoquinoline derivative nomifensine, which, in addition to being an effective inhibitor of norepinephrine uptake, proved to be approximately twice as active as benztropine in blocking the uptake of dopamine (Hunt et al., 1974), and it is claimed to exert therapeutic antidepressant activity.

The question whether the clinical antidepressant activity is more closely related to the effect of the drugs on noradrenergic or on serotonergic neurons is difficult to answer, as some of the antipsychotic drugs have also been reported to exert potent blocking effects on both systems (Lahti and Maickel, 1971; Tuomisto, 1974). In general, however, it appears that secondary amines cause predominantly an increase in the level of psychomotor activation and drive, whereas tertiary amines exert predominantly mood-elevating properties. It thus is possible that the former is associated with an increase in noradrenergic (blockade of norepinephrine uptake) and the latter with an increase in serotonergic (blockade of 5-HT uptake) activity (Carlsson et al., 1969a,b). If differences in the relative degree of inhibition of norepinephrine and 5-HT uptake are indeed of clinical significance, the availability of and controlled clinical trials with more selective inhibitors such as maproptiline (Ludiomil), nisoxetine, and fluoxetine (see Table 2) should provide a more definite answer to this problem. Thus, maproptiline is an antidepressant drug which does not interfere with the uptake of 5-HT in brain in vivo, only slightly inhibits its uptake in rat brain synaptosomal preparations in vitro, but exerts a potent inhibitory effect on the uptake of norepinephrine in several sympathetically innervated organs in the rat, including brain (Mâitre et al., 1971, 1974). Nisoxetine is also a specific inhibitor of norepinephrine uptake comparable in potency to that of secondary amines of tricyclic antidepressants, but unlike fluoxetine, to which it is structurally related, it does not affect uptake into 5-HT neurons (Fuller et al., 1975). Studies with fluoxetine suggest this drug to be a selective competitive inhibitor of the uptake of 5-HT (Fig. 4) into synaptosomes of rat brain comparable in its potency to chlorimipramine (Wong et al., 1975). Moreover, the drug is also a selective inhibitor of uptake of 5-HT in specific brain regions in vivo, and, interestingly, N-demethylation of fluoxetine to its primary amine does not alter either its potency or selectivity toward inhibiting uptake of 5-HT (Fig. 5).

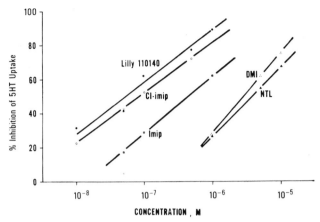

FIG. 4. Inhibition of 5-HT uptake into synaptosomes of rat brain by fluoxetine and tricyclic antidepressant drugs. Synaptosomes of 1 mg of protein were incubated in the presence of 10^{-7} M serotonin. Mean control values of 5-HT uptake were 6.13 ± 0.23 pmol/mg per 3 min. (Lilly 110140) Fluoxetine; (Cl-imip) chlorimipramine; (Imip) imipramine; (DMI) desipramine; (NTL) nortriptyline. From Wong *et al.* (1975).

3. MODE OF INTERACTION OF TRICYCLIC ANTIDEPRESSANTS WITH ADRENERGIC MECHANISMS

The predominant current view of the mode of action of tricyclic antidepressants is that this class of drugs enhances noradrenergic activity by blocking the reuptake of norepinephrine through the neuronal membrane in peripheral and central noradrenergic neurons (Axelrod *et al.*, 1961; Dengler

FIG. 5. Inhibition of the uptake of nor-epinephrine into rat hearts by tricyclic antidepressants and the ineffectiveness of fluoxetine and desmethylfluoxetine. [^{14}C]Norepinephrine at 5 μCi/kg was injected intravenously through the tail vein at 1 hr after the administration of each drug. The animals were sacrificed 30 min therafter and the hearts analyzed for [^{14}C]norepinephrine. (DMI) Desipramine; (IMIP) imipramine; (Cl-DMI) chlordesi-pramine; (Cl-IMIP) chlorimipramine; (110140) fluoxetine; (103947) desmethyl-fluoxetine. From Wong *et al.* (1975).

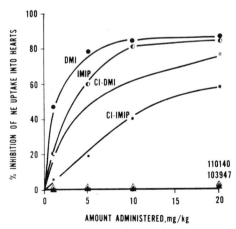

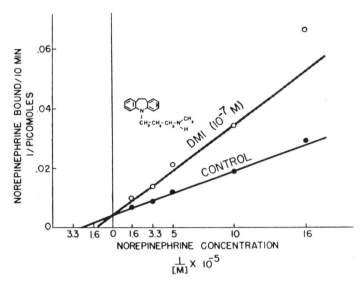

FIG. 6. Reciprocal plots of the relationship between rate of uptake of norepinephrine into aorta and the concentration of [³H]norepinephrine in the tissue bath in the presence and absence of desipramine (DMI). From Maxwell *et al.* (1969).

et al., 1961; Glowinski and Axelrod, 1965; Carlsson and Waldeck, 1965*a,b*; Giachetti and Shore, 1966), resulting in an increased availability of the physiologically active amine at postsynaptic receptor sites and in an increased concentration of the *O*-methylated metabolite of norepinephrine, normetanephrine. Tricyclic antidepressants act as competitive inhibitors (Fig. 6) of the high-affinity uptake mechanism (uptake$_1$) for norepinephrine (Berti and Shore, 1967; Maxwell *et al.*, 1969). Uptake$_1$ is a saturable process, stereochemically selective for 1-norepinephrine, and involves a sodium/potassium-dependent carrier system dependent on metabolic energy and on the functioning of the sodium/potassium-stimulated ATP-ase (Iversen, 1967, 1973; Bogdanski *et al.*, 1968; Bogdanski and Brodie, 1969).

Since MAO inhibitors are also known to antagonize the reserpine-like syndrome (Burns and Shore, 1961) and to increase normetanephrine, the possibility existed that tricyclic antidepressants might interfere with the oxidative deamination of norepinephrine and of other biogenic amines. Many studies have demonstrated, however, that tricyclic antidepressants do not block MAO *in vivo* (Pulver *et al.*, 1960; Pletscher and Gey, 1962; Sulser *et al.*, 1962, 1964), though the drugs have been shown to be very weak reversible MAO inhibitors *in vitro* (Wagner *et al.*, 1975).

The blockade of the high-affinity uptake of norepinephrine by tricyclic antidepressants can satisfactorily explain the potentiation of exogenous norepinephrine or of norepinephrine released by nerve stimulation, the antagonism of the reserpine-like syndrome with the resulting shift in autonomic activity which has been shown to depend on the availability of brain catecholamines (Sulser *et al.*, 1964) as well as on their rapid release from storage sites (Sulser and Soroko, 1965). The finding that reserpine-like drugs released more metaraminol (which is not a substrate of either MAO or COMT) from hearts after pretreatment with tricyclic antidepressants (Carlsson and Waldeck, 1965*a* Murad and Shore, 1966) can also be interpreted to be the consequence of blockade of the neuronal uptake mechanism. Studies by Giachetti and Shore (1966) have provided a convenient method for differentiating between the two amine-concentrating mechanisms (Carlsson and Waldeck, 1965*a,b*) and their sensitivity to drugs. Thus, a substance inhibiting the uptake of metaraminol may be presumed to act on the neuronal membrane pump (tricyclic antidepressants), while a drug not inhibiting the uptake of metaraminol but blocking the uptake of *m*-octopamine may be presumed to act on the intracellular storage mechanism (reserpine). Recently, evidence has been provided by Sulser *et al.* (1969) that tricyclic antidepressants exert a blocking action on norepinephrine reuptake in brain *in vivo* (Fig. 7). While the effects of tricyclic antidepressants on uptake mechanisms through the neuronal membrane represent the main site of action in adrenergic neurons, some studies have indicated that these drugs may also impair the intraneuronal amine-concentrating mechanism of storage vesicles. Thus, when slices of various brain areas (except caudate nucleus) were incubated with [³H]tyramine, it was found that desipramine given *in*

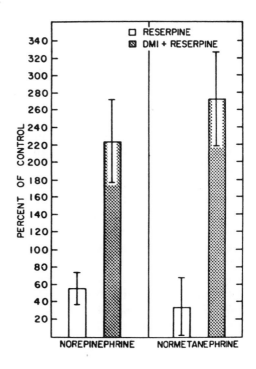

FIG. 7. Modification by desipramine of the effect of reserpine on the release of [³H]norepinephrine and [³H]normetanephrine into the perfusate from the hypothalamus. Desipramine (10 mg/kg i.p.) was administered 1 hr before reserpine (5 mg/kg i.p.). Results of the first postreserpine hour are expressed as a percentage of those for the desipramine control period ± S.E. Desipramine control mean [³H]norepinephrine, 4.25 ± 0.36 nCi/hr; [³H]normetanephrine, 0.5 ± 0.09 nCi/hr. From Sulser *et al.* (1969).

vivo or added *in vitro* inhibited the synthesis of [³H]octopamine but not the uptake, retention, and oxidative deamination of [³H]tyramine (Steinberg and Smith, 1970). Since desipramine does not inhibit dopamine-β-hydroxylase, the data may indicate that the drug prevented the uptake of [³H]tyramine into the storage granules where tyramine is converted by dopamine-β-hydroxylase to octopamine. Leitz (1970) studied the effect of desipramine on metaraminol-induced release of norepinephrine from heart slices and found that the tricyclic antidepressant reduced the release of norepinephrine to a much greater extent than it blocked the uptake of metaraminol. Since the release of norepinephrine and the uptake of metaraminol were stoichiometrically related, the results indicate that desipramine not only reduced the uptake of metaraminol but also acted within the neuron to prevent metaraminol from releasing norepinephrine.

While the interaction of tricyclic antidepressants with adrenergic (and serotoninergic) mechanisms is an established fact and can satisfactorily explain many of the pharmacologic actions, various aspects of drug interactions, and side effects of this group of drugs, the question arises whether or not these mechanisms contribute to or are responsible for the therapeutic efficacy in depressive illness. Clinical improvement requires treatment for weeks, whereas the pharmacologic effects of tricyclic antidepressants on adrenergic neurons, e.g., blockade of uptake of norepinephrine, occur within minutes or hours. It is thus of interest that differences in the turnover of norepinephrine following acute and chronic administration of tricyclic antidepressants have been reported (Schildkraut *et al.*, 1970, 1971). The turnover of the catecholamine in brain (as measured by the disappearance of [³H]norepinephrine from brain) was decreased after the acute administration of tricyclic antidepressants but increased during chronic treatment with these drugs. However, since the level of tritiated norepinephrine in brain was measured at one time only, it is difficult to accurately compute the turnover rate of the endogenous amine. Moreover, when *in vivo* turnover rates were estimated from the conversion of [¹⁴C]tyrosine to labeled catecholamines (Costa and Neff, 1970), it was found that chronic administration of tricyclic antidepressants actually decreases the turnover rate of norepinephrine in brain (Rosloff, 1975).

Although it cannot be assumed *a priori* that all tricyclic antidepressants have to elicit their therapeutic effect through one common mechanism, studies with a new tricyclic antidepressant, iprindole, have nevertheless further clouded the issue. Iprindole is a clinically effective tricyclic antidepressant (Ayd, 1969; Hicks, 1965; McClatchey *et al.*, 1967; Sterlin *et al.*, 1968; Rickels *et al.*, 1973), but, unlike imipramine-like drugs, this tricyclic antidepressant does not block the neuronal uptake of norepinephrine (Gluckman and Baum, 1969; Lemberger *et al.*, 1970; Lahti and Maickel, 1971; Freeman and Sulser, 1972; Rosloff and Davis, 1974) or of 5-HT (Ross *et al.*, 1971; Rosloff and Davis, 1974), and it does not alter the metabolism of norepinephrine (Freeman and Sulser, 1972) or its turnover when given

TABLE 6

Effect of Iprindole and Desipramine (DMI) on the Uptake and Metabolism of [³H]Norepinephrine in the Rat Heart[a]

Radioactivity measured	Control	Iprindole	DMI
Total radioactivity (TR)	100 ± 12	104 ± 5	10 ± 1[b]
[³H]Norepinephrine (NE)	100 ± 12	105 ± 5	7 ± 1[b]
[³H]Normetanephrine (NMN)	100 ± 12	126 ± 13	21 ± 2[b]
[³H]Deaminated catechol metabolites (DCM)	100 ± 15	92 ± 9	25 ± 3[b]
[³H]Deaminated O-methylated metabolites (DOM)	100 ± 6	89 ± 4	81 ± 3[c]

[a] Desipramine (10 mg/kg i.p.) and iprindole (10 mg/kg i.p.) were administered 90 min before intravenous injection of 100 μCi [³H]NE/kg. Animals were sacrificed 90 min after the administration of the labeled amine. The results are expressed as a percentage of the control values ± S.E.M. Control mean values: TR = 401 nCi; NE = 365 nCi; NMN = 12 nCi; DCM = 8 nCi; DOM = 15 nCi. $N = 6$. From Freeman and Sulser (1972).
[b] $p < 0.001$.
[c] $p < 0.05$.

chronically (Rosloff and Davis, 1974). In accordance with this lack of action of iprindole on amine-uptake mechanisms (Table 6), the drug does not potentiate the blood pressure response to norepinephrine or inhibit the pressure response to intravenous tyramine in human subjects (Fann *et al.*, 1972). Although such data do cast serious doubts on the general validity of the hypothesis that a blockade of the neuronal uptake mechanism of norepinephrine (or 5-HT or both) is a prerequisite for the antidepressant activity of tricyclic antidepressants, they do not rule out an interaction with noradrenergic mechanisms, e.g., at the receptor level (see Section 5). Iprindole, like other tricyclic antidepressants, potentiates the awakening effect of L-dopa in reserpinized mice (Ross *et al.*, 1971), which indicates that iprindole is able to potentiate the responses of catecholamines through a mechanism other than through inhibition of their uptake (Fig. 8). Studies by Ross *et al.* (1971) with opipramol point in the same direction. This tricyclic antidepressant also lacks inhibitory effects on the uptake of norepinephrine in mouse heart (Lahti and Maickel, 1971) and on norepinephrine and 5-HT in brain slices of the mouse, but potentiates the awakening effect of L-dopa in mice.

4. INTERACTION OF TRICYCLIC ANTIDEPRESSANTS WITH OTHER DRUGS

Stone *et al.* (1964) have shown that a number of tricyclic antidepressants (protriptyline, imipramine, amitriptyline, desipramine, nortriptyline) can

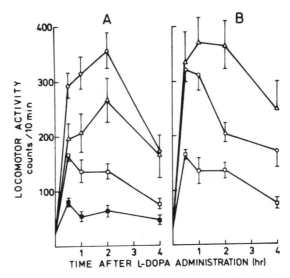

FIG. 8. Potentiation of the awakening effect of L-dopa in reserpinized mice. Reserpine (5 mg/ kg i.p.) was given 24 hr, the test drug 1 hr, and Ro 4-4602, a peripheral decarboxylase inhibitor (50 mg/kg i.p.), 30 min before L-dopa (100 mg/kg i.p.). (■) Controls, without Ro 4-4602; (□) controls, with Ro 4-4602; (△) iprindole; (○) iprindole: (A) 10 mg/kg i.p.; (B) 25 mg/kg i.p. From Ross *et al.* (1971).

prevent the adrenergic neuron blockade caused by guanethidine and reduce its depletion of catecholamines in peripheral organs. Since the guanethidine-induced postganglionic sympathetic blockade was prevented by prior administration of tricyclic antidepressants but could not be reversed, once established, it is likely that the drugs interfered with the uptake of guanethidine into the neuron, thus limiting its access to the norepinephrine storage sites. Carlsson and Waldeck (1965a,b) have demonstrated that tricyclic antidepressants do interfere with the uptake of hydrophilic amines (e.g., guanethidine and metaraminol) by blocking the transport mechanism localized in the cell membrane. The available evidence indicates that this is the same specialized transport system by which norepinephrine and other biogenic amines are taken up into neuron terminals. The blockade of this rather unspecific transport system through the neuronal membrane by tricyclic drugs has clinical consequences. For example, the antihypertensive effect of guanethidine, bethanidine, and debrisoquin can be nullified by the simultaneous administration of tricyclic antidepressants (Leishman *et al.*, 1963; Mitchell *et al.*, 1967, 1970). Pretreatment with a tricyclic antidepressant prevents the antihypertensive effect of guanethidine-like drugs. It is of interest that the administration of tricyclic antidepressants in the recommended dosage results in restoration of the blood pressure to or near the level prior to the institution of the antihypertensive therapy and that the effect persists after the drug is discontinued.

However, tricyclic antidepressants can enhance or prolong various behavioral effects elicited by amphetamine (Carlton, 1961; Stein and Seifter, 1961; Scheckel and Boff, 1964; Halliwell *et al.*, 1964; Sulser *et al.*, 1964). Typical examples are shown in Figs. 9 and 10. Sulser *et al.* (1966) first demonstrated that the potent action of desipramine in enhancing and prolonging the locomotor stimulation of amphetamine in the rat is associated with a striking increase in the concentration of amphetamine in brain. A number of investigators have since confirmed these data and have provided convincing evidence that this action of desipramine-like drugs is the consequence of an inhibition of the *para*-hydroxylation of amphetamine (Consolo

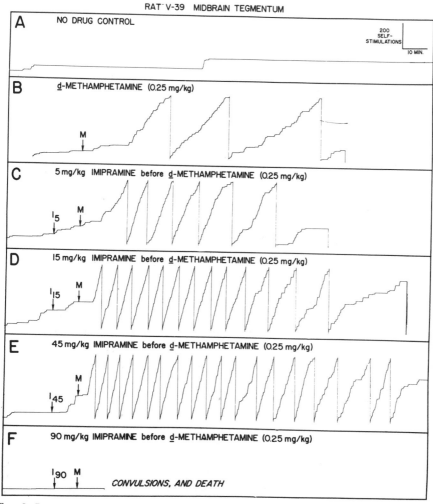

Fig. 9. Potentiation of the facilitating effect of methamphetamine on self-stimulation by various doses of imipramine. From Stein (1962).

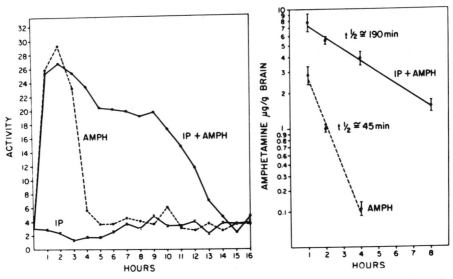

FIG. 10. Effect of iprindole on CNS stimulation elicited by *d*-amphetamine (*left*) and on the half-life of [³H]*d*-amphetamine in brain (*right*). CNS stimulation (locomotor and stereotyped activity) was measured in Williamson activity cages and is expressed as mean counts per hour. Vertical bars represent the standard deviation of the mean. *N* = 4–6. Iprindole (IP), 10 mg/kg i.p., was given 30 min before *d*-amphetamine or [³H]*d*-amphetamine (AMPH), 5 mg/kg. From Freeman and Sulser (1972).

et al., 1967; Valzelli *et al.*, 1967; Groppetti and Costa, 1969; Lewander, 1969). It could still be argued, however, that tricyclic antidepressants enhance the action of amphetamine by blocking the reuptake of catecholamines, which are released by increased amounts of amphetamine onto adrenergic receptor sites. Recent studies with iprindole have weakened this argument. This antidepressant shares with imipramine-like antidepressants the ability both to enhance and prolong various central actions of amphetamine and to markedly inhibit the metabolism of amphetamine (Fig. 10 and Table 7). This inhibition of the metabolism of amphetamine by iprindole appears to be the sole factor involved in the interaction of the two drugs because iprindole does not block the neuronal uptake of norepinephrine (see Table 6) or alter the metabolism of intraventrically administered [³H]norepinephrine (Freeman and Sulser, 1972). Thus, in animals pretreated with iprindole, the levels of amphetamine in brain and heart were increased manyfold over those of control animals and the concentration of *p*-hydroxynorephedrine formed from amphetamine was markedly reduced. Pretreatment with iprindole also reduced total *p*-hydroxyamphetamine (free and conjugated) in the urine to negligible amounts after the administration of amphetamine (Freeman and Sulser, 1972). *In vitro* studies to unravel the precise mechanism of this important drug interaction have been hampered because neither the *d* nor the *l* isomer of amphetamine is metabolized by microsomal preparations of rat liver (Dingell and Bass, 1969).

TABLE 7

Effect of Iprindole (IP) on P-Hydroxylation of Amphetamine (AMPH) and Accumulation of p-Hydroxynorephedrine (PHN) in Rat Brain[a]

Treatment	2 hr		8 hr		12 hr		24 hr	
	AMPH	PHN	AMPH	PHN	AMPH	PHN	AMPH	PHN
Saline + AMPH	962 ± 55	24 ± 3	60 ± 10	17 ± 1	27 ± 0.1	16 ± 1	5 ± 0.1	13 ± 0.8
IP + AMPH	6066 ± 132[b]	6 ± 4[c]	1309 ± 41[b]	3 ± 3[b]	689 ± 115[b]	3 ± 1[b]	41 ± 4[b]	1 ± 0.2[b]

[a] Iprindole (10 mg/kg i.p.) was given ½ hr prior to [^{3}H]dl-amphetamine (5 mg/kg i.p.). The animals were sacrificed at various times after the administration of amphetamine. $N = 4$–8. Results are expressed in ng/g ± S.E. From Freeman and Sulser (1972).
[b] $P < 0.001$.
[c] $P < 0.01$.

In contrast to the enhancement by tricyclic antidepressants of many central actions of amphetamine, peripheral effects of this indirectly acting sympathomimetic amine are reduced or blocked by tricyclic antidepressants (Sigg, 1959; Bonaccorsi and Hrdina, 1967; Schmitt and Schmitt, 1970). Since imipramine-like drugs inhibit the metabolism of amphetamine to p-hydroxyamphetamine and p-hydroxynorephedrine, it is conceivable that these hydroxylated metabolites might mediate the peripheral (e.g., cardiovascular) effects of amphetamine (Sulser and Sanders-Bush, 1970; Clay et al., 1971; Ross and Renyi, 1971). This hypothesis has been disproved, however, since the tricyclic antidepressant iprindole, which is a potent inhibitor of the aromatic hydroxylation of amphetamine (Freeman and Sulser, 1972), does not block the blood pressure response to amphetamine in the rat (Freeman and Sulser, 1975). Since low concentrations of amphetamine are transported into the noradrenergic neuron via the amine-transport mechanism of the cell membrane, tricyclic antidepressants obviously interfere with the uptake of amphetamine (Obianwu et al., 1968; Lundborg and Waldeck, 1971; Azzaro et al., 1974). The mechanism responsible for the differences in the interaction of tricyclic antidepressants with amphetamine in the peripheral (blockade of its action) and central sympathetic nervous system (enhancement of its action) remains to be elucidated.

Tricyclic antidepressants have since been shown to inhibit the metabolism of a number of other drugs, e.g., guanethidine (Mitchell et al., 1970), tremorine, oxotremorine, pentobarbital and hexobarbital (Kato et al., 1963; Sjöqvist et al., 1968; Shah and Lal, 1971), and propranolol (Shand and Oates, 1971).

5. EFFECT OF TRICYCLIC ANTIDEPRESSANTS ON ADAPTIVE REGULATION AT PRE- AND POSTSYNAPTIC SITES

The heuristic catecholamine hypothesis of affective disorders (Schildkraut, 1965; Schildkraut and Kety, 1967) is derived chiefly from studies on acute pharmacologic effects elicited by a number of clinically effective psychotropic drugs, including the tricyclic antidepressants, on synaptic mechanisms such as catecholamine storage, release, reuptake, and metabolism. The catecholamine hypothesis of affective disorders does not take into account, however, the discrepancy in the time course between biochemical and pharmacologic effects elicited by tricyclic antidepressants within minutes and hours and the clinical therapeutic action, which requires treatment for weeks. Segal et al. (1974) have recently reported adaptive changes in the activity of tyrosine hydroxylase, which are inversely correlated with prolonged changes in catecholamine-mediated neuron transmission following the chronic administration of reserpine and tricyclic antidepressants. Thus, repeated administration of desipramine for 8 days produced a significant decrease in the activity of tyrosine hydroxylase in the locus coeruleus and hippocampus–cortex area, but only a marginal decrease in the activity of the enzyme in the caudate nucleus, a predominantly dopaminergic area (Fig. 11). No significant change in enzyme activity was observed 24 hr following the administration of desipramine. Such adaptive changes in the biosynthetic capacity can explain the decrease in the level of norepinephrine observed following chronic (Schildkraut *et al.*, 1970, 1971; Roffler-Tarlov *et al.*, 1973) but not acute administration of tricyclic antidepressants (Sulser *et al.*, 1962, 1964). Such data are also compatible with the finding of a decreased turnover rate of norepinephrine following chronic administration of tricyclic antidepressants (Rosloff, 1975) and might explain the clinical findings that chronic treatment with tricyclic antidepressants does not reverse the low level of metabolites of biogenic amines in the CSF of endogenously depressed patients (Goodwin *et al.*, 1975).

In general, the activity of adrenergic neurons is regulatable by drugs by intraneuronal or interneuronal feedback mechanisms chiefly involving regulation of catecholamine synthesis (Weiner, 1970; Segal *et al.*, 1973; Costa *et al.*, 1974). Results from our laboratory have recently provided evidence for

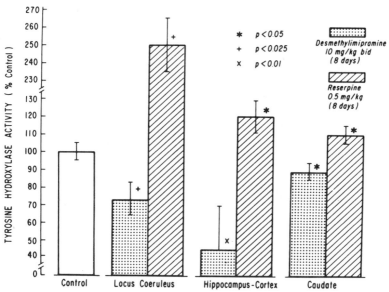

FIG. 11. Opposite effects of repeated administration of desmethylimipramine and of reserpine on tyrosine-hydroxylase activity in discrete brain regions of the rat. Each bar represents the mean percentage ± S.E.M. of corresponding controls. From Segal *et al.* (1974).

an additional regulatory mechanism in the CNS involving the noradrenergic adenylate cyclase receptor system that adapts its sensitivity to the neurotransmitter norepinephrine in a manner inversely related to the degree of its stimulation by the catecholamine (Vetulani *et al.*, 1976a). The administration of tricyclic antidepressants on a clinically more relevant time basis led to a marked reduction in the sensitivity of the cAMP-generating system to norepinephrine (Table 8) regardless of the action of the drugs on presynaptic sites (Vetulani *et al.*, 1976b). Thus, desipramine, a blocker of norepinephrine uptake, shares this effect with iprindole, which does not effect neuronal reuptake of the catecholamine or alter its metabolism or turnover. Moreover, this delayed action elicited by tricyclic antidepressants on noradrenergic receptor sensitivity is not related to the concentration of the tricyclic antidepressants in brain and appears to be a common mechanism of action of all clinically effective treatments for depression, including MAO inhibitors and electroconvulsive treatment (Vetulani and Sulser, 1975; Vetulani *et al.*, 1976a). The therapeutic action of tricyclic antidepressants may thus be related to the slowly developing adaptive changes in the sensitivity of the noradrenergic receptor system, rather than to their acute action on presynaptic sites. This interpretation is compatible with the recent suggestion by Segal *et al.* (1974) that "the depression prone patient has catecholamine receptors with heightened responsiveness." An adaptive reduction in this responsiveness by pharmacotherapy would then lead to clinical improvement in patients suffering from depression.

TABLE 8

Effect of Long-Term Treatment (4–8 Weeks) with Desipramine or Iprindole on the Response of the cAMP-Generating System in the Rat Limbic Forebrain to Norepinephrine[a]

Treatment	Time of sacrifice (hr)[b]	N	Basal level of cAMP (pmol/mg protein ± S.E.M.)	cAMP response to NE[c]	Percentage of control response
Control	1 or 24	15	17.8 ± 2.6	20.4 ± 2.7	100
Desipramine	1	12	20.5 ± 2.7	9.9 ± 3.5[d]	49
	24	14	16.6 ± 1.6	6.9 ± 2.1[e]	34
Iprindole	1	13	22.3 ± 3.6	9.4 ± 4.7[d]	46
	24	15	16.9 ± 1.5	7.9 ± 2.4[f]	38

[a] Desipramine and iprindole (hydrochlorides) were injected daily in a dose of 10 mg/kg i.p. The controls received saline. From Vetulani *et al.* (1976b).
[b] Time after last injection.
[c] Difference in the level of cAMP between the preparation exposed to 5 μM norepinephrine and that of the control preparation (corresponding hemisection).
[d] $P < 0.05$.
[e] $P < 0.001$.
[f] $P < 0.01$.

6. METABOLIC FATE OF TRICYCLIC ANTIDEPRESSANTS

Since imipramine is the prototype of the tricyclic antidepressants, its metabolism has been the object of a number of investigations. Herrmann and his associates (Herrmann et al., 1959; Herrmann and Pulver, 1960; Herrmann, 1963) demonstrated first that imipramine is metabolized by N-demethylation and hydroxylation with the subsequent formation of glucuronides (Fig. 12). Imipramine N-oxide has been isolated from the urine of patients who were treated with imipramine (Fishman and Goldenberg, 1962) and has been found to be a minor metabolite in the rat (Bickel and

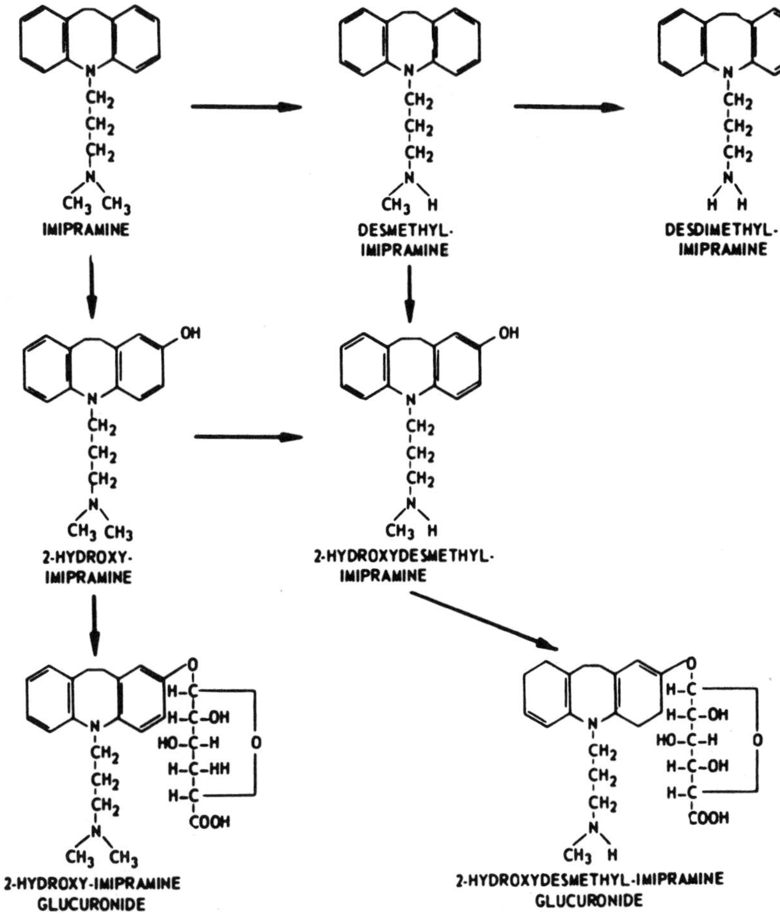

FIG. 12. Major pathways of imipramine metabolism. From Dingell et al. (1964).

Baggiolini, 1966). The identification of this metabolite is of some interest, as it has been postulated that N-oxides are intermediate products in the dealkylation of alkylamines (Fish *et al.*, 1956). Bickel *et al.* (1968) have demonstrated that imipramine-N-oxide is reduced to imipramine and to a minor degree demethylated to desipramine (DMI) by tissue homogenates or blood in the absence of added cofactors. Other investigators concluded, however, that imipramine-N-oxide may not be involved as an intermediate in the formation of desipramine from imipramine (Nakazawa, 1970). Gillette *et al.* (1961) isolated a metabolite of imipramine from rat brain and identified it as the secondary amine desipramine (DMI). Studies on the fate of imipramine labeled in one of the methyl groups with ^{14}C have confirmed the importance of demethylation in the metabolism of the drug (Bernhard and Beer, 1962). Considerable demethylation occurs with a number of other tertiary amines of tricyclic antidepressants (chlorimipramine, amitriptyline, trimeprimin), whereas this process is much less pronounced in the case of the corresponding desmethyl derivatives (Bickel *et al.*, 1967). A comprehensive study by Bickel and Weder (1968) revealed the presence of at least 14 metabolites in the rat following the administration of imipramine; the major metabolites were desipramine, imipramine-N-oxide, 2-hydroxyimipramine, 2-hydroxydesipramine, and their glucuronide conjugates.

Although demethylation and hydroxylation are the major pathways of imipramine metabolism, the relative contribution of each varies markedly from species to species. Dingell *et al.* (1962, 1964) have investigated the metabolism of imipramine in various species both *in vivo* and *in vitro*. While rat liver microsomal preparations metabolize the tertiary amine imipramine mainly to the secondary amine desipramine, which is slowly oxidized to other products, rabbit liver microsomes oxidize imipramine to 2-hydroxyimipramine and metabolize desipramine more rapidly than imipramine. These species differences in the metabolism of imipramine and desipramine by liver microsomes are reflected in the fate of the drugs *in vivo*. Rabbits and mice metabolize imipramine and desipramine at about the same rates. In rats, however, desipramine disappears more slowly than its tertiary amine imipramine. Consequently, desipramine accumulates in tissues of rats, but not in those of rabbits or mice, following the administration of imipramine. It is noteworthy that desipramine also accumulates in human tissues after the ingestion of imipramine (Dingell *et al.*, 1964).

Imipramine is metabolized mainly in the liver and to a very minor extent in lung and kidney (Minder *et al.*, 1971). Interestingly, Dingell and Sanders (1966) found that a transferase system which is present in the lungs of rabbits, but not in those of rats, can methylate desipramine to imipramine. Although this methylation of desipramine is a minor route of metabolism, it is conceivable that species differences in this metabolic pathway in nonhepatic tissues may work in concert with differences in the metabolism by liver microsomal enzymes.

Studies on the metabolic fate of amitriptyline have shown that N-demethylation and hydroxylation are also the major metabolic reactions for this tricyclic antidepressant (Hucker and Porter, 1961; Hucker, 1962; Cassano et al., 1965a,b). Imipramine and amitriptyline are hydroxylated, however, at different positions on the molecule. The hydroxylation of imipramine occurs mainly in the 2 position of the aromatic ring, forming phenolic metabolites, whereas amitriptyline is hydroxylated at the ethylene bridge, thus forming the alcoholic metabolites 10-hydroxy- and 10,11-dihydroxyamitriptyline. McMahon et al. (1963) have investigated the metabolism of the secondary amine nortriptyline. About 40% of the dose of the drug administered to rats undergoes hydroxylation at the 10 position of the ethylene bridge and is excreted in the urine as conjugates. Only a small percentage is N-demethylated to the primary amine, which is in agreement with the results obtained with the secondary amine of imipramine. 10-Hydroxynortriptyline and 10-hydroxydesmethylnortriptyline have also been identified in human urine, plasma, and CSF following treatment with nortriptyline (Hammar et al., 1971; Knapp et al., 1972). Although little is presently known about the metabolism of some of the newer tricyclic antidepressants, their structural similarity to imipramine and amitriptyline suggests that N-demethylation or hydroxylation or both would also be the major pathways of their metabolism.

7. SOME GENERAL CONSIDERATIONS ON N-DEMETHYLATION OF TRICYCLIC ANTIDEPRESSANTS

Since both pharmacologic and biochemical profiles of the secondary amines of tricyclic antidepressants differ quantitatively and qualitatively from those of the corresponding tertiary amines, any of the multitude of factors which are known to alter hepatic drug metabolism (Burns et al., 1965; Conney, 1967) could alter the observed response to this type of drug by altering the ratio of the tertiary to the secondary amine at the site of action. With regard to altering adrenergic function, the ultimate pharmacologic effect of a tricyclic antidepressant will thus depend on the relative potency of the parent drug and of its major metabolite in blocking the reuptake of norepinephrine into the neuron (enhanced noradrenergic response) and in blocking noradrenergic receptor sites (decreased noradrenergic response). Thus, Häefely et al. (1964) have shown that the tertiary amine of a dibenzocycloheptatriene derivative (RO-41577) decreases the effect of sympathetic nerve stimulation, while the corresponding secondary amine (RO-46011) enhances this response. Stone et al. (1964) have shown that the secondary amines desipramine, nortriptyline, and protriptyline are potent antagonists of the guanethidine-induced adrenergic neuron blockade, while the corresponding tertiary amines imipramine and amitriptyline, like the phenothiazine derivative chlorpromazine, failed to exhibit this antagonism. With regard to central noradrenergic mechanisms, Sulser et al. (1962) observed that the secondary amine desipramine prevented the reserpine-like syndrome elicited by RO-41284 when the levels of desipramine in brain were quite low. However, after relatively high doses of the tertiary amine imipramine were administered, a marked antagonism of the reserpine-like syndrome was observed only when the level of desipramine in brain was several times that of imipramine. Moreover, metabolism *in vivo* by *N*-demethylation will also substantially alter the potency of the drugs in blocking the uptake of serotonin and lead to desmethyl metabolites with more pronounced effects on the uptake of norepinephrine. As discussed earlier, the phenoxyphenyl propylamine derivative fluoxetine represents an exception to this rule (Fuller et al., 1975).

The marked differences between tertiary and secondary amines of tricyclic antidepressants in modifying noradrenergic or serotonergic neuronal systems, or both, may determine their clinical profile and their indication in retarded depressions (secondary amines) or depressions characterized by symptoms of anxiety and agitation (tertiary amines).

8. MISCELLANEOUS PHARMACOLOGIC EFFECTS OF TRICYCLIC ANTIDEPRESSANTS

The tricyclic antidepressants exert anticholinergic effects both peripherally and centrally (Domenjoz and Theobald, 1959; Sulser and Watts, 1960; Vernier et al., 1962; Halliwell et al., 1964; Gluckman and Baum, 1969) and thus show similarities to the structurally related phenothiazines and antihistaminic agents. In contrast to the rather weak peripheral anticholinergic effects of tricyclic antidepressants, the reserpine-induced increased central parasympathetic output (Bogdanski et al., 1961) is particularly sensitive to blockade by imipramine-like drugs, and this blockade appears to be central in origin (Sulser and Watts, 1960; Sulser et al., 1964). Since adrenergic synaptic mechanisms may exert an inhibitory effect on central parasympathetic activity, tricyclic antidepressants, may antagonize the reserpine-induced increase in parasympathetic activity by increasing the availability of norepinephrine in the vicinity of parasympathetic nuclei of the brain, thus increasing the noradrenergic inhibitory brake (Sigg and Sigg, 1967). Biochemically, desipramine has been reported to decrease the "bound" acetylcholine fraction in brain, while reserpine significantly increased the amount of "bound" acetylcholine in whole brain (Hrdina and Ling, 1973). However, there appears to be no correlation between antireserpine and central cholinolytic action elicited by tricyclic antidepressants, (Lapin, 1967; Metỹs and Metỹsova, 1967). While the anticholinergic properties of tricyclic antidepressants can satisfactorily explain many of the side effects observed in man (e.g., dry mouth, difficulty in accommodation), their role in the mechanism of therapeutic action is not clear.

Because of the structural similarity of tricyclic antidepressants to several potent antihistaminics, it is not surprising that the antihistaminic properties of certain tricyclic antidepressants are quite substantial (Domenjoz and Theobald, 1959; Vernier et al., 1962; Theobald et al., 1964), but the antihistamine potency of these drugs does not seem to parallel their clinical efficacy.

Karobath (1975) examined a number of tricyclic antidepressants as inhibitors of the dopamine-sensitive adenylate cyclase in a cell-free homogenate of rat brain striatum. Amitriptyline and doxepin were found to be potent inhibitors of this enzyme, about as potent as butyrophenones (Clement-Cormier et al., 1974; Karobath and Leitich, 1974), but less potent than antipsychotic drugs of the phenothiazine class. Interestingly, in slices of guinea pig cerebral cortex, tricyclic antidepressants have been reported to cause an enhanced accumulation of cAMP (Huang and Daly, 1972), an effect which these drugs share with antipsychotic and nonantipsychotic phenothiazine derivatives. Present evidence suggests that these compounds cause an enhanced accumulation of extracellular adenosine, which then stimulates the accumulation of cAMP. Tricyclic antidepressants have also been reported to inhibit the activity of phosphodiesterase in rat brain (McNeill and Muschek, 1970; Weinryb et al., 1972). The significance of these miscellaneous biochemical effects elicited by tricyclic antidepressants on adenylate cyclase–phosphodiesterase systems remains to be elucidated.

9. REFERENCES

AHTEE, L., and SAARNIVARA, L., 1971, The effect of drugs upon the uptake of 5-hydroxytryptamine and metaraminol by human platelets, J. Pharm. Pharmacol. 23:495–501.

AXELROD, J., WHITBY, L. G., and HERTTING, G., 1961, Effect of psychotropic drugs on the uptake of ³H-norepinephrine by tissues, Science 133:383–384.

AYD, F. J., 1969, Clinical evaluation of a new tricyclic antidepressant, iprindole, Dis. Nerv. Syst. 30:818–824.

AZZARO, A. J., ZIANCE, R. J., and RUTLEDGE, C. O., 1974, The importance of neuronal uptake of amines for amphetamine-induced release of ³H-norepinephrine from isolated brain tissue, J. Pharmacol. Exp. Ther. 189:110–118.

BABBINI, M., MISSERE, G., and TONINI, G., 1961, Imipramine, chlorpromazine and central nervous system stimulants, in: Techniques for the Study of Psychotropic Drugs (G. Tonini, ed.), pp. 89–90, Societa Tipografica Modenese, Modena.

BENESOVA, O., BOHDANECKI, Z., and VOTAVA, Z., 1962, Electro-physiological comparison of the action of imipramine and propazepine, Psychopharmacologia 3:423–431.

BERNHARD, K., and BEER, H., 1962, Aktivitäten der Exspirations Kohlensäure, des ZNS and anderer Organe nach Gaben von C^{14} Signiertem N-(γ-dimethylaminopropyl) iminodibenzyl (Tofranil) an Ratten und Hunde, *Helv. Physiol. Pharmacol. Acta* **20**:114–121.

BERTI, F., and SHORE, P. A., 1967, A kinetic analysis of drugs that inhibit the adrenergic neuronal membrane amine pump, *Biochem. Pharmacol.* **16**:2091–2094.

BESENDORF, H., STEINER, F. A., and HÜRLIMANN, A., 1962, Laroxyl, a new antidepressant with sedative effects, *Schweiz. Med. Wochenschr.* **92**:244–246.

BICKEL, M. H., 1968, Untersuchungen zur Biochemie und Pharmakologie dei Thymoleptica, in: *Progress in Drug Research* (E. Jucker, ed.), Birkhäuser Verlag, Basel and Stuttgart.

BICKEL, M. H., and BAGGIOLINI, M., 1966, The metabolism of imipramine and its metabolites by rat liver microsomes, *Biochem. Pharmacol.* **15**:1155–1169.

BICKEL, M. H., and WEDER, H. J., 1968, The total fate of a drug: Kinetics of distribution, excretion and formation of 14 metabolites in rats treated with imipramine, *Arch. Int. Pharmacodyn, Ther.* **173**:433–463.

BICKEL, M. H., FLÜCKIGER, M., and BAGGIOLINI, M., 1967, Vergleichende Demethylierung von Tricyclischen Psychopharmaka durch Rattenlebermikrosomen, *Arch. Pharmakol. Exp. Pathol.* **256**:360–366.

BICKEL, M. H., WEDER, H. J., and AEBI, H., 1968, Metabolic intercorrelations between imipramine, its N-oxide, and its desmethyl derivative in rat tissue *in vitro, Biochem. Biophys. Res. Commun.* **33**:1012–1018.

BOGDANSKI, D. F., and BRODIE, B. B., 1969, The effects of inorganic ions on the storage and uptake of H^3-norepinephrine by rat heart slices, *J. Pharmacol. Exp. Ther.* **165**:181–189.

BOGDANSKI, D. F., SULSER, F., and BRODIE, B. B., 1961, Comparative action of reserpine, tetravenazine and chlorpromazine on central parasympathetic activity, *J. Pharmacol Exp. Ther.* **132**:176–182.

BOGDANSKI, D. F., TISSARI, A., and BRODIE, B. B., 1968, The effects of inorganic ions on uptake, storage and metabolism of biogenic amines in nerve endings, in: *Psychopharmacology—A Review of Progress* (D. H. Efron, ed.), pp. 17–26, U.S. Government Printing Office, Washington, D.C.

BONACCORSI, A., and HRDINA, P., 1967, Interactions between desipramine and sympathomimetic agents on the cardiovascular system, in: *Antidepressant Drugs* (S. Garattini and M. N. G. Dukes, eds.), pp. 149–157, Excerpta Medica, Amsterdam.

BORELLA, L. E., HERR, F., and WOJDAN, A., 1969a, Prolongation of certain effects of amphetamine by chlorpromazine. *Can. J. Physiol. Pharmacol.* **47**:7–13.

BORELLA, L. E., PAQUETTE, R., and HERR, F., 1969b, The effect of some CNS depressants on the hypermotility and anorexia induced by amphetamine in rats, *Can. J. Physiol. Pharmacol.* **47**:841–847.

BRADLEY, P. B., and KEY, B. J., 1959, A comparative study of the effects of drugs on the arousal system of the brain, *Br. J. Pharmacol.* **14**:340–349.

BUNNEY, W. E., and DAVIS, J. M., 1965, Norepinephrine in depressive reactions, *Arch. Gen. Psychiatry* **13**:483–494.

BURNS, J. J., and SHORE, P. A., 1961, Biochemical effects of drugs, *Annu. Rev. Pharmacol.* **1**:79–104.

BURNS, J. J., CUCINELL, S. A., KOSTER, R., and CORNEY, A. H., 1965, Application of drug metabolism to drug toxicity studies, *Ann. N. Y. Acad. Sci.* **123**:273–286.

CAIRNCROSS, K. D., 1965, On the peripheral pharmacology of amitriptyline, *Arch. Int. Pharmacodyn. Ther.* **154**:438–448.

CARLSSON, A., and WALDECK, B., 1965a, Inhibition of ^{3}H-metaraminol uptake by antidepressive and related agents, *J. Pharm. Pharmacol.* **17**:243–244.

CARLSSON, A., and WALDECK, B., 1965b, Mechanism of amine transport in the cell membranes of the adrenergic nerves, *Acta Pharmacol. Toxicol.* **22**:293–300.

CARLSSON, A., FUXE, K., HAMBURGER, B., and LINDQVIST, M., 1966, Biochemical and histochemical studies on the effects of imipramine-like drugs and (+)-amphetamine on central and peripheral catecholamine neurons, *Acta Physiol. Scand.* **67**:481–497.

CARLSSON, A., CORRODI, H., FUXE, K., and HÖKFELT, T., 1969*a*, Effect of antidepressant drugs on the depletion of intraneuronal brain 5-hydroxytryptamine stores caused by 4-α-ethyl-metatyramine, *Eur. J. Pharmacol.* **5**:357–366.

CARLSSON, A., CORRODI, H., FUXE, K., and HÖKFELT, T., 1969*b*, Effect of antidepressant drugs on the depletion of intraneuronal brain 5-hydroxytryptamine stores caused by 4-α-dimethyl-metatyramine, *Eur. J. Pharmacol.* **5**:367–373.

CARLTON, P. L., 1961, Potentiation of the behavioral effect of amphetamine by imipramine, *Psychopharmacologia* **2**:364–376.

CASSANO, G. B., SJÖSTRAND, S. E., and HANSSEN, E., 1965*a*, Distribution and fate of C^{1} amitriptyline in mice and rats. *Psychopharmacologia* **8**:1–11.

CASSANO, G. B., SJÖSTRAND, S. E., and HANSSEN, E., 1965*b*, Distribution of C^{14} amitriptyline in the cat brain, *Psychopharmacologia* **8**:12–22.

CLAY, G. A., CHO, A. K., and ROBERFROID, M., 1971, Effect of diethylaminoethyl diphenyl-propylacetate hydrochloride (SKF 525A) on the norepinephrine depleting actions of *d*-amphetamine, *Biochem. Pharmacol.* **20**:1821–1831.

CLEMENT-CORMIER, Y. C., KEBABIAN, J. W., PETZOLD, G. L., and GREENGARD, P., 1974, Dopamine sensitive adenylate cyclase in mammalian brain: A possible site of action of antipsychotic drugs, *Proc. Natl. Acad. Sci. U.S.A.* **71**:1113–1117.

CONNEY, A. H., 1967, Pharmacological implications of microsomal enzyme induction, *Pharmacol. Rev.* **19**:317–366.

CONSOLO, S., DOLFINI, S., GARATTINI, S., and VALZELLI, L., 1967, Desipramine and amphetamine metabolism, *J. Pharm. Pharmacol.* **19**:253–256.

CORRODI, H., and FUXE, K., 1969, Decreased turnover in central 5-HT nerve terminals induced by antidepressant drugs of the imipramine type, *Eur. J. Pharmacol.* **7**:56–59.

COSTA, E., 1973, Pharmacological implications of the changes of brain monoamine turnover rates elicited by (+)-amphetamine and some related compounds, in: *Psychopharmacology, Sexual Disorders and Drug Abuse* (T. A. Ban *et al.*, eds.), pp. 637–658, North-Holland Publishing Co., Amsterdam.

COSTA, E., and GARATTINI, S., (eds.), 1970, *International Symposium on Amphetamines and Related Compounds*, Raven Press, New York.

COSTA, E., and NEFF, N. H., 1970, Estimation of turnover rates to study the metabolic regulation of the steady-state level of neuronal monoamines, in: *Handbook of Neurochemistry*, Vol. 4 (A. Lajtha, ed.), pp. 45–90, Plenum Press, New York.

COSTA, E., GARATTINI, S., and VALZELLI, L., 1960, Interactions between reserpine, chlorpromazine and imipramine, *Experientia* **16**:461–463.

COSTA, E., GUIDOTTI, A., and ZIVKOVIC, B., 1974, Short and long term regulation of tyrosine hydroxylase, *Adv. Biochem. Psychopharmacol.* **12**:161–175.

COYLE, J. T., and SNYDER, S. H., 1969, Catecholamine uptake by synaptosomes in homogenates of rat brain: Stereospecificity in different areas, *J. Pharmacol. Exp. Ther.* **170**:221–231.

D'ENCARNACACO, P. S., and ANDERSON, K., 1970, Effect of lithium pretreatment on amphetamine and DMI tetrabenazine produced psychomotor behavior, *Dis. Nerv. Syst.* **31**:494–496.

DENGLER, H., SPIEGEL, H. E., and TITUS, E. O., 1961, Effects of drugs on uptake of isotopic norepinephrine by cat tissues, *Nature (London)* **191**:816–817.

DINGELL, J. V., and BASS, A. D., 1969, Inhibition of the hepatic metabolism of amphetamine by desipramine, *Biochem. Pharmacol.* **18**:1535–1537.

DINGELL, J. V., and SANDERS, E., 1966, Methylation of desmethylimipramine by rabbit lung *in vitro*, *Biochem. Pharmacol.* **15**:599–605.

DINGELL, J. V., SULSER, F., and GILLETTE, J. R., 1962, Metabolism of imipramine in rats and rabbits, *Fed. Proc. Fed. Am. Soc. Exp. Biol.* **21**:184.

DINGELL, J. V., SULSER, F., and GILLETTE, J. R., 1964, Species differences in the metabolism of imipramine and desipramine, *J. Pharmacol. Exp. Ther.* **143:**14–23.

DOLFINI, E., TANSELLA, M., VALZELLI, L., and GARATTINI, S., 1969, Further studies on the interaction between desipramine and amphetamine, *Eur. J. Pharmacol.* **5:**185–190.

DOMENJOZ, R., and THEOBALD, W., 1959, Zur Pharmakologie des Tofranil, *Arch. Int. Pharmacodyn. Ther.* **120:**450–489.

FANN, W. E., DAVIS, J. M., JANOWSKY, D. S., KAUFMANN, J. S., GRIFFITH, J. D., and OATES, J. A., 1972, Effect of iprindole on amine uptake in man, Arch. Gen. Psychiatry **26:**158–162.

FISCHBACH, R., HARRER, G., and HARRER, H., 1966, Verstärkung der Noradrenalin-wirkung durch Psychopharmaka beim Menschen, *Arzneim. Forsch.* **2**(a):263–265.

FISH, M. S., SWEELEY, C. C., JOHNSON, N. M., LAWRENCE, E. P., and HORNING, E. C., 1956, Chemical and enzymic rearrangements of N,N-demethylamino acid oxides, *Biochim. Biophys. Acta* **21:**196–197.

FISHMAN, V., and GOLDENBERG, H., 1962, Identification of a new metabolite of imipramine, *Proc. Soc. Exp. Biol. Med.* **110:**187–190.

FREEMAN, J. J., and SULSER, F., 1972, Iprindole–amphetamine interactions in the rat: The role of aromatic hydroxylation of amphetamine in its mode of action, *J. Pharmacol. Exp. Ther.* **183:**307–315.

FREEMAN, J. J., and SULSER, F., 1975, The role of parahydroxylation of amphetamine in its peripheral mode of action, *J. Pharm. Pharmacol.* **27:**38–42.

FULLER, R. W., SNODDY, H. D., and MOLLOY, B. B., 1975, Blockade of amine depletion by nisoxetine in comparison to other uptake inhibitors, *Psychopharmacol. Res. Commun.* **1:**455–464.

FUXE, J., and UNGERSTEDT, U., 1968, Histochemical studies on the effect of (+)-amphetamine, drugs of the imipramine group and tryptamine on central intraventricular injection of catecholamines and 5-hydroxytryptamine, *Eur. J. Pharmacol.* **4:**135–144.

GARATTINI, S., GIACHETTI, A., TORI, A., PIERI, L., and VALZELLI, L., 1962, Effect of imipramine, amitriptyline and their monomethylderivatives on reserpine activity, *J. Pharm. Pharmacol.* **14:**509–514.

GIACHETTI, A., and SHORE, P. A., 1966, Studies *in vitro* of amine uptake mechanisms in heart, *Biochem. Pharmacol.* **15:**607–614.

GILLETTE, J. R., DINGELL, J. V., SULSER, F., KUNTZMAN, R., and BRODIE, B. B., 1961, Isolation from rat brain of a metabolic product, desmethylimipramine, that mediates the antidepressant activity of imipramine, *Experientia* **17:**417–418.

GLOWINSKI, J., and AXELROD, J., 1965, Effect of drugs on the uptake, release and metabolism of norepinephrine in the rat brain, *J. Pharmacol. Exp. Ther.* **149:**43–49.

GLUCKMAN, M. I., and BAUM, T., 1969, The pharmacology of iprindole, a new antidepressant, *Psychopharmacologia* **15:**169–185.

GOODWIN, F. K., SACK, R. L., and POST, R. M., 1975, Clinical evidence for neurotransmitter adaptation in response to antidepressant therapy, in: *Neurobiological Mechanisms of Adaptations and Behavior* (A. J. Mandell, ed.), pp. 33–45, Raven Press, New York.

GROPPETTI, A., and COSTA, E., 1969, Tissue concentrations of p-hydroxynorephedrine in rats injected with d-amphetamine: Effect of pretreatment with desipramine, *Life Sci.* **8:**653–665.

HÄEFELY, W., HÜRLIMANN, A., and THOENEN, H., 1964, Scheinbar paradoxe Beeinflussung von peripheren Noradrenalin Wirkungen durch einige Thymoleptica, *Helv. Physiol. Pharmacol. Acta* **22:**15–33.

HÄFLIGER, F., 1959, Chemistry of Tofranil, *Can. Psychiatry Assoc. J.* **4:**S69–S74.

HÄFLIGER, F., and BURCKHARD, V., 1964, Iminodibenzyl and related compounds, in: *Psychopharmacological Agents*, Vol. 1 (M. Gordon, ed.), pp. 35–101, Academic Press, New York.

HALLIWELL, G., QUINTON, R. M., and WILLIAMS, F. E., 1964, A comparison of imipramine, chlorpromazine and related drugs in various tests involving autonomic functions and antagonism of reserpine *Br. J. Pharmacol.* **23:**330–350.

HAMMAR, C. G., ALEXANDERSON, B., HOLMSTEDT, B., and SJÖQVIST, F., 1971, Gas chromatography–mass spectrometry of nortriptyline in body fluids of man, *Clin. Pharmacol. Ther.* **12:**496–505.

HERRMANN, B., 1963, Quantitative Methoden zur Untersuchung des Stoffwechsels von Tofranil, *Helv. Physiol. Pharmacol. Acta* **21:**402–408.

HERRMANN, B., and PULVER, R., 1960, Der Stoffwechsel des Psychopharmakons Tofranil, *Arch. Int. Pharmacodyn. Ther.* **126:**454–469.

HERRMANN, B., SCHINDLER, W., and PULVER, R., 1959, Paper chromatographic determination of metabolic products of Tofranil, *Med. Exp.* **1:**381–385.

HICKS, J. T., 1965, Iprindole, a new antidepressant for use in general office practice, *Ill. Med. J.* **128:**622–626.

HIMWICH, H. E., BRUNE, G., STEINER, W., and KOHL, H., 1964, A pharmacological study of terminal methyl groups in animals, *Adv. Biol. Psychiatry* **6:**196–207.

HORN, A. S., COYLE, J. T., and SNYDER, S. H., 1971, Catecholamine uptake by synaptosomes from rat brain: Structure–activity relationships of drugs with differential effects on dopamine and norepinephrine neurons, *Mol. Pharmacol.* **7:**66–80.

HRDINA, R. D., and LING, G. M., 1973, Effects of desipramine and reserpine on "free" and "bound" acetylcholine in rat brain, *J. Pharm. Pharmacol.* **25:**504–507.

HUANG, M., and DALY, J. W., 1972, Accumulation of cyclic adenosine monophosphate in incubated slices of brain tissue. 1. Structure–activity relationships of agonist and antagonists of biogenic amines and of tricyclic tranquilizers and antidepressants, *J. Med. Chem.* **15:**458–462.

HUCKER, H. B., 1962, Metabolism of amitriptyline, *Pharmacologist* **4:**171.

HUCKER, H. B., and PORTER, C. C., 1961, Studies on the metabolism of amitriptyline, *Fed. Proc. Fed. Am. Soc. Exp. Biol.* **20:**172.

HUNT, P., KANNENGIESSER, M. H., and RAYNAUD, J. P., 1974, Nomifensine: A new potent inhibitor of dopamine uptake into synaptosomes from rat brain corpus striatum, *J. Pharm. Pharmacol.* **26:**370–371.

IVERSEN, L. L., 1967, *The Uptake and Storage of Noradrenaline in Sympathetic Nerves,* Cambridge University Press, London.

IVERSEN, L. L., 1973, Neuronal and extraneuronal catecholamine uptake mechanisms, in: *Frontiers of Catecholamine Research* (E. Usdin and S. H. Snyder, eds.), pp. 403–408, Pergamon Press, New York.

IZQUIERDO, J. A., COUSSIO, J. D., and KAUMANN, A. J., 1962, Effect of imipramine on the pressor responses to the afferent vagal stimulation in reserpinized dogs, *Arch. Int. Pharmacodyn. Ther.* **135:**303–310.

JORI, A., and GARATTINI, S., 1965, Interaction between imipramine-like agents and catecholamine induced hyperthermia, *J. Pharm. Pharmacol.* **17:**480–488.

KAROBATH, M. E., 1975, Tricyclic antidepressive drugs and dopamine sensitive adenylate cyclase from rat brain striatum, *Eur. J. Pharmacol.* **30:**159–163.

KAROBATH, M. E., and LEITICH, H., 1974, Antipsychotic drugs and dopamine stimulated adenylate cyclase prepared from corpus striatum of rat brain, *Proc. Natl. Acad. Sci. U.S.A.* **71:**2915–2918.

KATO, R., CHIESARA, E., and VASSANELLI, P., 1963, Mechanism of potentiation of barbiturates and meprobamate actions by imipramine, *Biochem. Pharmacol.* **12:**357–364.

KLERMAN, G. L., and COLE, J. O., 1965, Clinical pharmacology of imipramine and related antidepressant compounds, *Pharmacol. Rev.* **17:**101–141.

KNAPP, D. R., GAFFNEY, T. E., McMAHON, R. E., and KIPLINGER, G., 1972, Studies of human urinary and biliary metabolites of nortriptyline with stable isotope labeling, *J. Pharmacol. Exp. Ther.* **180:**784–790.

KUHN, R., 1957, Über die Behandlung depressiver Zustände mit einem Iminodibenzylderivat (G-22355), *Schweiz. Med. Wochenschr.* **87:**1135–1140.

KUHN, R., 1958, The treatment of depressive states with G-22355 (imipramine hydrochloride), *Am. J. Psychiatry* **115**:459–464.

KULKARNI, A. S., and BOCKNIK, S. E., 1973, Interaction of Ro 4-1284 with doxepin, amitriptyline and desmethylimipramine on mouse avoidance behavior, *Eur. J. Pharmacol.* **22**:59–63.

LAHTI, R. A., and MAICKEL, R. P., 1971, The tricyclic antidepressants—Inhibition of norepinephrine uptake as related to potentiation of norepinephrine and clinical efficacy, *Biochem. Pharmacol.* **20**:482–486.

LAPIN, I. P., 1967, Comparison of antireserpine and anticholinergic effects of antidepressants and of central and peripheral cholinolytics, in: *Antidepressant Drugs* (S. Garattini and M. N. G. Dukes, eds.), pp. 266–278, Excerpta Medica, Amsterdam.

LEISHMAN, A. W. D., MATTHEW, H. L., and SMITH, A. J., 1963, Antagonism of guanethidine by imipramine, *Lancet* **1**:112.

LEITZ, F. H., 1970, Mechanisms by which amphetamine and desipramine inhibit the metaraminol-induced release of norepinephrine from sympathetic nerve endings in rat heart, *J. Pharmacol. Exp. Ther.* **173**:152–157.

LEMBERGER, L., SERNATINGER, E., and KUNTZMAN, R., 1970, Effect of desmethylimipramine, iprindole and DL-erythro-α-(3,4-dichlorophenyl)-β-(*t*-butylamino) propanol HCl on the metabolism of amphetamine, *Biochem. Pharmacol.* **11**:3021–3028.

LEW, C., and IVERSEN, S. D., 1971, Effects of imipramine, desipramine, and monoamine oxidase inhibitors on the metabolism and psychomoter stimulant actions of *d*-amphetamine in mice, *Eur. J. Pharmacol.* **14**:351–359.

LEWANDER, T., 1969, Influence of various psychoactive drugs on the *in vivo* metabolism of *d*-amphetamine in the rat, *Eur. J. Pharmacol.* **6**:38–44.

LIDBRINK, P., TOUSSAN, G., and FUXE, K., 1971, The effect of imipramine-like drugs and antipsychotic drugs on uptake mechanisms in the central noradrenaline and 5-hydroxytryptamine neurons, *Neuropharmacology* **10**:521–536.

LOEW, D., 1964, Untersuchungen über die aminpotenzierenden Wirkungen von antidepressiv wirkenden Stoffen am Kaninchen, *Med. Exp.* **11**:333–351.

LUNDBORG, P., and WALDECK, B., 1971, On the mechanism of amphetamine induced release of reserpine-resistant ^{3}H-noradrenaline and ^{3}H-α-methylnoradrenaline, *Acta Pharmacol. Toxicol.* **30**:339–347.

MÂITRE, L., STAEHELIN, M., and BEIN, H. J., 1971, Blockade of noradrenaline uptake by 34276-Ba, a new antidepressant drug, *Biochem. Pharmacol.* **20**:2169–2186.

MÂITRE, L., WALDMEIER, P. C., BAUMANN, P. A., and STAEHELIN, M., 1974, Effect of maproptiline, a new antidepressant drug, on serotonin uptake, *Adv. Biochem. Psychopharmacol.* **10**:297–304.

MARTIN, W. R., RIEHL, J. L., and UNNA, K. R., 1960, Chlorpromazine. III. The effects of chlorpromazine and chlorpromazine sulfoxide on vascular responses to 1-epinephrine and levarterenol, *J. Pharmacol. Exp. Ther.* **130**:37–45.

MATUSSEK, N., and RÜTHER, E., 1965, Wirkungsmechanismus der Reserpin—Umkehr mit Desmethylimipramine, *Med. Pharmakol. Exp.* **12**:217–225.

MAXWELL, R. A., KEENAN, P. D., CHAPLIN, E., ROTH, B., and ECKHARDT, S. B., 1969, Molecular features affecting the potency of tricyclic antidepressants and structurally related compounds as inhibitors of the uptake of tritiated norepinephrine by rabbit aortic strips, *J. Pharmacol. Exp. Ther.* **166**:320–329.

McCLATCHEY, W. T., MOFFAT, T., and IRVINE, G. M., 1967, A double blind study of Wy 3263 versus imipramine and placebo, *J. Ther. Clin. Res.* **1**:13–19.

McMAHON, R. E., MARSHALL, F. J., CULP, H. W., and MILLER, W. M., 1963, The metabolism of nortriptyline-*N*-methyl-C^{14} in rats, *Biochem. Pharmacol.* **12**:1207–1217.

McNEILL, J. H., and MUSCHEK, L. D., 1970, Inhibition of brain phosphodiesterase by tricyclic antidepressants, *Clin. Res.* **18**:625–629.

MEDUNA, L. J., ABOOD, L. G., and BIEL, J. H., 1961, N(8-Methyl-aminopropyl)-iminodibenzyl: A new antidepressant, *J. Neuropsychiatry* **2**:232–238.

MEEK, J., and WERDINIUS, B., 1970, 5-Hydroxytryptamine turnover decreased by the antidepressant drug chlorimipramine, *J. Pharm. Pharmacol.* **22**:141–143.

MEEK, J., FUXE, K., and ANDÉN, N. E., 1970, Effect of antidepressant drugs of the imipramine type on central 5-hydroxytryptamine neurotransmission, *Eur. J. Pharmacol.* **9**:325–332.

METYŠ, J., and METYŠOVA, J., 1967, Relationships between antireserpine and central cholinolytic effects of imipramine-like antidepressants, in: *Antidepressant Drugs* (S. Garattini and M. N. G. Dukes, eds.), pp. 255–265, Excerpta Medica, Amsterdam.

MILLER, K. W., FREEMAN, J. J., DINGELL, J. V., and SULSER, F., 1970, On the mechanism of amphetamine potentiation by iprindole, *Experientia* **26**:863–864.

MINDER, R., SCHNETZER, F., and BICKEL, M. H., 1971, Hepatic and extrahepatic metabolism of the psychotropic drugs chlorpromazine, imipramine and imipramine-*N*-oxide, *Naunyn-Schmiedebergs Arch. Pharmakol.* **268**:334–347.

MITCHELL, J. R., ARIAS, L., and OATES, J. A., 1967, Antagonism of the antihypertensive action of guanethidine sulfate by desipramine HCl, *J. Am. Med. Assoc.* **202**:973–976.

MITCHELL, J. R., CAVANAUGH, J. H., ARIAS, L., PETTINGER, W. A., and OATES, J. A., 1970, Guanethidine and related agents. III. Antagonism by drugs which inhibit the norepinephrine pump in man, *J. Clin. Invest.* **49**:1596–1604.

MONNIER, M., and KRUPP, P., 1959, Elektrophysiologische Analyse der Wirkungen verschiedener Neuroleptica (Chlorpromazin, Reserpin, Tofranil, Meprobamat), *Schweiz. Med. Wochenschr.* **89**:430–433.

MÜLLER, J. C., PRYOR, W. W., GIBBONS, J. E., and ORGAIN, E. S., 1955, Depression and anxiety occurring during Rauwolfia therapy, *J. Am. Med. Assoc.* **159**:836–839.

MURAD, J. E., and SHORE, P. A., 1966, Association between biochemical and behavioral actions of tricyclic antidepressants, *Int. J. Neuropharmacol.* **5**:299–304.

NAKAZAWA, K., 1970, Studies on the demethylation, hydroxylation and *N*-oxidation of imipramine in rat liver, *Biochem. Pharmacol.* **19**:1363–1369.

OBIANWU, H. O., STITZEL, R., and LUNDBORG, P., 1968, Subcellular distribution of ³H-amphetamine and ³H-guanethidine and their interaction with adrenergic neurons, *J. Pharm. Pharmacol.* **20**:585–594.

OSBORNE, M., 1962, Interaction of imipramine with sympathomimetic amines and reserpine, *Arch. Int. Pharmacodyn. Ther.* **138**:492–504.

OSBORNE, M., and SIGG, E. B., 1960, Effects of imipramine on the peripheral autonomic system, *Arch. Int. Pharmacodyn. Ther.* **129**:273–289.

PLETSCHER, A., and GEY, K. F., 1962, Action of imipramine and amitriptyline on cerebral monoamines as compared with chlorpromazine, *Med. Exp.* **6**:165–168.

PULVER, R., EXER, B., and HERRMANN, B., 1960, Einige Wirkungen des *N*(γ-dimethylaminopropyl)-imino dibenzyl-HCl und seiner Metabolite auf den Stoffwechsel von Neurohormonen, *Arzneim.-Forsch.* **10**:530–533.

RICKELS, K., CHUNG, H., CSANALOSI, I., SABLOSKY, W., and SIMON, T., 1973, Iprindole and imipramine in non-psychotic depressed outpatients, *Br. J. Psychiatry* **123**:329–339.

ROFFLER-TARLOV, S., SCHILDKRAUT, J. J., and DRASKOCZY, R. R., 1973, Effects of acute and chronic administration of desmethylimipramine on the content of norepinephrine and other monoamines in the rat brain, *Biochem. Pharmacol.* **22**:2923–2926.

ROSLOFF, B. N., 1975, Studies on mechanism of action of tricyclic antidepressant drugs, using iprindole as a tool, Ph.D. thesis, Graduate School, Vanderbilt University.

ROSLOFF, B. N., and DAVIS, J. M., 1974, Effect of iprindole on norepinephrine turnover and transport, *Psychopharmacologia* **40**:53–64.

ROSS, S. B., and RENYI, A. L., 1967, Inhibition of the uptake of tritiated catecholamines by antidepressant and related agents, *Eur. J. Pharmacol.* **2**:181–186.

ROSS, S. B., and RENYI, A. L., 1969, Inhibition of the uptake of tritiated 5-hydroxytryptamine in brain tissue, *Eur. J. Pharmacol.* **7**:270–277.

ROSS, S. B., and RENYI, A. L., 1971, Uptake and metabolism of β-phenethylamine and tyramine in mouse brain and heart slices, *J. Pharm. Pharmacol.* **23**:276–279.

Ross, S. B., Renyi, A. L., and Ogren, S. O., 1971, A comparison of the inhibitory activities of iprindole and imipramine on the uptake of 5-hydroxytryptamine and noradrenaline in brain slices, *Life Sci.* **10:**1267–1277.

Ross, S. B., Renyi, A. L., and Ögren, S. O., 1972, Inhibition of the uptake of noradrenaline and 5-hydroxytryptamine by chlorphentermine and chlorimipramine, *Eur. J. Pharmacol.* **17:**107–112.

Ryall, R. W., 1961, Effects of cocaine and antidepressant drugs on the nictitating membrane of the cat, *Br. J. Pharmacol.* **17:**339–357.

Salama, A. I., Insalaco, J. R., and Maxwell, R. A., 1971, Concerning the molecular requirements for the inhibition of the uptake of racemic ^{3}H-norepinephrine into rat cerebral cortex slices by tricyclic antidepressants and related compounds, *J. Pharmacol. Exp. Ther.* **178:**474–481.

Schaeppi, U., 1960, Beeinflussung der Reizübertragung im peripheren Sympatheticus durch Tofranil, *Helv. Physiol. Pharmacol. Acta.* **18:**545–562.

Scheckel, C. L., and Boff, E., 1964, Behavioral effects of interacting imipramine and other drugs with *d*-amphetamine, cocaine and tetrabenazine, *Psychopharmacologia* **5·**198–208.

Schildkraut, J. J., 1965, The catecholamine hypothesis of affective disorders: A review of supporting evidence, *Am. J. Psychiatry* **122:**509–522.

Schildkraut, J. J., and Kety, S. S., 1967, Biogenic amines and emotion, *Science* **156:**21–30.

Schildkraut, J. J., Schanberg, S. M., Breese, G. R., and Kopin, I. J., 1969, Effects of psychoactive drugs on the metabolism of intracisternally administered serotonin in rat brain, *Biochem. Pharmacol.* **18:**1971–1978.

Schildkraut, J. J., Winokur, A., and Applegate, C. W., 1970, Norepinephrine turnover and metabolism in rat brain after long term administration of imipramine, *Science* **168:**867–869.

Schildkraut, J. J., Winokur, A., Dreskoczy, P. R., and Hensle, J. H., 1971, Changes in norepinephrine turnover in rat brain during chronic administration of imipramine and protriptyline: A possible explanation for the delay in onset of clinical antidepressant effects, *Am. J. Psychiatry* **27:**72–79.

Schmitt, H., and Schmitt, H., 1966, Inhibition de l'hypertension reserpinique postamphetaminique par les substances antidepressives du group de 1'-imipramine, *C. R. Soc. Biol.* **160:**303–306.

Schmitt, H., and Schmitt, H., 1970, Interactions between reserpine and amphetamine on blood pressure, in: *Amphetamines and Related Compounds* (E. Costa and S. Garattini, eds.), pp. 531–550, Raven Press, New York.

Schubert, J., Nyback, H., and Sedvall, J., 1970, Effect of antidepressant drugs on accumulation and disappearance of monoamines formed *in vivo* from labelled precursors in mouse brain, *J. Pharm. Pharmacol.* **22:**136–139.

Segal, D. S., Knapp, S., Kuczenski, R., and Mandell, A. J., 1973, Effects of environmental isolation on behavior and regional rat brain tyrosine hydroxylase and tryptophan hydroxylase activity, *J. Behav. Biol.* **1:**1–8.

Segal, D. S., Kuczenski, R., and Mandell, A. J., 1974, Theoretical implications of drug-induced adaptive regulations for a biogenic amine hypothesis of affective disorder, *Biol. Psychiatry* **9:**147–159.

Shah, H. C., and Lal, H., 1971, The potentiation of barbiturates by desipramine in the mouse: Mechanism of action, *J. Pharmacol. Exp. Ther.* **179:**404–409.

Shand, D. G., and Oates, J. A., 1971, Metabolism of propranolol by rat liver microsomes and its inhibition by phenothiazine and tricyclic antidepressant drugs, *Biochem. Pharmacol.* **20:**1720–1723.

Shaskan, E. G., and Snyder, S. H., 1970, Kinetics of serotonin accumulation into slices from rat brain: Relationship to catecholamine uptake, *J. Pharmacol. Exp. Ther.* **175:**404–418.

Sheard, M. H., Zolovick, A., and Aghajanian, G. K., 1972, Raphe neurons: Effect of tricyclic antidepressant drugs, *Brain Res.* **43:**690–694.

Sigg, E. B., 1959, Pharmacological studies with Tofranil, *Can. Psychiatry Assoc. J.* **4:**S75–S85.

SIGG, E. B., 1968, Tricyclic thymoleptic agents and some newer antidepressants, in: *Psychopharmacology—A Review of Progress* (D. H. Efron, ed.), pp. 655–669, U. S. Government Printing Office, Washington, D.C.

SIGG, E. B., and SIGG, T. D., 1967, Adrenergic modulation of central function, in: *Antidepressant Drugs* (S. Garatini and M. N. G. Dukes, eds.), pp. 172–178, Excerpta Medica, Amsterdam.

SIGG, E. B., SOFFER, L., and GYERMEK, L., 1963, Influence of imipramine and related psychoactive agents on the effect of 5-hydroxytryptamine and catecholamines on the cat nictitating membrane, *J. Pharmacol. Exp. Ther.* **142**:13–20.

SJÖQVIST, R., HAMMER, W., SCHUMACHER, H., and GILLETTE, J. R., 1968, The effect of desmethylimipramine and other "anti-tremorine" drugs on the metabolism of tremorine and oxotremorine in rats and mice, *Biochem. Pharmacol.* **17**:915–934.

SNYDER, S. H., and COYLE, J. T., 1969, Regional difference in H^3-norepinephrine and H^3 dopamine uptake into rat brain homogenates, *J. Pharmacol. Exp. Ther.* **165**:78–86.

SNYDER, S. H., TAYLOR, K. M., COYLE, J. T., and MEYERHOFF, J. L., 1972, The role of brain dopamine in behavioral regulation and the actions of psychotropic drugs, in: *Current Concepts of Amphetamine Abuse*, pp. 3–16, U.S. Government Printing Office, Washington, D.C.

SPENGLER, J., and WASER, P., 1969, Der Einfluss verschiedener Pharmaka auf den Futterkonsum von albino Ratten im akuten Versuch, *Arch. Exp. Pathol. Pharmakol.* **237**:171–177.

STEIN, L., 1962, New methods for evaluating stimulants and antidepressants, in: *Psychosomatic Medicine* (J. H. Nodine and J. H. Moyer, eds.), pp. 297–311, Lea & Febiger, Philadelphia.

STEIN, L., and SEIFTER, J., 1961, Possible mode of antidepressant action of imipramine, *Science* **134**:286–287.

STEIN, L., and WISE, C. D., 1973, Amphetamine and noradrenergic reward pathways, in: *Frontiers in Catecholamine Research* (E. Usdin and S. H. Snyder, eds.), pp. 963–968, Pergamon Press, New York.

STEINBERG, M. I., and SMITH, C. B., 1970, Effects of desmethylimipramine and cocaine on the uptake, retention and metabolism of H^3-tyramine in rat brain slices, *J. Pharmacol. Exp. Ther.* **173**:176–192.

STEINER, W. G., and HIMWICH, H. E., 1963, Effects of antidepressant drugs on limbic structures of rabbit, *J. Nerv. Ment. Dis.* **137**:277–284.

STERLIN, C., LEHMANN, H. E., and OLIVEROS, R. F., 1968, A preliminary investigation of Wy-3263 versus amitriptyline in depressions, *Curr. Ther. Res.* **10**:576–582.

STONE, C., PORTER, C., STAVORSKI, J., LUDDEN, C., and TOTARO, J., 1964, Antagonism of certain effects of catecholamine depleting agents by antidepressants and related drugs, *J. Pharmacol. Exp. Ther.* **144**:196–204.

SULSER, F., and BASS, A. D., 1968, Pharmacodynamic and biochemical considerations of the mode of action of reserpine-like drugs, in: *Psychopharmacology—A Review of Progress* (D. H. Efron, ed.), pp. 1065–1076, U.S. Government Printing Office, Washington, D.C.

SULSER, F., and BICKEL, M. H., 1962, On the role of brain catecholamines in the antireserpine action of desmethylimipramine, *Pharmacologist* **4**:178.

SULSER, F., and BRODIE, B. B., 1961, On mechanism of the antidepressant action of imipramine, *Biochem. Pharmacol.* **8**:48.

SULSER, F., and DINGELL, J. V., 1968, Potentiation and blockade of the central action of amphetamine by chlorpromazine, *Biochem. Pharmacol.* **17**:634–636.

SULSER, F., and SANDERS-BUSH, E., 1970, Biochemical and metabolic considerations concerning the mechanism of action of amphetamine and related compounds, in: *Psychotomimetic Drugs* (D. H. Efron, ed.), pp. 83–94, Raven Press, New York.

SULSER, F., and SANDERS-BUSH, E., 1971, Effect of drugs on amines in the CNS, *Annu. Rev. Pharmacol.* **11**:209–230.

SULSER, F., and SOROKO, F., 1965, On the role of rate of brain norepinephrine release in the antibenzoquinolizine action of desipramine, *Psychopharmacologia* 8:191–200.

SULSER, F., and WATTS, F., 1960, On the anti-reserpine actions of imipramine (Tofranil), in: *Techniques for the Study of Psychotropic Drugs* (G. Tonini, ed.), pp. 85–87, Societa Tipographica Modenese, Modena.

SULSER, F., WATTS, J., and BRODIE, B. B., 1962, On the mechanism of antidepressant action of imipramine-like drugs, *Ann. N. Y. Acad. Sci.* 96:279–286.

SULSER, F., BICKEL, M. H., and BRODIE, B. B., 1964, The action of desmethylimipramine in counteracting sedation and cholinergic effects of reserpine-like drugs, *J. Pharmacol. Exp. Ther.* 144:321–330.

SULSER, F., OWENS, M. L., and DINGELL, J. V., 1966, On the mechanism of amphetamine potentiation by desipramine (DMI), *Life Sci.* 5:2005–2010.

SULSER, F., OWENS, M. L., NORWICH, M. R., and DINGELL, J. V., 1968, The relative role of storage and synthesis of brain norepinephrine in the psychomotor stimulation evoked by amphetamine or by desipramine and tetrabenazine, *Psychopharmacologia* 12:322–332.

SULSER, F., OWENS, M. L., STRADA, S. J., and DINGELL, J. V., 1969, Modification by desipramine of the availability of norepinephrine released by reserpine in the hypothalamus of the rat, *J. Pharmacol. Exp. Ther.* 168:272–282.

THEOBALD, W., BÜCH, O., KUNZ, H., MORPURGO, C., STENGER, E. G., and WILHELMI, G., 1964, Comparative pharmacological studies with Tofranil, Pertofran and Ensidon, *Arch. Int. Pharmacodyn. Ther.* 148:560–596.

THEOBALD, W., BÜCH, O., and KUNZ, H., 1965, Vergleichende Untersuchungen über die Beeinflussung vegetativer Funktionen durch Psychopharmaka im akuten Tierversuch, *Arzneim.-Forsch.* 15:117–125.

THOENEN, H., HÜRLIMANN, A., and HÄEFELY, W., 1964, Mode of action of imipramine and 5-(3'-methylamino propyliden)-dibenzo[a,e]-cyclohepta[1,3,5]trienhydrochloride (Ro 4-6011), a new antidepressant drug, on peripheral adrenergic mechanisms, *J. Pharmacol. Exp. Ther.* 144:405–414.

TODRICK, A., and TAIT, A. C., 1969, The inhibition of human platelets 5-hydroxytryptamine uptake by trycyclic antidepressive drugs. The relation between structure and potency, *J. Pharm. Pharmacol.* 21:751–762.

TUOMISTO, J., 1974, A new modification for studying 5-HT uptake by blood platelets: A re-evaluation of tricyclic antidepressants as uptake inhibitors, *J. Pharm. Pharmacol.* 26:92–100.

VALZELLI, L., CONSOLO, S., and MORPURGO, C., 1967, Influence of imipramine-like drugs on the metabolism of amphetamine, in: *Antidepressant Drugs* (S. Garattini and M. N. G. Dukes, eds.), pp. 61–69, Excerpta Medica, Amsterdam.

VERNIER, V. G., 1961, The pharmacology of antidepressant agents, *Dis. Nerv. Syst.* 12:1–7.

VERNIER, V. G., 1966, Pharmacological evidence of mode of action of antidepressant non-MAO drugs from behavioral and electrophysiological studies, in: *Antidepressant Drugs of Non-MAO Inhibitor Type* (D. H. Efron and S. S. Kety, eds.), pp. 78–99, U.S. Government Printing Office, Washington, D.C.

VERNIER, V. G., HANSON, H., and STONE, C., 1962, The pharmacodynamics of amitriptyline, in: *Psychosomatic Medicine* (J. H. Nodine and L. H. Moyer, eds.), pp. 683–690, Lea & Febiger, Philadelphia.

VETULANI, J., and SULSER, F., 1975, Action of various antidepressant treatments reduces reactivity of noradrenergic cyclic AMP generating system in limbic forebrain, *Nature (London)* 257:495–496.

VETULANI, J., STAWARZ, R. J., and SULSER, F., 1976a, Adaptive mechanisms of the noradrenergic cyclic AMP generating system in the limbic forebrain of the rat: Adaptation to persistent changes in the availability of norepinephrine, *J. Neurochem.* 27:661–666.

VETULANI, J., STAWARZ, R. J., DINGELL, J. V., and SULSER, F., 1976b, A possible common mechanism of action of antidepresant treatments: Reduction in the sensitivity of the noradrenergic cyclic AMP generating system in the rat limbic forebrain, *Naunyn-Schmiedebergs Arch. Pharmacol.* **293**:109–114.

WAGNER, L. A., GAHUDI, H. N., GREEN, R. D., and CLARK, D. E., 1975, *In vitro* and *in vivo* studies on the monoamine oxidase (MAO) inhibitory properties of desmethylimipramine (DMI), *Pharmacologist* **17**:289.

WATTS, J. S., and REILLY, J., 1966, The effect of desmethylimipramine on the activity of certain benzoquinolizines, *Arch. Int. Pharmacodyn. Ther.* **159**:251–257.

WEINER, N., 1970, Regulation of norepinephrine biosynthesis, *Annu. Rev. Pharmacol.* **10**:273–290.

WEINRYB, I., CHASIN, M., FREE, C. A., HARRIS, D. N., GOLDENBERG, H., MICHEL, I. M., PARK, V. S., PHILIPS, M., SAMANIEGO, S., and HESS, S. M., 1972, Effects of therapeutic agents on cyclic AMP metabolism *in vitro, J. Pharm. Sci.* **61**:1556–1567.

WONG, D. T., BYMASTER, F. P., HORNG, F. S., and MOLLOY, B. B., 1975, A new selective inhibitor for uptake of serotonin into synaptosomes of rat brain: 3-(*p*-Trifluoromethyl-phenoxy)-*N*-methyl-3-phenylpropylamine, *J. Pharmacol. Exp. Ther.* **193**:804–811.

5

TRICYCLIC AND MONOAMINE-OXIDASE-INHIBITOR ANTIDEPRESSANTS: CLINICAL USE

David J. Kupfer and Thomas P. Detre

1. INTRODUCTION

Depression, despite the availability of a wide range of biological, pharmacological and psychological therapies, remains a major health problem. The social and economic cost, together with the immense personal and family suffering caused by this recurrent illness have stimulated a number of comparative studies to identify effective treatments. Although progress has undoubtedly been made and hundreds of reports on controlled and uncontrolled clinical trials, and review articles and chapters have been written on this subject (Cole, 1964; Cole and Davis, 1975), information regarding efficacy and choice of antidepressant drug management is surprisingly scant.

That the antidepressant activity of the tricyclics and the MAOIs was discovered accidentally is not just of historical interest; it is also a statement on the current state of the art. Neuropharmacology is still in its infancy. The pharmacologist can study and alter the structure of drugs but cannot, as yet, predict with precision whether a drug will have an ameliorative effect on specific target symptoms. The mode of action of these antidepressants is also on very tenuous ground. We do not have even testable hypotheses as to why the drugs used in the treatment of depression are also effective in a variety of unrelated conditions ranging from asthma and enuresis to chronic pain

David J. Kupfer and Thomas P. Detre • Department of Psychiatry, University of Pittsburgh School of Medicine, and Western Psychiatric Institute and Clinic, Pittsburgh, Pennsylvania.

syndromes (Section 10). Nor do the biological theories of depression have a substantial impact on the classification of affective disorders. Attempts to correlate clinical psychopathological changes or even adverse effects with plasma levels have not yielded very encouraging results. The criteria used for diagnosis, severity of illness, and for defining improvement are inconsistent, and thus the conclusions about outcome and treatment are tentative at best.

Classification systems which have been used for the diagnostic, prognostic, and treatment decisions in affective disorders range from typological models describing discrete discontinuous disease entities to dimensional models assuming a continuum of symptomatology (Strauss, 1973; Klein, 1974). Of the two most widely accepted dichotomous models, one is based on the endogenous/reactive dichotomy and the other on the psychotic/neurotic dichotomy.

Endogenous depressions have been described as episodes occurring most frequently in subjects with obsessive premorbid personality 40 years of age or older with a history of previous mild "attacks." The onset of symptoms is gradual and characterized by sleep continuity disturbances, early morning awakenings, diurnal fluctuations of mood and activity (both of which tend to be more markedly depressed in the morning than in the evening), decreased libido, and impaired appetite with weight loss (Kiloh et al., 1962; Carney et al., 1965; Rosenthal and Klerman, 1966; Rosenthal and Gudeman, 1965). In contrast, the nonendogenous or reactive episodes are said to be precipitated by stressful events and tend to occur in the first three decades of life in subjects with a premorbid personality characterized by hysteroid features, immaturity, feelings of inadequacy and self-pity, irritability, hypochondriasis, and obsessionality. The onset of symptoms is sudden, and the course shows great variability. Typically there is initial insomnia (difficulty falling asleep), and unlike endogenous depressions, mood and activity tend to be more depressed in the evening (Hamilton and White, 1959; Watts, 1957). Critics of this method of classification have pointed out, however, that even if the relationship between stress and the onset of depression could be documented, the judgment of what constitutes a significant precipitating event would have to be highly subjective since over 70% of all depression can be linked to some kind of stressful event.

The psychotic/neurotic dichotomy, the other well-accepted classification schema for affective diseases (Ascher, 1951/52; Mapother, 1926), is supported by evidence that is even shakier than the endogenous/reactive one. It is generally agreed that "neurotic" and "psychotic" refer to different degrees of severity, but adequate definitions of these terms are lacking. First of all, the label "psychotic" implies the presence of an altered ideational process, but it is often nearly impossible to judge at which point self-derogatory views held by a patient are of sufficient intensity to be labeled delusional. Secondly, in many cases, the label neurotic depression is applied to patients who can survive without hospitalization, but this group too is probably a heterogeneous collection of subjects, some of whom are seen early in the course of their illness, others who managed to avoid hospitalization because of an unusually supportive social environment, and yet others whose illnesses are actually mild.

Still another classification schema distinguishes between primary and secondary depression. Robins and Guze (1972), who first proposed this classification, defined primary affective disorder as occurring in individuals with no previous psychiatric disorder (or only episodes of depression or mania), and secondary affective disorder as that which is superimposed on a preexisting psychiatric illness other than depression or mania (Robins and Guze, 1972; Guze *et al.*, 1971; Woodruff *et al.*, 1974). The concept of secondary depression has considerable merit, provided the criteria are sufficiently broad to include depressions occurring in association with toxic, infectious, or exhaustive states (those which may be found following the chronic use of or withdrawal from alcohol and other general CNS depressants, narcotic analgesics or stimulants, or following major surgical procedures and other life-threatening medical conditions). One ambiguity of this classification schema is exemplified by the fact that once a patient receives a diagnosis, for example, of obsessive neurosis, subsequent affective episodes are classified as secondary, even if there has been a period of several years between episodes and the patient is no longer considered to be neurotic. Furthermore, it is at this point not yet known: (1) whether and how many of these patients so diagnosed had a proclivity for depressive symptoms in the past; (2) whether the occurrence of secondary depression means that such episodes will arise in the future only when provoked by similar causes; and (3) whether the treatment response to either tricyclics, MAOI, lithium carbonate, or other drugs is in any way different in secondary depression from treatment response observed with such drugs in primary depression.

Practically all the typologies currently in use also differentiate between "retarded" and "agitated" depression. Since, however, all depressed patients are retarded with regard to thinking, decision-making, and other goal-directed activities, this dichotomization is defensible only if it is restricted to statements regarding the level of motor activity which, much like sleep, is notoriously difficult to measure by observation alone.

Perhaps the most satisfactory approach toward classification has its historical roots in the work of Kraeplin (1921) and has recently been espoused by Leonhard *et al.* (1962), Angst (1966), Perris (1966), and Winokur *et al.* (1969), who distinguish two rather specific genetically determined syndromes: recurrent bipolar cyclic disorder with both manic and depressive phases and a unipolar syndrome which, with the rare exception of unipolar manic illness, presents as recurrent depression (Perris, 1966). Because bipolar and unipolar types can be differentiated in terms of genetic and family history, biochemical and psychophysiological factors, as well as response to certain drugs (Perris, 1971; Kupfer *et al.*, 1975*a*), this classification system is eminently suitable for psychobiological studies.

The strategy adopted in our clinical and research activity is to some extent a synthesis of the clinical trial and clinical practice models (Kupfer *et al.*, 1973, 1975*b*) and emphasizes objectively measurable psychobiologic traits. We differentiate between two major subtypes of depression: (1) the anxious/ hyperactive type (Table 1) is the type most frequently encountered in recurrent unipolar depressions and is characterized by a major sleep continuity disturbance marked by intermittent wakefulness and early morning awakening and increased psychomotor activity; (2) the anergic/hypoactive type of depression (Table 2) occurs primarily but not exclusively in bipolar disorders and is characterized by profound anergia, significant decrease in psychomotor activity; sleep, rather than being discontinuous or decreased, tends to be unchanged or even increased although some difficulty in falling asleep, particularly in younger subjects, may be present. As in the typical anxious/hyperactive group, libido is impaired in the anergic/hypoactive group, but not as dramatically; anorexia, on the other hand, is rarely prominent in the anergic/hypoactive group, indeed, approximately 40% of these patients gain weight while depressed (Kupfer and Foster, 1975). In approximately one third of bipolar patients and in the so-called circular form of manic-depressive disease, the depressive phase is often accompanied by hyperactivity and sleep loss rather than anergia–hypoactivity, and thus these groups should be regarded as "pseudo-bipolar" since from a psychobiological point of view there is no true polarity.

This method of classification preserves the differentiation between unipolar and bipolar as well as primary and secondary affective disorder, but it does away with the retarded vs. agitated, reactive/endogenous, delusional/ nondelusional, neurotic/psychotic dichotomizations. Severity is defined simply in terms of associated impairments in social functioning rather than the presence or absence of delusion or the "need" for hospitalization for it has been repeatedly shown that a decision in favor of inpatient care is often a function of lack of available social support.

Obviously, whatever classification system is used, the natural history regarding the age of onset, number and duration of depressive episodes, the cycle length (i.e., time from the beginning of one episode to the beginning of the next one) are essential both for the management of a given episode and the decision regarding indications for maintenance treatment. After reviewing the charts of more than 1000 hospitalized depressives over a 20-year

TABLE 1

Type	Anxious-Hyperactive Group
Primary	1. Unipolar (including all typical and the abortive juvenile form)
Secondary	1. Depression following abuse of alcohol and other general CNS-depressant states 2. Depression following abuse of narcotic analgesics (including chronic pain syndromes)

TABLE 2

Type	Anergic–Hypoactive Group
Primary	1. Bipolar phasic type circular-cyclothymic circular mixed 2. Unipolar II anergic, atypical
Secondary	1. Postpsychotic depression 2. Depression associated with toxic-infectious exhaustive states 3. Depression following amphetamine abuse including other congeners and cocaine

period, Angst *et al.* (1973) concluded that: (1) the mean age at first onset is significantly lower (30 years) for bipolar than for unipolar disease (43 years); (2) while single episodes in both types are rare and recurrence is the rule, the number of episodes are limited with the mean number being somewhat higher in bipolar (8–9) than in unipolar disease (5–6); (3) the average duration of treated episodes is relatively short (up to three months duration) and shows little intraindividual variations; (4) cycle length tends to decrease from episode to episode in both types, but remains somewhat longer in unipolar (37 months between episode one and two, 22 months between episode two and three) than in bipolar (33 months between episode one and two, 20 months between episode two and three) depression.

Unfortunately, the majority of controlled studies had been completed prior to the nosological advances and thus do not differentiate between unipolar/bipolar or primary/secondary depressions. As a result, while the value of tricyclic and MAOI antidepressants is reasonably well documented, their relative efficacy in the treatment and prophylaxis of different subtypes is on far less secure foundations. Finally, there are only a very few controlled trials comparing drug treatments with psychotherapy or studying the additive effect psychotherapy may have when administered concurrently with drug treatment. The lack of adequate data here is particularly striking given that up to 95% of all depressive episodes occur in patients who were never hospitalized and managed with some form of psychotherapy alone or in combination with drug treatment.

Since all that any effective treatment can achieve is to improve on the "odds" given by the natural history of the disorder in question, neither the diagnostic nor the treatment decision can be based solely on the presenting psychological and somatic symptoms, but must include data on heredity, premorbid personality, character structure, and life history (Bornstein *et al.*, 1973). A severely ill young depressed patient may be easily labeled as schizophrenic on the basis of "end-stage symptoms," unless data on the temporal development of the disorder is obtained. The first attack of depression appearing postsurgically in a patient who had a robust premorbid personality and only one distant relative with a mood disorder is likely to have a different course in treatment than a depressive syndrome developing in a person whose family tree is loaded with recurrent affective disorders. Psychological symptoms which form the basis of most classification systems improvised for drug studies are particularly misleading because symptoms even in the same patient tend to change as he or she moves through the different developmental stages of life.

In order to avoid redundancy, we have not described in this chapter the biochemical models of depression nor the manner in which classification systems developed on these models relate to the efficacy of antidepressants. Suffice it to say that while there is some data to support such a biochemically based classificatory system, these studies are based on too few patients with too much contradictory information and thus it would be premature to comment on the validity and applicability of such a strategy to clinical practice (Fawcett, 1975).

2. TRICYCLIC ANTIDEPRESSANTS: CLINICAL STUDIES

A comprehensive review by Morris and Beck (1974) showed that in 85 controlled trials comparing 93 treatment groups, tricyclic antidepressants were superior to placebo in 60 (40 inpatient and 20 outpatient), indistinguishable in 31 (25 inpatient and 6 outpatient) but in no case was placebo superior in a controlled investigation. To put it simply, 65–70% of all patients who need pharmacotherapy for a depressive episode and meet admission criteria for a controlled clinical investigation are likely to benefit from an adequate dose of a tricyclic antidepressant. Whether tricyclic antidepressants are as effective for outpatients (assumed to be less severely ill) as for inpatients is still debated. Although Angst (1970) argues that tricyclic antidepressants have a greater overall efficacy in inpatients, Morris and Beck did not find any differences in treatment response between inpatients and outpatients. This dispute probably cannot be resolved until the role of attrition is adequately evaluated, which in turn requires a comparison of improvement rates in mildly depressed patients who dropped out of the study with patients who completed the trial.

Actually, there is very little known as to what type of depression is most likely to respond to tricyclics and even less regarding the choice of tricyclic drugs. Kiloh *et al.* (1962) and others noted that patients with features of endogenous depression, particularly when premorbid personality is of a hysterical, irritable, and hypochondriacal type, respond much less favorably. Using a four-class typology to predict response to tricyclics, Paykel (1972) concluded that "psychotic depressives" (patients rated globally as severely ill, but not necessarily "delusional") improve most, anxious depressives the least, and hostile or young depressives with personality disorder somewhere in between.

Since controlled comparisons among the tricyclic compounds have shown that imipramine or amitriptyline are not superior to other tricyclics, stated preferences of one type of tricyclic antidepressant over another are based primarily on clinical impressions (Hippius, 1972). Amitriptyline is said to be more "sedative" and allegedly also more effective in the treatment of "agitated" patients than imipramine. However, as pointed out earlier, the judgment on agitation is not based on any objective evidence. Furthermore, the superiority of amitriptyline might simply be a function of a greater milligram per milligram potency (10–15%) of amitriptyline over imipramine. The same methodological objections apply to the other claims that protriptyline or desmethyl derivatives of amitriptyline and imipramine (nortriptyline and desipramine) tend to be more stimulating and thus should be used in the treatment of "retarded" depression. Nor, for that matter, is there any evidence that doxepin, one of the newer antidepressants has any advantages over either imipramine or amitriptyline in the treatment of "anxious" depression, a term also not further defined (Grof, et al., 1974; Hollister, 1974) (see Table 3). Of two other tricyclics (trimipramine or chlorimipramine) not yet marketed in the United States and less well studied, chlorimipramine has been found effective in some patients who seemed refractory to other tricyclics (Rickels et al., 1974; McClure et al., 1973).

When methods for measuring plasma levels of several tricyclic compounds became available, it was assumed that plasma level concentrations accurately reflect concentrations at the receptor site. Attempts to correlate drug effects with plasma levels have been only partially successful, however (Braithwaite et al., 1972). Burrows (1972), while failing to find a linear relationship between clinical response and plasma nortriptyline levels, reported that a significant relationship could be found when variations of plasma nortriptyline levels within each patient were correlated with their

TABLE 3
Tricyclic Drugs and Their Approximate Effective Dose Ranges

Drug			Effective dose range (mg/day)
Generic name	Trade name	Dosage form	
Imipramine	Tofranil Presamine	Oral or i.m.	150–300
Amitriptyline	Elavil	Oral or i.m.	150–300
Desipramine	Norpramin Pertofran	Oral	150–250
Nortriptyline	Aventyl	Oral	50–100
Protriptyline	Vivactyl	Oral	10–60
Doxepin	Sinequan	Oral	75–200

respective mood scores. Discouraging results also produced appealing, but not yet well-substantiated, supplemental hypotheses such as the so-called "therapeutic window" (Asberg, 1974a). In two studies using nortriptyline, it was noted that maximum nortriptyline antidepressant effect was present when plasma levels ranged between 50 and 170 ng/ml, but very high levels were associated with a decreased and at times a deleterious clinical effect (Asberg, 1974b; Kragh-Sorensen et al., 1973). Since patients with "endogenous depression" require high dosages to produce remissions and since the administration of standard doses of imipramine and nortriptyline are associated with low plasma levels and a high relapse rate (Glassman et al., 1975), it is unclear what dosage should be administered and what plasma levels ought to be maintained both to avoid the dilemma implied in the "therapeutic window" concept and at the same time maintain a prophylactic effect (Kragh-Sorensen et al., 1974).

On the other hand, certain adverse effects seem to correlate satisfactorily with the plasma levels of tricyclics both in depressed patients and in nondepressed volunteers (Asberg et al., 1970). ECG conduction disturbances, for instance, occur with plasma levels exceeding 200 ng/ml nortriptyline. A contrast between impressive and consistent interindividual variation and minimal intraindividual variation lends support to the notion that while environmental factors, among them concomitant treatment with other drugs, can affect the plasma levels, the kinetics of these drugs are to some extent under genetic control. Whether genetic differences in the pharmacokinetics of the tricyclics are independent of or related to the genetic factors which predispose to affective disease is as yet unknown.

3. ADVERSE EFFECTS OF TRICYCLIC ANTIDEPRESSANTS

Given that the majority of untreated depressed patients complain of dry mouth, indigestion, sluggishness, and other somatic symptoms, which are then automatically ascribed to the drugs, it is essential that an inventory of these somatic symptoms be taken prior to the initiation of treatment (Figure 1) (Busfield et al., 1962; Kupfer and Detre, 1971). Furthermore, what constitutes an adverse effect depends on the therapeutic goals. For example, the sedative qualities of tricyclic agents can be quite effective in alleviating insomnia and agitation (Schulterbrandt et al., 1974).

The most frequent and prominent side effects represent an extension of the drug's pharmacologic activity and can be considerably ameliorated by proper management (Table 4) (Medical Letter, 1975a,b; Detre and Jarecki, 1971). Foremost among these is the pronounced anticholinergic activity which is manifested in antimuscarinic (atropinic) effects: blurring of vision (cycloplegia with a loss of accommodation, myopia); acute glaucoma, dryness

F-KDS-2-71

KDS™-2*

USE A NO. 2 PENCIL.   PLEASE ANSWER EVERY ITEM BY SHADING EITHER YES OR NO   DO NOT MARK IN SHADED AREA

| JAN | FEB | MAR | APR | MAY | | JUN | JUL | AUG | SEP | OCT |
| NOV | DEC | | | DATE | | 71 | 72 | 73 | 74 | 75 |

FACILITY CODE

SEX OF PATIENT: MALE ===   FEMALE ===

MARK ONE: AM ===   PM ===   EVENING ===   NIGHT ===

IF ANYBODY HAS PRESCRIBED MEDICATION FOR YOU DURING THE LAST WEEK, PLEASE MAKE SURE YOU REPORT IT.

DO YOU HAVE ANY OF THE FOLLOWING SYMPTOMS?		SYMPTOM	IF YES, DOES IT MAKE YOU VERY UNCOMFORTABLE?		DO YOU HAVE ANY OF THE FOLLOWING SYMPTOMS?		SYMPTOM	IF YES, DOES IT MAKE YOU VERY UNCOMFORTABLE?	
YES	NO	DROWSINESS	YES	NO	YES	NO	DECREASED APPETITE	YES	NO
YES	NO	STIFFNESS OF MUSCLES IN LEGS OR ARMS	YES	NO	YES	NO	SKIN RASH	YES	NO
					YES	NO	BLOODY URINE	YES	NO
YES	NO	VAGINAL DISCHARGE	YES	NO	YES	NO	JAUNDICE (YELLOW DISCOLORATION OF SKIN OR EYES)	YES	NO
YES	NO	SHORTNESS OF BREATH	YES	NO					
YES	NO	BLEEDING GUMS	YES	NO	YES	NO	FEVER	YES	NO
YES	NO	TREMORS OR "SHAKES"	YES	NO	YES	NO	DIFFICULTY STARTING URINATION	YES	NO
YES	NO	DIFFICULTY IN SWALLOWING	YES	NO	YES	NO	FREQUENT URGE TO URINATE	YES	NO
YES	NO	SPASMS OF NECK OR TONGUE	YES	NO	YES	NO	INABILITY TO URINATE	YES	NO
YES	NO	RESTLESSNESS, INABILITY TO BE STILL	YES	NO	YES	NO	LACK OF ENERGY	YES	NO
					YES	NO	IRREGULARITY OR ABSENCE OF MENSTRUAL PERIOD	YES	NO
YES	NO	ITCHING	YES	NO					
YES	NO	POOR MEMORY	YES	NO	YES	NO	NOSEBLEED	YES	NO
YES	NO	DIZZINESS	YES	NO	YES	NO	WEAKNESS IN LEGS OR ARMS	YES	NO
YES	NO	CLUMSINESS	YES	NO	YES	NO	DARK URINE	YES	NO
YES	NO	COLD HANDS OR FEET	YES	NO	YES	NO	PAINS OR CRAMPS IN THE ABDOMEN	YES	NO
YES	NO	NUMBNESS OR TINGLING OF LEGS OR ARMS	YES	NO					
					YES	NO	SWELLING OF BREASTS	YES	NO
YES	NO	FAINTING SPELLS	YES	NO	YES	NO	HISSING NOISES IN EARS	YES	NO
YES	NO	LOSS OF HAIR	YES	NO	YES	NO	FLUID DISCHARGE FROM BREAST	YES	NO
YES	NO	BLURRED VISION	YES	NO	YES	NO	DIFFICULTY MAINTAINING SEXUAL EXCITEMENT	YES	NO
YES	NO	HEADACHE	YES	NO					
YES	NO	NERVOUSNESS	YES	NO	YES	NO	DIFFICULTY IN REACHING ORGASM	YES	NO
YES	NO	NAUSEA OR VOMITING	YES	NO	YES	NO	INCREASED SWEATING	YES	NO
YES	NO	DIFFICULTY GETTING OR MAINTAINING AN ERECTION	YES	NO	YES	NO	EDEMA (SWELLING) OF LEGS	YES	NO
					YES	NO	UNSTEADY GAIT (POOR BALANCE)	YES	NO
YES	NO	DIFFICULTY IN EJACULATING	YES	NO	YES	NO	TEARING EYES	YES	NO
YES	NO	DIARRHEA	YES	NO	YES	NO	SLURRED SPEECH	YES	NO
YES	NO	CONSTIPATION	YES	NO	YES	NO	PAINFUL SORES INSIDE MOUTH	YES	NO
YES	NO	DRY MOUTH AND THROAT	YES	NO	YES	NO	RAPID OR POUNDING HEART BEAT	YES	NO
YES	NO	INCREASED SALIVATION	YES	NO	YES	NO	INCREASED APPETITE	YES	NO
YES	NO	NASAL STUFFINESS	YES	NO	YES	NO	INCREASED THIRST	YES	NO
YES	NO	NIGHTMARES	YES	NO	YES	NO	CRAMPS IN LEGS OR ARMS	YES	NO
YES	NO	CHILLS	YES	NO	YES	NO	CHEST PAIN	YES	NO
YES	NO	IRREGULAR HEART BEAT	YES	NO	YES	NO	BACK PAIN	YES	NO
YES	NO	COUGH	YES	NO	YES	NO	PAINFUL INTERCOURSE	YES	NO

*This KDS Form was developed by David J. Kupfer, M.D. & Thomas P. Detre, M.D.   IBM M63482   Copyright ©1971, KDS SYSTEMS, INC.   ALL RIGHTS RESERVED.

FIG. 1. Inventory form for somatic symptoms of depression.

of the mouth, sweating, urinary retention (found especially in elderly males with prostatic hyperplasia), constipation, and rarely paralytic ileus. Many of these *autonomic* effects can be alleviated by neostigmine bromide (15 mg once or twice a day). Aggravation of symptoms of hiatus hernia secondary to the anticholinergic effect of the drug on the esophageal sphincter was reported

TABLE 4
Adverse Effects of Tricyclic Antidepressants

Allergic:	Cholestatic jaundice
	Rashes
	Bone marrow depression
Autonomic:	Blurring of vision
	Acute glaucoma
	Dryness of the mouth
	Sweating
	Urinary retention
	Paralytic ileus
Cardiovascular:	Hypotension
	Heart block
	Tachycardia and other arrhythmias
Central nervous system:	Drowsiness
	Tremors
	Epileptiform seizures
	Peripheral neuropathy
Neuroendocrine:	Galactorrhea
	Amenorrhea
	Excessive weight gain
	Loss of libido
Psychotoxic:	Dysmnesia
	Mood switch

recently (Tyber, 1975), but this is very infrequent. If loss of accomodation is a cause of discomfort, a prism of +0.5–1.5 diopter can be prescribed. The hazards of acute glaucoma have been exaggerated for this complication occurs almost exclusively in narrow-angle glaucoma which is congenital and represents only 5% of all cases. Ideally an ophthalmologic examination should be performed prior to treatment with tricyclics, but given the rarity of this complication and the high additional cost, it is justified only when the history or the symptoms elicited in the course of treatment warrant such a referral. Probably a tricyclic which produces fewer anticholinergic side effects will be marketed in the future. Jacobsson *et al.* (1974), measuring levels of salivation and accommodation, have already reported that imipramine-*N*-oxide is less troublesome than imipramine.

The most frequent *cardiovascular* effects consist of (orthostatic) hypotension, tachycardia, occasional heart block, and various arrhythmias, particularly in patients with preexisting cardiac disease. The drug also has a direct (toxic) effect on cardiac muscle with prolongation of the PR interval and widening of the QRS complex which in turn may produce bundle branch or even complete heart block (see p. 210). Since orthostatic hypotension may cause dizziness and result in injuries, elderly patients (and when possible their families) should always be given careful instructions to avoid getting up suddenly or negotiating stairs. All patients should be told to "dangle" their legs on the edge of the bed for 30 sec prior to arising.

While less frequent than that reported with phenothiazines, the administration of tricyclics has been associated with such *neuroendocrine* effects as galactorrhea and amenorrhea in women, loss of libido in men, and excessive weight gain in both sexes. The excessive weight gain is one of the major reasons for noncompliance, particularly during long-term maintenance treatment. Although the effect of tricyclics on fatty acid metabolism and glucose regulation is under active investigation, the pathophysiology of excessive weight gain is still unknown.

The most common *central nervous system* effects are drowsiness and, somewhat less frequently, rather coarse tremors especially in the upper extremities which do not respond to antiparkinsonian agents. Epileptiform seizures in patients without prior history of seizure disorder and a normal pretreatment EEG has been described in some cases, particularly when the dose of the imipramine or amitriptyline is above 150 mg daily (Petti and Campbell, 1975). Peripheral neuropathy (usually peroneal palsy) has been reported but is very rare. While a finer tremor occurring in about 10% of the elderly patients is believed to be a mild extrapyramidal syndrome secondary to presumed dopaminergic blockade in the striatum, certain symptoms of parkinsonism (motor retardation, dysarthria) tend to ameliorate on the tricyclic regimen, possibly due to the antimuscarinic properties of these drugs. Characteristically some degree of tolerance to many of the side effects develops within two weeks, but tremor and occasionally drowsiness will persist as long as the patient is receiving the drug.

Psychotoxic effects of the tricyclic compounds usually take one of two forms. Most frequent is the dysmnesic type of syndrome which can range in severity from transient forgetfulness for recent details to a full-blown "atropinic" delirium with flushed skin, marked disorientation, incoherence, ataxic gait, dysarthria, hallucinations and a fluctuating level of consciousness, and at times myoclonic or grand mal seizures. These symptoms are said to be reversible by intramuscular administration of 0.5–2 mg physostigmine (Snyder et al., 1974).

The "nonorganic" type of psychotoxic effect consists of a marked switch in mood from withdrawal and depression to euphoria. Although it was at first assumed that this switch occurs primarily in patients who actually have a bipolar disease, there is some evidence to suggest a direct drug effect which thus will occur in unipolar patients as well. Unlike the acceleration of a switch process already in progress seen in bipolar patients which then persists even after the tricyclics are reduced or discontinued, these drug-induced hypomanic states subside within two or three days after the drug is stopped.

Allergic and idiosyncratic reactions are rare. Cholestatic jaundice, similar to that associated with phenothiazine administration, which subsides upon discontinuation of the drug, as well as various types of rashes (generalized urticaria or a discrete maculopapular erythema) and increased photosensitivity have also been reported but are rare. For patients with sensitive skin sunscreens containing 5% PABA formulations are recommended as the most effective nonopaque sunscreen (e.g., Presun) (*Medical Letter,* 1974*b*). Even less frequent and usually promptly reversible following discontinuation of the drug are the hemopoietic reactions such as bone-marrow depression and agranulocytosis.

Less well known but quite common are symptoms of withdrawal which occur when patients receive the equivalent of 150 mg of imipramine or more for two months or longer. Symptoms begin usually within 96 hr following abrupt discontinuation and consist of nausea, vomiting, diarrhea, cramps, chills, as well as insomnia and anxiety. Since gradual withdrawal can usually prevent or mitigate the discomfort, treatment consists of readministering the dose the patient was originally receiving and then instituting a gradual withdrawal schedule over a period of 10–14 days.

An overdosage of a tricyclic antidepressant generally produces a clinical picture dominated by marked anticholinergic activity; mydriasis, ataxia, confusion, clonic or athetoid movement; and in severe cases, coma with myoclonic seizures, respiratory depression, and hyperpyrexia (Goel and Shanks, 1974). Cardiovascular complications include hypotension, rhythm abnormalities, prolongation of the PR and PRS intervals and changes in the ST-T waves of the ECG, conduction defect atrial and ventricular flutter, and in severe cases congestive heart failure. Patients should be scrupulously monitored because plasma levels may remain elevated for several days after intoxication and may be partially responsible for severe arrhythmias and the sudden cardiac arrest occurring three to six days following overdose, and sometimes when a patient is no longer comatose. A reasonable estimate of the severity of a tricyclic overdose can also be obtained within the first 24 hr by measuring the duration of the QRS complex which, in turn, correlates with plasma levels (1000 ng/ml when the QRS is equal to or greater than 100 ms) (Spiker *et al.*, 1975). Quinidine, digitalis, or epinephrine should definitely not be used in the management of cardiovascular complications due to the overdosage. Some clinicians recommend propranolol and lidocaine, but the majority of severe overdose cases have been successfully managed with neostigmine methylsulfate given intramuscularly or by slow intravenous injection. The initial dose is 1–2 mg which can be repeated within 20–30 min as necessary (Snyder *et al.*, 1974; Burks *et al.*, 1974). In addition to the routine life-support measures, gastric aspiration may be attempted early in the course if the patient is not comatose.

Interaction with other drugs that enhance the effects of the tricyclic antidepressants can also be the cause of severe adverse effects, or conversely tricyclics may produce additivity with or even potentiation of other drug effects (*Medical Letter,* 1975*a,b*). Although these interactional effects may be secondary to tricyclic blockade of the cholinergic receptors or perhaps the ability of these compounds to inhibit uptake of norepinephrine by the presynaptic neuron, a wide variety of other mechanisms may also be involved. Concurrent administration of barbiturates appears to reduce the antidepressive effect of tricyclics, presumably by the induction of microsomal enzymes. Guanethidine's antihypertensive effect is lessened when the tricyclics are administered, an effect which may be the result of uptake blockade at the target site.

The most frequently reported interactional effect in the psychiatric literature is that produced by the concomitant or consecutive administration of MAOIs and tricyclics (Section 9). Concurrent administration of tricyclics and sympathomimetic amines (such as amphetamines, epinephrine, isoproterenol, methylphenidate, and the like) can augment the amine pressor effects, even to the point of causing a hypertensive crisis (Teychenne *et al.*, 1975). Drug interaction with phenothiazines, tryptophan, or thyroid preparations seems to increase the antidepressive effect of the tricyclics (see p. 223), and tricyclics tend to enhance the effects of all oral hypoglycemic agents. Since, in addition to those mentioned, numerous other interactional effects have been reported, the clinician must rely on an updated drug information system and consider each case treated with an antidepressant concomitantly with other drugs a "therapeutic trial."

4. MAOI: CLINICAL STUDIES

Although the efficacy of MAOI in the treatment of depression has been demonstrated in controlled trials (Table 5), it is generally felt that MAOIs do not produce the same rate of improvement as the tricyclics (Morris and Beck, 1974). Of the MAOIs currently available, the FDA has approved phenelzine (a hydrazine MAOI) and tranylcypromine (a nonhydrazide MAOI) for treatment of depression. Twelve studies comparing MAOIs and imipramine showed that tranylcypromine was as effective as imipramine in three, while imipramine was more effective than phenelzine in five out of nine and comparable in the other four studies. Of the MAOIs not actively marketed or withdrawn (such as isocarboxazid, niamide, iproniazid, phreniprazine, and tryptamine), none seems clearly superior to placebo and certainly not to imipramine or other tricyclics. Including only the two currently approved

TABLE 5
Monoamine Oxidase Inhibitors and Their Approximate Effective Dose Ranges

Drug		Dosage form	Effective dose range (mg/day)
Generic name	Trade name		
Tranylcypromine	Parnate	Oral	20–40
Isocarboxazid	Marplan	Oral	20–60
Phenelzine	Nardil	Oral	45–75

FDA drugs, the overall success of the various MAOIs over placebo is 61%, tranylcypromine being somewhat more effective than phenelzine. It should be pointed out, however, that the majority of controlled studies used inadequate dosages. Phenelzine in doses of 60 mg daily is probably both effective and safe while phenelzine 45 mg daily, the dosage generally recommended, is only marginally effective. These clinical impressions are in agreement with laboratory data (Robinson et al., 1973) since platelet MAO inhibition of at least 90% seems to correlate with a favorable phenelzine response in an outpatient population of neurotic or atypical depressives.

Whether there are specific indications for MAOIs is still an open question. For instance, amitriptyline was more effective than phenelzine in depressed outpatients (Kay et al., 1973), but phenelzine seemed superior to placebo in "anxious" depressive states (Robinson et al., 1973; Ravaris et al., 1976). There are also a number of uncontrolled investigations, originating with Sargent (1961) and West and Dally (1959), which suggest that MAOIs are indicated for so-called atypical depressions characterized by chronic fatigue, anhedonia, phobic anxiety, and somatic complaints rather than the typical endogenous features. Raskin (1974), reviewing the findings of a collaborative study sponsored by NIMH, concluded that phenelzine at 45 mg/day may be indicated for patients with an "atypical" depression. Phenelzine responders in this trial were mainly women with "hysterical" phobia and obsessive/compulsive symptoms, who also had low emotional withdrawal scores and rated themselves more as extroverts than as introverts. Klein and Davis (1969) identified a group of female patients with somewhat similar characteristics who, in their euthymic phase, are flamboyant and histrionic but respond in a catastrophic fashion to stress by sudden depression, hostility, irritability and withdrawal, oversleeping, repeated naps during the day, and overeating. In this study treatment with MAOI produced prompt improvement in mood, the overeating and oversleeping subsided, and maintenance treatment appeared to have a prophylactic effect against the sudden mood shifts. Results from another group of uncontrolled clinical trials (Himmelhoch et al., 1972; O'Regan, 1974) suggest that the MAOIs are the treatment of choice for depressed patients unresponsive to tricyclics who show marked hypersomnia, decreased levels of psychomotor activity, and frequently excessive eating and weight gain, thus giving some support to the contention that the MAOIs are "energizers." Since the majority of these hypersomnic depressives who benefit from MAOI suffer from bipolar disease (Detre et al., 1972), it is possible that the unipolar–bipolar differentiation may be relevant not only for choosing the appropriate drug for maintenance therapy, but also for the treatment of the acute episode.

Methods for predicting clinical response include platelet MAO inhibition and REM sleep suppression (Akindele et al., 1970; Dunleavy and Oswald, 1973), but neither of these should be regarded as "specific," as these effects can be observed in all subjects who receive MAOI in sufficient doses regardless of whether a mood disorder is present. On even less firm ground is the claim that the rapidity with which hydrazide MAO inhibitors are inactivated by acetylation can be used to screen patients who would respond to a hydrazide MAOI. One investigation (Johnstone and Marsh, 1973) reported significantly greater clinical improvement during phenelzine treatment in "slow" acetylators than in "fast" acetylators, but these findings have not been confirmed.

5. ADVERSE EFFECTS OF THE MAOIs

The most prominent "side effect" of MAOI (Table 6), the hypertensive crisis, is in fact not even a side effect but an interactional effect, since it occurs almost exclusively when the person who is treated with one of the MAOIs ingests certain foods or drugs. The hypertensive crisis is characterized by a flushed face, occipital headache, neck stiffness, nausea, vomiting, and photophobia; intracranial bleeding occurs, but it is infrequent. Cole and Davis (1975) have estimated one death per 100,000 patients treated with tranylcypromine was caused by such hypertensive crisis. Since these reactions occur after the ingestion of ripe cheeses and other food stuffs containing appreciable amounts of tyramine and since the effects of sympathomimetic amines such as tyramine are potentiated by MAOI, it was assumed that other amines or drugs influencing amine metabolism such as the tricyclic antidepressants or amine-containing foods could also precipitate them.

In 1964, Bethune found that 8.4% of patients treated with MAOI experienced a hypertensive crisis, but this percentage dropped to 3.3% after the appropriate dietary precautions had been observed. Since, as Raskin

TABLE 6
Adverse Effects of Monoamine Oxidase Inhibitors

Autonomic:	Dry mouth
	Constipation
	Flushing
	Urinary retention
	Restlessness
Cardiovascular:	Hypotension
	Ankle and periorbital edema
Central nervous system:	Tremor
	Hyperreflexia
	Parasthesias
	Seizures
Psychotoxic:	Mood switch
	Allergy
	Skin reaction
	Hepatitis
	Red/green color blindness

(1972) showed, none of the 110 patients treated with phenelzine suffered hypertensive crises when on a low-tyramine diet, it is important to provide verbal instructions as well as copies of a list of food stuffs and drugs to be avoided to all patients treated with MAOI, warn the patient to report taking MAOI prior to undergoing medical, surgical, and dental procedures, and prescribe them for outpatients only when there is reasonable certainty that the patient alone or with the help of family can follow the necessary precautions. This dietary list should include: any sympathomimetic agents (including over-the-counter cold remedies and diet pills), certain ripe cheeses (especially edam, cheddar), broad bean, yogurt, yeast preparations, avocado, pickled herring, chicken livers, meat extracts, canned figs, raisins, soy sauce, chocolate, beer, chianti, and sherry.

The majority of adverse effects associated with MAOI are similar to those associated with the administration of tricyclics. The *autonomic* side effects consist of dry mouth, constipation, dizziness, restlessness, postural hypotension, and occasionally flushing and urinary retention. Aside from hypotension, other vascular effects include ankle and periorbital edema, both of which respond to diuretics. *Central nervous system* effects unrelated to drug interaction occur rarely and usually consist of tremor, hyperreflexia, paresthesias, but MAOIs even in subjects without a prior history can provoke seizures.

Rapid conversion of a retarded depressive state to a manic excited state is the most significant *psychotoxic* effect and occurs primarily in patients with personal or family histories of bipolar disease. Sudden-onset severe insomnia, especially following the administration of tranylcypromine in anergic depressed patients, usually marks the beginning of this drug-induced switch toward hypomania. Other CNS effects reported include exacerbation of somatic symptoms as well as cases of confusional states particularly in patients over 45. The majority of *allergic* and idiosyncratic reactions associated with MAOI administration occurred with the drugs introduced in the early 1960s. While skin reactions, especially maculopapular rashes, are occasionally reported with the MAOIs currently in use, red/green blindness with optic atrophy occurred exclusively with pheniprazine (hydrazine MAOI), since withdrawn from the market. Cases of severe hepatotoxicity, including yellow degeneration of the liver, were reported in the early sixties, leading to the removal of iproniazid and of a number of other MAOIs. Neither phenelzine nor tranylcypromine, however, tend to cause hepatitis. Abrupt withdrawal does not cause clinically significant symptoms, although rebounds from REM suppression are observable on sleep EEG records within a week following withdrawal (Wyatt *et al.*, 1971*b*).

Overdosage caused by ingestion of MAOIs is characterized primarily by hyperpyrexia, respiratory depression, and marked postural hypotension, although hypertension may also be present (Spiker *et al.*, 1975). Of particular importance is the observation that manifestations of overdosage may not be apparent until 12 hr after the drug ingestion and may then persist for at least one week after ingestion of the last dose. Utmost conservatism is recommended in the management of patients, because drugs that are likely to be useful in combatting overdosage tend to be potentiated by the MAOIs. For sedation, phenothiazines are quite effective, but alpha-adrenergic blocking agents (such as phentolamine or regitine) are the treatment of choice for hypertension associated with the overdosage (or for that matter the treatment of a hypertensive crisis) since this syndrome mirrors the clinical manifestations associated with pheochromocytoma. Acidification of the urine is said to hasten the excretion of phenelzine; hemodialysis has been used in severe cases, but it is of questionable value.

Reports that the combination of an MAOI plus a tricyclic agent tend to produce hyperpyrexia, convulsions, restlessness, muscle twitching, and even death has led to the view that a washout period of 1–3 weeks is necessary before a patient is switched from an MAOI to a tricyclic antidepressant. This chain of events turned out to be relatively rare even when such a combined regimen was administered continuously over a period of weeks or months to depressed patients (Section 9). Hyperpyrexic syndromes have been also described following the concomitant administration of meperidine and MAOI. Since hyperpyrexia is the earliest warning signal, baseline temperatures should be obtained and patients carefully watched and treatment promptly discontinued as soon as the temperature begins to rise above normal. Of the great variety of agents that MAOIs are known to potentiate, hypoglycemic agents, anticholinergic drugs, as well as the CNS depressant effects of narcotic analgesics should be mentioned, as these drugs tend to be used most frequently in the age group which is also most likely to suffer from severe mood disorders. Finally an enhanced pressor response following the simultaneous administration of levadopa with MAOI has been reported recently (Teychenne *et al.*, 1975). Since drug interactional effects are extremely difficult to predict, patients receiving MAOI should be carefully monitored whenever an additional drug is prescribed.

6. TREATMENT OF THE ACUTE EPISODE

Assuming that the criteria for the diagnosis for depression have been met and there are no contraindications to administering a tricyclic antidepressant, one should begin with 50–75 mg h.s. in a single dose. Although in large-scale studies clinical effects could not be identified during the initial 14–21 days, on closer observation discrete changes are noticeable in the majority of patients within 3–10 days after treatment begins. Haskell *et al.* (1975), for instance, recently showed a marked improvement of suicidal feelings, insomnia, and anorexia within one week in depressed outpatients, while improvement in work functioning and interests, retardation, and pessimism and hopelessness was more gradual. These changes are worthy of attention, particularly when treatment other than tricyclics was already used in the course of the episode in question or the patient is so agitated or determined to commit suicide that only a very limited trial is justified before ECT is considered. Given the differences in severity of the disorder and the possibility that an individual may be overly sensitive to the effects of tricyclics, if the patient tolerates the test dose of 50–75 mg h.s. for two days, and if there is no complicating medical problem and the patient is below age 65, then the dose can be increased 25 mg daily up to 150 mg. If no improvement is seen after one week and the patient continues to tolerate the drug well, it should be raised to and kept at the 200-mg dose daily for one week; if there is still little or no improvement, the dose may be raised to 250 mg daily for yet another week before discontinuing it. In general when adverse effects on higher dose schedules drown out ameliorative effects on mood, it is best to treat the patient with reduced dosages rather than discontinue the drug altogether.

The view shared by some clinicians that "neurotic" patients improve on lower dosage than psychotic patients has not been well documented, although milder episodes tend to improve faster whether treated or not. Low-dose responders probably represent a different group of patients who are chronically anxious and periodically have some depressive symptoms. In any case, it is questionable whether the dosage schedules for outpatients should be different than for inpatients except perhaps in those instances where, because of limited but definite response to 200 mg, a higher dose is contemplated. Parenteral administration is allegedly more rapidly effective, but it is usually not necessary and should be reserved for patients who are unable to cooperate. When tricyclics are administered intramuscularly, the equivalent dose of parenterally administered drugs should be 25% lower than the oral dose.

Recently clinicians have begun to advocate that most if not all psychotropic medication should be administered in a single dose in the evening near bedtime since simplifying dosage schedules increases compliance without increasing the incidence of orthostatic hypotension or confusional states (Ayd, 1974; Goldberg *et al.*, 1974). Patients suffering from agitation and insomnia furthermore may benefit from a substantial bedtime dose because the drowsiness produced by the drug facilitates sleep without interfering with daytime activities. Up to what dose levels the single bedtime dose is safe is unclear, but 150 mg seems to be well tolerated. Whether fluctuations in plasma levels produced by a single daily dose alters treatment response or not and if so what the frequency of administration should then be is as yet unanswered. In any case, there is no justification for prescribing the more costly sustained release forms (such as imipramine pamoate) since tricyclics have a long half-life and act in a cumulative fashion (Mendels and Digiacomo, 1973).

Although carefully controlled studies are not yet available, clinical observation suggests that the onset of action of the MAOIs is much faster than that of the tricyclics. Accordingly it is possible to prescribe and evaluate the effectiveness of that drug regimen in less than the usual 3–4 week treatment period required for tricyclics. Most clinicians familiar with these drugs recommend initial doses of phenelzine 30–45 mg and tranylcypromine 20–30 mg, and increase these doses after three to four days to 60–90 mg and 30–60 mg, respectively, until remission of the symptoms has been achieved, at which time the dose is gradually reduced and the drug eventually stopped altogether. As mentioned earlier (p. 212) this practice is consistent with reports that correlate degree of enzyme inhibition with clinical effectiveness.

Unlike the tricyclics where all or most of the dose is administered h.s., MAOIs are usually given in divided doses because of the tendency of MAOIs to precipitate insomnia. Gradual reduction of the duration of sleep, on the other hand, signals a favorable response for patients who fall into the category of atypical anergic depressives who complain about sleepiness throughout the day and whose sleep tends to be prolonged or at least unchanged. Reduction of sleepiness is usually followed by increased normalization of motor activity and improved mood.

The treatment of children with severe or recurrent depression is controversial (Ossofsky, 1974; Drotar, 1974). The view that all depressions in childhood are reactive is widely held, and many clinicians believe that the endogenous type of unipolar and bipolar disease does not make its appearance prior to adolescence. It should be pointed out, however, that the duration of episode as well as the symptoms are age related and thus episodes prior to adolescence tend to be shorter and last for days to weeks instead of months or years. The clinical picture is characterized by physical complaints (particularly of abdominal pain and headache), poor school performance, withdrawal, negativism, increased dependency, and sleep and appetite disturbance rather than the typical symptoms seen in later years. In one of the very few controlled single-blind studies available, Weinberg *et al.* (1973) diagnosed 45 of 72 children on the basis of impaired school performance and behavioral problems somewhat arbitrarily as depression; he found that the 19 patients treated with tricyclics significantly improved compared either to the nontreated or the nondepressed controls. The results have been supported by Ossofsky's analysis (1974) of her open trial of imipramine for 220 children treated for "depression." Guidelines for appropriate doses are lacking, but if the drug schedules used in the treatment of enuretic children can be accepted, 50–100 mg daily of imipramine or its equivalent seems appropriate. Restoration of sleep, appetite, school functioning, and social activities to their premorbid levels can be used to determine the duration of pharmacotherapy.

7. PROPHYLAXIS

Evidence presented regarding the prophylactic action of maintenance chemotherapy in recurrent affective disorders is quite convincing. Yet this prophylactic activity must be understood in a more restricted sense; antidepressants cannot induce remission or prevent relapse in an absolute sense (Table 7). To be sure, the impact of undesirable mood changes is mitigated: patients receiving maintenance therapy require hospitalization less frequently and continue to function better in their work and family than those who do not, but antidepressants do not actually prevent recurrences.

The extent to which the three types of drugs used for maintenance therapy, namely, the tricyclics, the MAOIs, and lithium, are effective can be deduced by analyzing the results of controlled trials. In an NIMH/VA collaborative study which compared imipramine and lithium in maintenance treatment (Prien *et al.*, 1973), the relative effectiveness of lithium over imipramine seemed to be determined by the frequency of manic episodes rather than on the type of affective disorders. The conclusions reached, however, must still be considered tentative both because the number of patients studied was small (less than 100) and because, given the episodic nature of this syndrome and the rather long interval between the episodes (on the average 30 months between the first and second) (Angst *et al.*, 1973), a follow-up period of two years is obviously inadequate. Furthermore, since the majority of relapses in this trial occurred in the first four months of treatment and since the average duration of episodes was approximately 3–4 months, relapses may have occurred simply because the patients were put prematurely on a lower maintenance dose and not because the drugs failed to "prevent" the onset of the new episode. Perhaps this explains why another conclusion of this study, that certain residual symptoms (such as anxiety, mild depression, or feelings of guilt) at discharge predicts failure of maintenance treatment, was not supported by Mindham *et al.* (1973) (Medical Research Council), who on the contrary found that patients with such residual symptoms derived more benefit than patients who had a full remission prior to entering the study. Klerman *et al.* (1974), after comparing the Boston/New Haven study with the MRC and the VA investigations, concluded that tricyclic antidepressants have an established role in the prevention of relapse in depressed patients of the unipolar type, even when the group contains a

TABLE 7
Maintenance Treatment of Depression: Tricyclic Antidepressants

	Relapse rate		
	VA-NIMH Study[a]	MRC Study[b]	Boston–New Haven Study[c]
Tricyclic group	48%	22%	12%
Placebo group	90%	55%	36%

[a] Prien *et al.* (1973).
[b] Mindham *et al.* (1973).
[c] Klerman *et al.* (1974).

significant percentage of "neurotic" patients. However, the Boston/New Haven study consisted primarily of female ambulatory unipolar patients with at most one previous episode of depression who, within the course of the initial uncontrolled phase, received amitriptyline; as a result two-thirds of the patients were asymptomatic or only mildly ill when entering the maintenance phase. Other placebo controlled studies which show amitriptyline to be effective in preventing depressive episodes have similar shortcomings as none of these trials extended beyond nine months.

Besides the small sample size and the short duration of maintenance trials, lack of sufficient attention to compliance is also a limiting factor. The conventional methods to assure compliance are notoriously unreliable. Tricyclics are known to produce a number of somatic symptoms (p. 206) or intensify a preexisting one, which in turn augments the patient's discomfort. Since many of these undesirable effects reach their peak in the first 10–14 days of treatment and before the beneficial ones are experienced, it is likely that at least some patients relapse simply because they do not take the drug as prescribed or do not take the drug at all. Furthermore, if patients were armed with more definitive information with regard to the effectiveness of maintenance treatment, they would then be better able to weigh the cost and risk of relapse against the cost and risk of prolonged maintenance chemotherapy.

Whether tricyclics can be recommended as an effective form of mainte-nance therapy following a course of ECT is unclear, particularly when such a recommendation implies that these drugs can be helpful even though ECT was required to produce a remission. Kay *et al.* (1970) confirmed early results reported by Seager and Berg in 1962 that, in contrast to diazepam maintenance, amitriptyline maintenance prevents relapses in post-ECT patients. However, since the natural course of depressive episodes is longer than the usual course of ECT (8–12 treatments over 2–3 weeks), the finding that symptomatic improvement achieved with ECT can be maintained with tricyclics may only prove that patients who would have benefited from these drugs to begin with continued to do so and thus can hardly be regarded as evidence that maintenance therapy with tricyclics is the treatment of choice for patients who respond to ECT alone. On the other hand, ECT may still be the treatment of choice: (1) whenever the patient's response to drug therapy is poor or idiosyncratic; (2) when there are nonpsychiatric complications which render administration of drugs hazardous; (3) when the patient is too ill to cooperate; and (4) in the rare condition called by Kraeplin a mixed state where manic and depressive symptoms appear simultaneously, a clinical presentation which is seen primarily, although not exclusively, in bipolar patients who develop an episode during the immediate postpartum period (Herzog and Detre, 1974).

With regard to the prophylactic use of MAOI, little is known that is based on systematic investigation. Given that response to MAOI tends to be quick and that the type of patient who benefits is likely to be completely well between episodes, there is little justification for maintaining patients on MAOI beyond 3–4 months unless, on the basis of prior history, it is known that the patient's episode tends to last longer. Should symptoms reoccur treatment can be administered again without delay and before the patient's level of functioning deteriorates to the point where the symptoms are incapacitating or hospitalization becomes necessary.

8. INTERACTIVE EFFECTS OF TRICYCLIC AGENTS AND SOCIOTHERAPY

The combination of drugs and psychotherapy is probably far more often prescribed, particularly for the milder forms of depression, than drug therapy alone, yet little is known of the effects of psychotherapy vs. pharmacotherapy or the interactional effects of the two treatment modes. The results of the Boston/New Haven collaborative group (Paykel *et al.*, 1975), which compared amitriptyline and psychotherapy alone or in combination on 150 depressed outpatients over a period of eight months of maintenance follow-up treatment, showed that while the social adjustment of the "high" contact group (one hour weekly) was significantly better (improved work performance, reduction of interpersonal friction, and anxious rumination) than the "low" contact group (15 min monthly), psychotherapy benefited primarily those depressed women who improved on amitriptyline in the first place. The quantity or "intensity" of the casework type of psychotherapy did not significantly protect against recurrence of depression (Weissman *et al.*, 1974). Similar conclusions were reached by Covi (1974), who compared "active treatment" consisting of three medication conditions (amitriptyline, diazepam, and placebo) and two social therapies (weekly group therapy or biweekly supportive contact), but noted that the effects of group therapy became evident only after a considerable lag period. Friedman (1975) compared the effects of amitriptyline and marital therapy, amitriptyline and minimal contact, placebo and marital therapy, and placebo and minimal contact. In this study too, drug effects were superior to the effects of marital therapy with regard to the patient's symptomatic condition, but marital therapy was superior to drug therapy with regard to the patient's participation and performance of family role tasks and other parameters in the patient's relationship with the spouse, suggesting that the marital therapy has an additive rather than a simple interactional effect with amitriptyline. It should be noted that in none of these trials was the method of psychotherapy clearly defined nor are there any studies where specific target-symptom-oriented psychotherapy was used.

9. COMBINED DRUG TREATMENTS

Attempts to treat cases refractory to both tricyclics and MAOIs have led to a number of clinical trials using combinations of pharmacological treatments (Ananth and Ruskin, 1974; Levine and Raskin, 1974). Although several of these combinations will be briefly discussed, the reader should be aware that most of these studies were uncontrolled and the indications proposed are based solely on clinical impressions.

Investigators, especially British psychiatrists, recommend a combination of MAOI and tricyclics for patients who fail to respond to either one of these drugs alone, but in the United States clinicians shy away from using these drugs together because of the potentially fatal (primarily the hypertensive and hyperpyretic episodes—"drug fever" or "malignant hyperpyrexia") complications. More recently, however, Schuckit *et al.* (1971), after surveying the charts of 350 outpatients, concluded that the hazards are highly exaggerated and that the toxic reactions described probably resulted from overdosages or occurred when the tricyclic agent was administered parenterally. Spiker and Pugh (1976), after a thorough review of 200 cases, have come to the same conclusion, noting that there were no strokes or deaths resulting from the use of an MAOI–tricyclic antidepressant regimen, and only 12 patients had their medication stopped because of adverse reactions, with the most troublesome side effect being orthostatic hypotension rather than hypertension. In their experience such combined treatment is efficacious in refractory depressions, and they recommend that tricyclics (amitripytline) should be administered first in doses of 20–50 mg h.s., followed several days later by an MAOI (either 15 mg phenelzine or 10 mg tranylcypromine). The two drugs should then be increased slowly over a preiod of 2–3 weeks until a dose equivalent to 150 mg amitriptyline and 45 mg phenelzine is reached.

Since phenothiazines alone have been repeatedly shown in controlled trials to be effective, particularly in "agitated" depressions, clinicians used them for some time in combination with antidepressants. When tricyclics alone were compared with the combination of phenothiazines and tricyclics (amitriptyline, perphenazine), the two drugs together were not more effective than tricyclics alone in the treatment of (anxious, nonpsychotic) depression (Rickels *et al.*, 1972; Hollister *et al.*, 1966). It has been suggested that phenothiazine should be given first to control agitation and diminish delusional thinking, then be followed by a tricyclic in the treatment of psychotic depression; when (after 10–14 days) the effects of the antidepressants become noticeable, the phenothiazine should be gradually tapered. A fixed combination of the tricyclic and a phenothiazine is rarely justified for it reduces the flexibility of administering the two drugs independently and thus (Kotin *et al.*, 1973) may even contribute to inadequate treatment for depression.

In some combinations, the additional drug has mild to moderate stimulant or antidepressant properties itself. Such is the case when dextroamphetamine or methylphenidate is given together with an antidepressant. Pharmacologically, in addition to blocking norepinephrine re-uptake, dextroamphetamine inhibits hepatic drug-metabolizing enzymes, increasing tricyclic plasma levels, and thus the combination might well produce a more immediate amelioration. But here again there are no double-blind studies documenting such an effect.

Still another combination used mostly in the treatment of recurrent depression is maintenance therapy using lithium carbonate in combination with either MAOI or tricyclics. The claim that lithium enhances rather than antagonizes the therapeutic effect of the tricyclic antidepressants has been tested in one double-blind investigation. While recommending that depressed patients suitable for long-term prophylactic lithium maintenance should be started on lithium, Lingjaerde et al. (1974) could only show marginally better results by adding lithium to the tricyclic regimen. Still others feel that tricyclics are contraindicated in the acute treatment of anergic, bipolar depression and believe that the combination with lithium does not hasten recovery.

In two patients unresponsive to previous treatment, Zall (1971) reported success with a combination of isocarboxazid and lithium. In 1972, Himmelhoch et al. (1972) reported that a group of hypersomnic depressed patients, who had failed to respond to treatment with tricyclic antidepressants, responded well to combined treatment with lithium carbonate and tranylcypromine. Since some of the patients suffered from unipolar rather than bipolar recurrent depressions, it was suggested that this form of treatment might be indicated in all depressions associated with hypersomnia.

In an uncontrolled clinical trial (Kupfer and Detre, unpublished data), tricyclic antidepressants administered concomitantly with lithium carbonate seemed to produce improvement in bipolar patients with the anxious–hyperactive type of depression while bipolar patients with the anergic–hypoactive type of depression who did poorly on lithium alone benefited from MAOI. Thus it is the severity and type of depression exhibited by patients in the depressive phase of manic-depressive disease which seems to determine the indications for the choice of concomitant treatment with antidepressant drugs.

These preliminary results are consistent with the typology presented earlier (p. 202) that, given the psychobiologic features of the typical and atypical depressions, the tricyclics and MAOIs affect both motor activity and sleep in a predictable manner: tricyclics will reduce motor activity and increase sleep efficiency beginning with the first night of drug administration; monoamine oxidase inhibitors such as tranylcypromine, on the other hand, produce an antidepressant effect in the anergic atypical depression by increasing motor activity without prolonging sleep time.

Continued search for the "right" combination has led to clinical experiments with vitamins, amino acids, and hormones. Since subnormal folate levels have been reported in depressed patients, it was felt that folic acid supplements might enhance the therapeutic activity of the antidepressants, particularly the tricyclic compounds. Similarly, the impression that depressed women who were on oral contraceptives improved dramatically on pyridoxine led to the speculation that there is perhaps a pyridoxine-responsive subgroup. The possible antidepressant activity of tryptophan, a serotonin precursor, alone or in combination with antidepressants has received considerable attention since serotonin depletion has been implicated in the pathogenesis of a subgroup of depressives. While rapid recovery following the administration of tranylcypromine (or nialimide) and tryptophan was observed in one uncontrolled trial (Ayuso Gutierrez and Lopez-Ibor, 1971), in another the combination of tricyclics and tryptophan in unipolar patients (Shaw *et al.*, 1972) was no better than tricyclics alone. Thyroid hormone, particularly T3 (triiodothyronine), was also considered a potential "accelerator." Originally, Prange *et al.* (1970) reported that the addition of small doses of T3 (25 μg/day) enhanced imipramine's antidepressant activity. Although confirmed by others (Coppen *et al.*, 1972; Wheatley, 1972), a failure by Feighner *et al.* (1972) to replicate the results led to a partial recanting by the original group which now recommends that T3 can accelerate the action of imipramine only in depressed women (Prange, 1975). TSH and TRH, as well as a variety of steroid hormones, have also been used as adjuncts to the tricyclic regimen, but the results are unconvincing.

10. OTHER USES OF THE ANTIDEPRESSANTS

10.1. Neurotic Disorders

Antidepressants have been found useful in a relatively rare "anxiety–depersonalization syndrome," originally described by Roth (Roth and Myers, 1969), as well as in an adult-panic reaction (Klein, 1964). Tricyclics, however, do not seem to have an effect on anticipatory anxiety, the discomfort experienced by many chronically anxious patients when confronted with novel situations. Given the naturally occurring fluctuations and relatively long (weeks, months) symptom-free intervals, these treatment trials were too short in duration to be considered definitive. High doses (300–400 mg) of imipramine seem to mitigate obsessive compulsive symptoms to a surprising degree, but again no controlled studies are available (Cammer, 1973).

10.2. Antidepressants in the So-Called Psychosomatic Disorders

The tricyclic compounds (e.g., amitriptyline) have been found effective in the treatment of such varied conditions as tension headache, migraine, asthma, and chronic pain syndromes. In a double-blind trial amitriptyline (h.s. dosages 10–60 mg) exerted a prophylactic effect on migraine attacks by reducing the number of attacks with a short warning and short duration, regardless of severity (Gomersall and Stuart, 1973). Amitriptyline alone and concomitantly with low doses of perphenazine have been used successfully in the treatment of face and lower back pain (Taub, 1975). The regimen seems particularly effective when chronic pain is associated with symptoms and clinical features that are also found in depression (the reason why these syndromes are often referred to as "depression equivalent"): (1) pain is relatively well localized rather than diffused; (2) no organic basis for the symptoms can be found; (3) a mood disorder precedes, accompanies, or follows the onset of pain; (4) complaints reoccur periodically; (5) there is a diurnal pattern (worse in the morning); and (6) a sleep disturbance is present (Detre and Jarecki, 1971).

10.3. Narcolepsy

Advances in the understanding of narcolepsy and the identification of its various subtypes, especially the REM-sleep onset type, stimulated trials with a variety of drugs known to affect the various "components" of sleep (Guilleminault *et al.*, 1974). In addition to psychomotor stimulants which long have been considered the treatment for narcolepsy, the tricyclics such as imipramine or desimipramine (75–150 mg) were found to abort the cataplectic attack, but had little effect on sleep attacks. Another tricyclic clomipramine (not yet marketed in the United States) in doses of 75 mg daily is said to be the most potent drug for the control of cataplexy. A tricyclic, together with amphetamine or one of its congeners (such as methylphenidate), has been used with considerable success in controlling all but the daytime sleep attacks in narcoleptic patients. The property of MAOI to suppress REM sleep completely suggested its use for the prevention of sleep attacks. At the present, however, MAOI is not routinely recommended (Wyatt *et al.*, 1971a) nor is the simultaneous administration of a tricyclic and MAOI, although the latter combination at least theoretically should provide the greatest protection against all four symptoms of narcolepsy.

10.4. Disorders of Childhood

The effectiveness of tricyclics in disorders of childhood ranging from school phobia and hyperactivity to enuresis has been documented in controlled trials. Since there is increasing evidence that children receiving imipramine in doses above 4–5 mg/kg show ECG changes similar to those seen in adults (Martin and Zaug, 1975; Winsberg *et al.*, 1975) and since it is also difficult to measure or predict what indirect effect the chronic administration of imipramine in children has on growth and development, most clinicians recommend that pharmacotherapy should be used only if other treatment efforts have failed (Hayes *et al.*, 1975).

10.5. Phobia

Amitriptyline has been used in dosages of 100–200 mg daily in the treatment of school phobia (Gittleman-Klein and Klein, 1972). In the one controlled study, amitriptyline was superior to placebo, especially six weeks after the clinical trial began. Other investigators have recommended MAOI in the treatment of phobic depressive children, although the latter were never subjected to a controlled trial.

10.6. Hyperactivity

Recent studies show that imipramine has been found almost as effective as amphetamine or methylphenidate (Rapoport et al., 1974; Quinn and Rapoport, 1975; Waizer et al., 1974), and the improvement occurs within hours of the first administration rather than weeks as in the case of depression. Tricyclics cause more acute side effects, particularly drowsiness, but less anorexia than methylphenidate (Greenberg et al., 1975). As stated earlier, since both groups of drugs may effect growth and maturation (Safer et al., 1972), which drug is ultimately chosen depends on the child's tolerance of the particular regimen.

10.7. Enuresis

Imipramine is the only tricyclic drug "approved" for use in enuresis in children more than six years of age, but other tricyclic drugs are about equally effective (Arnold and Ginsberg, 1974; Walker et al., 1974; Medical Letter, 1974a). The drug's anticholinergic activity on the bladder is probably the mechanism responsible for the improvement, but other as yet unidentified effects on the central nervous system may also play some role. The dose used is between 10 and 75 mg h.s., depending on the size of the child and clinical response. Given the potential hazards of long-term administration, alternative methods (such as various forms of behavior modification) should be tried first.

11. CURRENT PRACTICES AND FUTURE NEEDS

Confronted with a depressed patient whose illness seems severe enough to require some sort of biological treatment, the clinician may proceed by prescribing a tricyclic antidepressant before trying MAOI, lithium, or ECT, simply because tricyclics have been shown to be more effective and less intrusive than other modes of treatment; or he may decide to find guidelines which would help him to choose a treatment that is most likely to succeed in a given case.

Understandably, the strategy used by the clinician to evaluate the patient's progress is very different from the strategy of a double-blind clinical trial aimed to assess the efficacy of a particular drug. Unconcerned about whether the drug, the suggestion of giving a pill, or some other favorable change in the patient's support system is responsible for improvement, all the clinician needs to do is to make a global assessment of the treatment course based on his own observations and the information he receives from the patient or the family. Furthermore, since the clinician's task is to maximize the patient's cooperation, whenever necessary he will manipulate the patient's environment or use additional drugs even if such a combination adds little beyond some additional comfort for the patient; for instance, rather than waiting out the usual lag period, he may decide to use a phenothiazine or a benzodiazepine along with tricyclics to promote sleep in the first week or two of treatment.

A word of caution is in order. Much of what can be said about the treatment of depression is based on clinical trials on patients with moderately severe or severe forms of affective disorders or is reported by experienced clinicians who rarely come in contact with the mildest manifestations of this disease. Information regarding mild depressions, which represent the overwhelming majority of affective disorders, is still in an anecdotal stage and has little to do with the low level of technology and methodological sophistication that has characterized psychiatry for many decades. Historically, patients with mild depression failed to fascinate phenomenologically minded clinicians, and such patients were usually referred to psychotherapists who were primarily treatment oriented and rarely kept detailed records on presenting symptoms, life history, premorbid personality structure, and family history.

Finally, since depression is a self-limiting illness with a high spontaneous recovery and high placebo-response rate, and since by removing the patient from sources of conflict a hospital may by itself have a significant impact on patient recovery, it has been suggested (Raskin, 1974) that withholding medication entirely or using medication sparingly for the mildly depressed hospitalized patient may be one of the acceptable treatment choices. The data on which these recommendations are based is weak, however; the clinical description of these hospitalized "neurotic" patients is lacking in detail. Maybe some or even the majority of patients who find temporary refuge in the hospital from stressful life events and respond to placebo do have long-standing personality disorders with some depressive symptoms and thus suffer from a secondary rather than a primary depression. It is also conceivable, of course, that some mildly depressed hospitalized patients, much like patients with mild essential hypertension who become normotensive while in a structured and protective setting, become symptomatic again when re-exposed to the stresses and strains of everyday life.

12. REFERENCES

ANANTH, J., and RUSKIN, R., 1974, Treatment of intractable depression, *Int. Pharmacopsychiatry* **9:**218–229.

ANGST, J., 1966, Zur Atiologie und Nosologie endogener depressiver, *Psychosen. Monogr. Neurol. Psychiatr.* **112**:1–118.

ANGST, J., 1970, Clinical aspects of imipramine, in: *Tofranil,* Verlag Stamp Ai and Cie, AG, Berne.

ANGST, J., BAASTRUP, P., GROF, P., HIPPIUS, H., POLDINGER, W., and WEIS, P., 1973, The course of monopolar depression and bipolar psychoses, *Psychiatr. Neurol. Neurochir.* **76**:489–500.

AKINDELE, M. O., EVANS, J. I., and OSWALD, I., 1970, Monoamine oxidase inhibitors, sleep and mood, *Electroenceph. Clin. Neurophysiol.* **29**:47–56.

ARNOLD, S. J., and GINSBURG, A., 1974, Enuresis: Treatment with imipramine, *J. Am. Med. Assoc.* **228**:289–290.

ASBERG, M., 1974a, Individualization of treatment with tricyclic compounds, *Med. Clin. North Am.* **58**:1083–1091.

ASBERG, M., 1974b, Plasma nortriptyline levels-relationship to clinical effects, *Clin. Pharmacol. Ther.* **16**:215–229.

ASBERG, M., CRONHOLM, B., SJOQVIST, F., and TUCK, D., 1970, Correlation of subjective side effects with plasma concentrations of nortriptyline, *Br. Med. J.* **4**:18–21.

ASCHER, E., 1951/52, A criticism of the concept of neurotic depression, *Am. J. Psychiatry* **108**:901–908.

AYD, F. J., 1974, Single daily dose of antidepressants, *J. Am. Med. Assoc.* **230**:263–264.

AYUSO GUTIERREZ, J. L., and LOPEZ-IBOR ALINO, J. J., 1971, Tryptophan and an MAOI (Nialamide) in the treatment of depression. A double-blind study, *Int. Pharmacopsychiatry* **6**:92–97.

BETHUNE, H. C., BURRELL, R. H., CULPAN, R. H., and OGG, G. J., 1964, Vascular crisis associated with monoamine oxidase inhibitors, *Am. J. Psychiatry* **121**:245–248.

BORNSTEIN, P. E., CLAYTON, P. J., HALIKAS, J. A., MAURICE, W. L., and ROBINS, E., 1973, The depression of widowhood after thirteen months, *Br. J. Psychiatry* **122**:561–566.

BRAITHWAITE, R. A., GOULDING, R., THEANO, G., BAILY, J., and COPPEN, H., 1972, Plasma concentration of amitriptyline and clinical response, *Lancet* **1**:1297–1300.

BURKS, J. S., WALKER, J. E., RUMACK, B. H., and OTT, T. E., 1974, Tricyclic antidepressant poisoning and reversal of coma, choreoathetosis, and myoclonus by physostigmine, *J. Am. Med. Assoc.* **230**:1405–1407.

BURROWS, G. D., DAVIES, B., and SCOGGINS, B. A., 1972, Plasma concentration of nortriptyline and clinical response in depressive illness, *Lancet* **2**:619–623.

BURROWS, G. D., SCOGGINS, B. A., TURECEK, L. R., and DAVIES, G., 1974, Plasma nortriptyline and clinical response, *Clin. Pharmacol. Ther.* **16**:639–644.

BUSFIELD, B. L., SCHNELLER, P., and CAPRA, D., 1962, Depressive symptom or side effect? A comparative study of symptoms during pretreatment and treatment periods of patients on three antidepressant medications, *J. Nerv. Ment. Dis.* **134**:339–345.

CAMMER, L., 1973, Antidepressants as a prophylaxis against depression in the obsessive compulsive person, *Psychosomatics* **14**:201–206.

CARNEY, M. W. P., ROTH, M., and GARSIDE, R. F., 1965, The diagnosis of depressive syndromes and the prediction of ECT response, *Br. J. Psychiatry* **111**:659.

COLE, J. O., 1964, The therapeutic efficacy of antidepressant drugs: A review, *J. Am. Med. Assoc.* **190**:448–455.

COLE, J. O., and DAVIS, J. M., 1975, in: *Antidepressant Drugs* (A. M. Freedman, H. I. Kaplan, and B. J. Sadock, eds.), pp. 1941–1956, Williams and Wilkins, Baltimore.

COPPEN, A., WHYBROW, P. C., NORGUERA, R., MAGGS, R., and PRANGE, A. J., 1972, The comparative antidepressant value of L-tryptophan and imipramine with and without attempted potentiation by L-liothyronine, *Arch. Gen. Psychiatry* **26**:234–241.

COVI, L., LIPMAN, R. S., DEROGATIS, L. R., SMITH, J. E., and PATTISON, J. H., 1974, Drugs and group psychotherapy in neurotic depression, *Am. J. Psychiatry* **131**:191–198.

DETRE, T. P., and JARECKI, H. G., 1971, *Modern Psychiatric Treatment,* J. B. Lippincott, Philadelphia.

DETRE, T. P., HIMMELHOCH, J., SWARTZBURG, M., ANDERSON, C. M., BYCK, R., and KUPFER, D. J., 1972, Hypersomnia and manic-depressive disease, *Am. J. Psychiatry* **128:**1303–1305.

DROTAR, D., 1974, Concern over the categorization of depression in children, *J. Pediatr.* **85:**290–291.

DUNLEAVY, D. L., and OSWALD, I., 1973, Phenelzine, mood response, and sleep, *Arch. Gen. Psychiatry* **28:**353–356.

FAWCETT, J., 1975, Biochemical and neuropharmacological research, in: *Depression and Human Existence* (E. J. Anthony and T. Benedek, eds.), pp. 21–52, Little Brown and Company, Boston.

FEIGHNER, J. P., KING, L. J., SCHUCKIT, M. A., CROUGHAN, J., and BRISCOE, W., 1972, Hormonal potentiation of imipramine and ECT in primary depression, *Am. J. Psychiatry* **128:**1230–1238.

FRIEDMAN, A. S., 1975, Interaction of drug therapy with marital therapy in depressive patients, *Arch. Gen. Psychiatry* **32:**619–637.

GITTELMAN-KLEIN, R., and KLEIN, D. R., 1972, School phobia: Diagnostic consideration in the light of imipramine effects in drugs, development, in: *Cerebral Function* (W. L. Smith, ed.), pp. 200–223, Charles C. Thomas, Springfield, Illinois.

GLASSMAN, A. H., KANTOR, S. J., and SHOSTAK, M., 1975, Depression, delusions and drug response, *Am. J. Psychiatry* **132:**716–719.

GOEL, K. M., and SHANKS, R. A., 1974, Amitriptyline and imipramine poisoning in children, *Br. Med. J.* **1:**261–263.

GOLDBERG, H. L., FINNERTY, R. J., NATHAN, L., and COLE, J. O., 1974, Doxepin in a single bedtime dose in psychoneurotic outpatients, *Arch. Gen. Psychiatry* **31:**513–517.

GOMERSALL, J. D., and STUART, A., 1973, Amitriptyline in migraine prophylaxis, *J. Neurol. Neurosurg. Psychiatry* **36:**684–690.

GREENBERG, L. M., YELLIN, A. M., SPRING, C., and METCALF, M., 1975, Clinical effects of imipramine and methylphenidate in hyperactive children, *Int. J. Ment. Health* **4:**144–156.

GROF, P., SAXENA, B., CANTOR, R., KAIGLE, L., HETHERINGTON, D., and HAINES, T., 1974, Doxepin versus amitriptyline in depression: A sequential double-blind study, *Curr. Ther. Res.* **16:**470–476.

GUILLEMINAULT, C., CARSKADON, M., DEMENT, W. C., 1974, On the treatment of rapid eye movement narcolepsy, *Arch. Neurol.* **30:**90–93.

GUZE, S. B., WOODRUFF, R. A., and CLAYTON, P. J., 1971, Secondary affective disorder: A study of 95 cases, *Psychol. Med.* **1:**426–428.

HAMILTON, M., and WHITE, J. M., 1959, Clinical syndromes in depressive states, *J. Ment. Sci.* **105:**985.

HASKELL, D. S., DIMASCIO, A., and PRUSOFF, B., 1975, Rapidity of symptom reduction in depressions treated with amitriptyline, *J. Nerv. Ment. Dis.* **160:**24–33.

HAYES, T. A., PANITCH, M. L., and BARKER, E., 1975, Imipramine dosage in children: A comment on "imipramine and electrocardiographic abnormalities in hyperactive children," *Am. J. Psychiatry* **132:**546–547.

HERZOG, A., and DETRE, T., 1974, Postpartum psychoses, *Dis. Nerv. Syst.* **35:**231–236.

HIMMELHOCH, J. M., DETRE, T. P., KUPFER, D. J., SWARTZBURG, M., and BYCK, R., 1972, Treatment of previously intractable depressions with tranylcypromine and lithium, *J. Nerv. Ment. Dis.* **155:**216–220.

HIPPIUS, H., 1972, The current status of treatment for depression, in: *Depressive Illness, Diagnosis, Assessment, Treatment* (P. Keilholz, ed.), pp. 49–58, H. Huber, Bern.

HOLLISTER, L. E., 1974, Doxepin hydrochloride, *Ann. Intern. Med.* **81:**360–363.

HOLLISTER, L. E., OVERALL, J. E., and JOHNSON, M. H., 1966, Amitriptyline alone and combined with perphenazine in newly admitted depressed patients, *J. Nerv. Ment. Dis.* **142:**460–469.

JACOBSSON, L., GLITTERSTAM, K., and PALM, U., 1974, Objective assessment of anticholinergic side effects of tricyclic antidepressants, *Acta Psychiatr. Scand. Suppl.* **255**:47–53.

JOHNSTONE, E. C., and MARSH, W., 1973, Acetylator status and response to phenelzine in depressed patients, *Lancet* **1**:567–570.

KAY, D. W. K., FAHY, T., and GARSIDE, R. F., 1970, A seven-month double-blind trial of amitriptyline and diazepam in ECT treated depressed patients, *Br. J. Psychiatry* **117**:667.

KAY, D. W. K., GARSIDE, R. F., and FAHY, T. J., 1973, A double-blind trial of phenelzine and amitriptyline in depressed out-patients. A possible differential effect of the drugs on symptoms, *Br. J. Psychiatry* **123**:63–67.

KILOH, L. G., and GARSIDE, R. F., 1963, The independence of neurotic depression and endogenous depression, *Br. J. Psychiatry* **109**:451.

KILOH, L. G., BALL, J. R. B., and GARSIDE, R. F., 1962, Prognostic factors in treatment of depressive states with imipramine, *Br. Med. J.* **1**:1225–1227.

KLEIN, D. F., 1964, Delineation of two-drug responsive anxiety syndromes, *Psychopharmacologia* **5**:397.

KLEIN, D. F., 1974, Endogenomorphic depression. A conceptual and terminological revision, *Arch. Gen. Psychiatry* **31**:447–454.

KLEIN, D. F., and DAVIS, J. M., 1969, *Diagnosis and Drug Treatment of Psychiatric Disorders,* Williams and Wilkins, Baltimore.

KLERMAN, G. L., DIMASCIO, A., WEISSMAN, M., PRUSOFF, B., and PAYKEL, E. S., 1974, Treatment of depression by drugs and psychotherapy, *Am. J. Psychiatry* **131**:186–191.

KOTIN, J., POST, R. M., and GOODWIN, F. K., 1973, Drug treatment of depressed patients referred for hospitalization, *Am. J. Psychiatry* **130**:1139–1141.

KRAEPLIN, E., 1921, *Manic Depressive Insanity and Paranoia,* E. S. Livingstone, Edinburgh.

KRAGH-SORENSEN, P., HANSEN, C. E., and ASBERG, M., 1973, Plasma levels of nortriptyline in the treatment of endogenous depression, *Acta Psychiatr. Scand.* **49**:444–456.

KRAGH-SORENSEN, P., HANSEN, C. E., LARSEN, N. E., NAESTOFT, J., and HVIDBERG, E. F., 1974, Long-term treatment of endogenous depression with nortriptyline with control of plasma levels, *Psychol. Med.* **4**:174–180.

KUPFER, D. J., and DETRE, T. P., 1971, Once more. . .on the extraordinary side effects of drugs, *Clin. Pharmacol. Ther.* **12**:575–582.

KUPFER, D. J., and FOSTER, F. G., 1975, The sleep of psychotic patients: Does it all look alike? in: *Biology of the Major Psychoses: A Comparative Analysis* (D. X. Freedman, ed.), pp. 143–159, Raven Press, New York.

KUPFER, D. J., DETRE, T. P., and HIMMELHOCH, J., 1973, Classification of depression. A guide for the clinician. Symposium: Advances in the Treatment of Affective Disturbances, Rutgers University, New Brunswick, New Jersey.

KUPFER, D. J., PICKAR, D., HIMMELHOCH, J. M., and DETRE, T. P., 1975*a*, Are there two types of unipolar depression?, *Arch. Gen. Psychiatry* **32**:886–891.

KUPFER, D. J., FOSTER, F. G., DETRE, T. P., and HIMMELHOCH, J., 1975*b*, Sleep EEG and motor activity as indicators in affective states, *Neuropsychobiology* **1**:296–303.

LEONHARD, K., KORFF, I., SCHULZ, H., 1962, Temperament in families with monopolar and bipolar phasic psychoses, *Psychiatr. Neurol. (Basel)* **143**:416.

LEVINE, J., and RASKIN, A., 1974, Predicting treatment responsiveness–resistiveness in a population of depressed patients, *Pharmakopsychiatrie* **7**:217–222.

LINGJAERDE, O., EDLUND, A. H., GORMSEN, C. A., GOTTFRIES, C. G., HAUGSTAD, A., HERMANN, I. L., HOLLNAGEL, P., MAKIMATTILA, A., RASMUSSEN, K. E., REMVIG, J., and ROBAK, O. H., 1974, The effect of lithium carbonate in combination with tricyclic antidepressants in endogenous depression. A double-blind, multicenter trial, *Acta Psychiatr. Scand.* **50**:233–242.

LOPEZ-IBOR ALINO, J. J., AYUSO GUTIERREZ, J. L., and MONTEJO IGLESIAS, M. L., 1973, Tryptophan and amitriptyline in the treatment of depression, *Int. Pharmacopsychiatry* **8**:145–151.

MAPOTHER, E., 1926, Discussion on manic-depressive psychosis, *Br. Med. J.* **2**:872–879.

MARTIN, G. I., and ZAUG, P. J., 1975, Electrocardiographic monitoring of enuretic children receiving therapeutic doses of imipramine, *Am. J. Psychiatry* **132**:540–542.

McCLURE, D. J., LOW, G. L., and GENT, M., 1973, Clomipramine HCl—a double-blind study of a new antidepressant drug, *Can. Psychiatr. Assoc. J.* **18**:403–408.

MEDICAL LETTER, 1974*a*, Imipramine for enuresis, *Med. Lett.* **16**:22–24.

MEDICAL LETTER, 1974*b*, Sunscreen, *Med. Lett.* **16**:60.

MEDICAL LETTER, 1975*a*, Antidepressant drugs, *Med. Lett.* **17**:1–3.

MEDICAL LETTER, 1975*b*, Adverse interactions of drugs, *Med. Lett.* **17**:17.

MENDELS, J., and DIGIACOMO, J., 1973, The treatment of depression with a single daily dose of imipramine pamoate, *Am. J. Psychiatry* **130**:1022–1024.

MINDHAM, R. H. S., HOWLAND, C., and SHEPHERD, M., 1973, An evaluation of continuation therapy with tricyclic antidepressants in depressive illness, *Psychol. Med.* **3**:5–17.

MORRIS, J. B., and BECK, A. T., 1974, The efficacy of antidepressant drugs, *Arch. Gen. Psychiatry* **30**:667–674.

O'REGAN, J. B., 1974, Hypersomnia and MAOI antidepressants, *Can. Med. Assoc. J.* **111**:213.

OSSOFSKY, H. J., 1974, Endogenous depression in infancy and childhood, *Comp. Psychiatry* **15**:19–25.

PAYKEL, E. S., 1972, Depressive typologies and response to amitriptyline, *Br. J. Psychiatry* **120**:147–156.

PAYKEL, E. S., DIMASCIO, A., HASKELL, D., and PRUSOFF, B. A., 1975, Effects of maintenance amitriptyline and psychotherapy on symptoms of depression, *Psychol. Med.* **5**:66–77.

PERRIS, C., 1966, A study of bipolar (manic-depressive) and unipolar recurrent depressive psychoses, *Acta Psychiatr. Scand.* **42** (Suppl. 194):1–188.

PERRIS, C., 1971, Personality patterns in patients with affective disorders, *Acta Psychiatr. Scand.* **47**:43–50.

PETTI, T. A., and CAMPBELL, M., 1975, Imipramine and seizures, *Am. J. Psychiatry* **132**:538–540.

PRANGE, A. J., 1975, Pharmacotherapy of depression, in: *The Nature and Treatment of Depression* (F. F. Flach and S. C. Draghi, eds.), pp. 255–269, John Wiley & Sons, New York.

PRANGE, A. J., WILSON, I. C., KNOX, A., McCLANE, T. K., and LIPTON, M. A., 1970, Enhancement of imipramine by thyroid stimulating hormone: Clinical and theoretical implications, *Am. J. Psychiatry* **127**:191–199.

PRIEN, R. F., KLETT, C. J., and CAFFEY, E. M., 1973, Lithium carbonate and imipramine in prevention of affective episodes, *Arch. Gen. Psychiatry* **29**:420–425.

QUINN, P. O., and RAPOPORT, J. L., 1975, One-year follow-up of hyperactive boys treated with imipramine or methylphenidate, *Am. J. Psychiatry* **132**:241–245.

RAPOPORT, J. L., QUINN, P. O., BRADBARD, G., RIDDLE, K. D., and BROOKS, E., 1974, Imipramine and methylphenidate treatments of hyperactive boys, *Arch. Gen. Psychiatry* **30**:789–793.

RASKIN, A., 1972, Adverse reactions to phenelzine: Results of a nine hospital depression study, *J. Clin. Pharmacol.* **12**:22–25.

RASKIN, A., 1974, A guide for drug use in depressive disorders, *Am. J. Psychiatry* **131**:181–185.

RASKIN, A., SCHULTERBRANDT, J. G., REATIG, N., and McKEON, J. J., 1970, Differential response to chlorpromazine, imipramine, and placebo, *Arch. Gen. Psychiatry* **23**:164–173.

RAVARIS, C. L., NIES, A., ROBINSON, D. S., IVES, J. O., LAMBORN, K. R., and KORSON, L., 1976, A multiple dose, controlled study of phenelzine in depression-anxiety states, *Arch. Gen. Psychiatry* **33**:347–350.

RICKELS, K., HUTCHINSON, J. C., WEISE, C. C., CSANALOSI, I., CHUNG, M. R., and CASE, W., 1972, Doxepin and amitriptyline-perphenazine in mixed anxious-depressed neurotic outpatients: A collaborative study, *Psychopharmacologia* **23**:305–318.

RICKELS, K., WEISE, C. C., CSANALOSI, I., CHUNG, H. R., FELDMAN, H. S., RESENFELD, H., and

WHALEN, E. M., 1974, Clomipramine and amitriptyline in depressed outpatients. A controlled study, *Psychopharmacologia* **34**:361–376.

ROBINS, E., and GUZE, S. B., 1972, Classification of affective disorders: The primary-secondary, the endogenous-reactive, and the neurotic-psychotic concepts, in: *Recent Advances in the Psychobiology of Depressive Illnesses* (T. A. Williams, M. M. Katz, and J. A. Shield, eds.), U.S. Gov't. Printing Office, Washington, D.C.

ROBINSON, D. S., NIES, A., RAVARIS, C. L., and LAMBORN, K. R., 1973, The monoamine oxidase inhibitor, phenelzine, in the treatment of depressive-anxiety states, *Arch. Gen. Psychiatry* **29**:407–413.

ROSENTHAL, S., and GUDEMAN, J., 1967, The self-pitying constellation in depression, *Br. J. Psychiatry* **113**:485–489.

ROSENTHAL, S. H., and KLERMAN, G. L., 1966, Content and consistency in the endogenous depressive pattern, *Br. J. Psychiatry* **112**:471–484.

ROTH, M., and MYERS, D. H., 1969, Anxiety neuroses and phobic states: II. Diagnosis and management, *Br. Med. J.* **1**:559–562.

SAFER, D., ALLEN, R., and BART, E., 1972, Depression of growth in hyperactive children on stimulant drugs, *N. Engl. J. Med.* **287**:217–220.

SARGENT, W., 1961, Drugs in the treatment of depression, *Br. Med. J.* **1**:225–227.

SCHUCKIT, M., ROBINS, E., and FEIGHNER, J., 1971, Tricyclic antidepressants and monoamine oxidase inhibitors: Combination therapy in the treatment of depression, *Arch. Gen. Psychiatry* **24**:509–514.

SCHULTERBRANDT, J. G., RASKIN, A., and REATIG, N., 1974, True and apparent side effects in a controlled trial of chlorpromazine and imipramine in depression, *Psychopharmacologia* **38**:303–317.

SEAGER, C. P., and BIRD, R. L., 1962, Imipramine with electrical treatment in depression: A controlled trial, *J. Ment. Sci.* **108**:704–707.

SHAW, D. M., JOHNSON, A. L., and MACSWEENEY, D. A., 1972, Tricyclic antidepressants and tryptophan in unipolar affective disorder, *Lancet* **2**:1245.

SNYDER, B. D., BLONDE, L., MCWHIRTER, W. R., 1974, Reversal of amitriptyline intoxication by physostigmine, *J. Am. Med. Assoc.* **230**:1433–1434.

SPIKER, D. G., and PUGH, D. D., 1976, Combining tricyclic and monoamine oxidase inhibitor antidepressants, *Arch. Gen. Psychiatry* **33**:828–830.

SPIKER, D. G., WEISS, A. N., CHANG, S. S., RUWITCH, J. F., and BIGGS, J. T., 1975, Tricyclic antidepressant overdose: Clinical presentation and plasma levels, *Clin. Pharmacol. Ther.* **18**:539–546.

STRAUSS, J., 1973, Diagnostic models and the nature of psychiatric disorder, *Arch. Gen. Psychiatry* **29**:445–449.

TAUB, A., 1975, Factors in the diagnosis and treatment of chronic pain, *J. Autism Child. Schizoph.* **5**:1–12.

TEYCHENNE, P. F., CALNE, D. B., LEWIS, P. J., and FINDLEY, L. J., 1975, Interactions of levodopa with inhibitors of monoamine oxidase and L-aromatic amino acid decarboxylase, *Clin. Pharmacol Ther.* **18**:273–277.

TYBER, M. A., 1975, The relationship between hiatus hernia and tricyclic antidepressants: A report of five cases, *Am. J. Psychiatry* **132**:652–653.

WAIZER, J., HOFFMAN, S. P., POLIZOS, P., and ENGELHARDT, D. M., 1974, Outpatient treatment of hyperactive school children with imipramine, *Am. J. Psychiatry* **131**:587–591.

WALKER, R. D., DETURE, F. A., FENNELL, R. S., and RICHARD, G. A., 1974, Enuresis, diagnosis and management, *J. Fla. Med. Assoc.* **61**:861–864.

WATTS, C. A. H., 1957, The mild endogenous depression, *Br. J. Med.* **1**:4–8.

WEINBERG, W. A., RUTMAN, J., SULLIVAN, L., PENICK, E. C., and DIETZ, S. G., 1973, Depression in children referred to an educational diagnostic center: Diagnosis and treatment. Preliminary report, *J. Pediatr.* **83**:1065–1072.

WEISSMAN, M. M., KLERMAN, G. L., PAYKEL, E. S., PRUSOFF, B., and HANSON, B., 1974,

Treatment effects on the social adjustment of depressed patients, *Arch. Gen. Psychiatry* **30:**771–778.

WEST, E. D., and DALLY, T. J., 1959, Effects of iproniazid in depressive syndromes, *Br. Med. J.* **1:**1491–1494.

WHEATLEY, D., 1972, Potentiation of amitriptyline by thyroid hormone, *Arch. Gen. Psychiatry* **26:**229–233.

WHYBROW, P. C., COPPEN, A., PRANGE, A. J., NOGUERA, R., and BAILEY, J. E., 1972, Thyroid function and the response to *l*-iothyronine in depression, *Arch. Gen. Psychiatry* **26:**242–245.

WINOKUR, G., CLAYTON, P. J., and REICH, T., 1969, *Manic-Depressive Illness*, C. V. Mosby, St. Louis, Missouri.

WINSBERG, B. G., GOLDSTEIN, S., YEPES, L. E., and PEREL, J. M., 1975, Imipramine and electrocardiographic abnormalities in hyperactive children, *Am. J. Psychiatry* **132:**542–545.

WOODRUFF, R. A., GOODWIN, J. W., and GUZE, S. B., 1974, *Psychiatric Diagnosis*, pp. 3–24, Oxford University Press, New York.

WYATT, R. J., FRAM, D. H., BUCHBINDER, R., and SNYDER, F., 1971a, Treatment of intractable narcolepsy with a monoamine oxidase inhibitor, *New Engl. J. Med.* **285:**987–991.

WYATT, R. J., FRAM, D., KUPFER, D. J., and SNYDER, F., 1971b, Total prolonged drug-induced rapid eye movement sleep suppression in anxious-depressed patients, *Arch. Gen. Psychiatry* **24:**145–155.

ZALL, H., 1971, Lithium carbonate and isocarboxazid—an effective drug approach in severe depression, *Am. J. Psychiatry* **127:**136–139.

6

LITHIUM PHARMACOLOGY AND PHYSIOLOGY

Nelson Howard Hendler

1. INTRODUCTION

The use of lithium in psychiatry has followed a slow evolutionary path since Cade's first published report in 1949 (Cade, 1970). From 1949 to 1968 only 70 papers were published on the use of lithium in psychiatric patients (Kline, 1969). The way has been strewn with many hypotheses relating to the efficacy, mechanism of action, pharmacology, and toxicity of lithium. From this melange of data one can derive some basic principles which are critical to the proper interpretation of original articles, and using these precepts as a framework, one can construct a coherent body of information from one that originally seems so contradictory.

Many caveats must constantly be considered in evaluating the impact and validity of any article on lithium. The first and most apparent of these is the fact that acute lithium administration does not produce the same effects as chronic lithium dosage, and studies must be differentiated on this basis. Additionally, studies of lithium physiology done in normal control patients cannot be readily compared to studies in manic or depressed patients because of a difference in electrolyte metabolism seen in affective disorders. Also, despite some similarities, the differences between human and animal studies relating to pharmacology, physiology, and toxicity are apparent.

More subtle factors to be considered are variations between intracellular, serum, urine, and cerebrospinal fluid levels of lithium and how these affect

Nelson Howard Hendler • Department of Neurological Surgery and Department of Psychiatry and the Behavioral Sciences, The Johns Hopkins University School of Medicine, and The Johns Hopkins Hospital, Baltimore, Maryland.

various hormones and enzymes. A different affinity for lithium exists between some organs as does distinct variability within certain areas of an organ. Even if one carefully analyzes lithium's effect on homogenous cells, there are variabilities that exist within subcellular fragments, so that studies done on brain slices must be further differentiated to specific areas of the brain, and still further delineated based on the level of cellular functioning examined, i.e., membrane action potential, presynaptic vesicles, enzymatic degradation, synaptic transmission, or synthesis of various synaptic transmitters.

Armed with this conceptual framework, hopefully one can become more critical in the assessment and interpretation of the myriad number of articles about lithium now appearing in the world literature.

2. HISTORICAL REVIEW

2.1. Discovery in Basic Chemistry

A. Arfvedson is generally credited for the discovery of the alkali metal lithium in either 1817 or 1818, by separating sodium compounds from the mineral petalite (Schou, 1957; Kline, 1969). The name lithion (later lithia) was given to this new metal by Arfvedson's professor and mentor Baron Jons Jakob Berzelius (Kline, 1969), who himself discovered thorium in 1829 and biliverdin in 1840 (Garrison, 1929). Sir Humphrey Davy (1788–1829) who isolated sodium, potassium, calcium, and magnesium (Garrison, 1929), is also credited with isolating the free metal of lithium (Kline, 1969). In 1855, the metal was produced in quantity by R. Bunsen and A. Matthiessen from the chloride (Kline, 1969, 1973).

2.2. History of Clinical Uses

Kline traces the use of "alkali springs" in the treatment of psychiatric disorders to Soranus of Ephesus [Kline, 1969, biographer of Hippocrates, and second-century (A.D.) authority on obstetrics, gynecology, bandaging, and nutrition (Garrison, 1929)]. A fifth-century African physician from Numidia, Caelius Aurelianus (Kline, 1969), credited Soranus for the use of certain mineral waters for treating mental disorders and was himself considered to have evolved the "most sensible and humane treatment of insanity in antiquity . . ." (Garrison, 1929).

The modern-day application of lithium in medicine began with Lipowitz (1841), Ure (1844), and Garrod (1859) (Schou, 1957), when it was used to treat gout, rheumatism, uremia, and renal calculi (Kline, 1969). However, the presence of potassium and sodium *in vivo* negated lithium's *in vitro* effects of dissolving uric acid and urate deposits, thus eliminating it from the medical armamentarium (Kline, 1973). Lithium again crept into clinical use when Squires (1908) reported lithium bromide was effective against epilepsy (Kline, 1969, 1973; Cade, 1970); to date, this is still a controversial although perhaps valid observation (Gershon and Yuwiler, 1960; Erwin *et al.*, 1973). Culbreth, in 1917, reported lithium bromide was the most hypnotic of the bromides (Kline, 1969) and Wier, Mitchell, and Fontan used LiBr as a sleeping draught (Gershon and Yuwiler, 1960).

The medical use of lithium again waned until the classic report of Cade (1949), in which he treated "psychotic excitement" with lithium citrate. However, within a year of Cade's article, there was a report in the medical literature of death due to lithium (Roberts, 1950). At the same time lithium was enjoying a widespread popularity as a salt substitute, being the saltiest of the alkali metal chlorides (Geldard, 1953). Unfortunately the very patients who were using lithium chloride were those in whom lithium use would be counterindicated today—people who were taking sodium-depleting diuretics, had restricted sodium intake, and suffered from advanced renal or cardiac disease. Additionally, Dr. John H. Talbott found most cases of toxicity occurred when the self-administered dosages exceeded what would normally be considered unsafe dosages today (Kline, 1973). This bad publicity again sent lithium underground.

2.3. Present Uses

Kline (1973) credits "the persistence of Schou and the insistence of Gershon" for preventing the total disappearance of the use of lithium from psychiatry. Other early researchers in the psychiatric use of lithium were Trautner, Noack, Ashburner, Carrere, Pochard, Deschamps, Denis, Deshaies, Despinoy, Dontriaux, Landry, de Romeuf, Duc, Maurel, Giustino, Glesinger, Lafon, Margulies, Reyss-Brion, Giambert, Swadon, Chanoit, Teulie, Follin, Begoin (Schou, 1957), and later Baastrup, Mosketi, Vojtechovsky, and Andreani (Kline, 1973), most of whom confirmed Cade's original discovery. Since lithium's first clinical trial with manic excitement, other applications have been suggested. Gershon and Yuwiler (1960) mention possibilities of lithium treatments for epilepsy, premenstrual tension, sociopathic personalities, and postpuerperal mania. It has been effective in endogenous depression (Fieve *et al.*, 1968; Mendels *et al.*, 1972; Mendels, 1973), alcoholism (Kline *et al.*, 1974), schizoaffective schizophrenia (Angst *et al.*, 1970), periodic catatonia (Gjessing, 1967), aggressive behavior (Sheard, 1971; Demers, 1975) and cyclothymic personalities (Dyson and Mendels, 1968).

Lithium usage even now has found favor with the nonpsychiatric community again, albeit in a very esoteric application. White and Fetner's (1975) article, entitled "Treatment of the Syndrome of Inappropriate Secretion of Antidiuretic Hormone with Lithium Carbonate," is the case in point. However, discussion of the present and future uses of lithium in psychiatry is most comprehensively covered in the next chapter, authored by Gershon and Shopsin, and is best left to these two noted authorities. The concern of this chapter will be the attempt to explain where, how, and why lithium works.

3. BASIC CHEMISTRY AND BIOPHYSICS

3.1. Basic Properties

Lithium is an element of the alkali metal group, which includes sodium, potassium, rubidium, and cesium (Schou, 1957). These group IA metals have an ascending order in the size of the radius of each cation—beginning with lithium, 0.60 Å; sodium, 0.95 Å; potassium, 1.33 Å; rubidium, 1.48 Å; and ending with cesium, 1.69 Å (Williams, 1973). Lithium has an atomic number of 3, an atomic weight of 6.940, and a specific gravity of 0.534 (Schou, 1957). Lithium has a strong affinity for water (Kline, 1969), and this hygroscopic property makes it the most soluble of the alkali metal (group IA) chlorides (Schou, 1957; Williams, 1973). However, when lithium combines with water, the radius of the *hydrated* lithium ion is the largest of the group IA metals, while cesium has the smallest hydrated radius (Schou, 1957). The heavy hydration of lithium affects its mobility in water, thus giving it the lowest ionic conductivity (Williams, 1973). Schou (1957) also notes the *ionic* radius has the reverse order, i.e., lithium, 1.20 Å; sodium, 1.90 Å; and potassium, 2.66 Å (Swanson and Stahl, 1972). Lithium also has the greatest preference for small anions and those with a high charge, and this preference declines as one ascends through the group IA alkali metals, again ending with cesium (Williams, 1973).

The biological impact of the preceding statistics becomes most apparent when one compares lithium, not to the group IA monovalent alkali metal group, but rather to the group IIA divalent cation family. Several authors (Schou, 1957; Williams, 1973; Birch, 1974) have noted the similarities between the chemical properties of lithium and magnesium. The most striking of these is the radius of the simple ion, i.e., lithium 0.60 Å and magnesium 0.65 Å (Williams, 1973), and the atomic radius of 1.33 Å and 1.36 Å, respectively (Birch, 1974). The similarity continues when one considers the ionizing potential (Schou, 1957), the weak affinity for nitrogen, the preference for anions with a small radius or high charge, and the occurrence in nature, not as a chloride, but as a silicate (Williams, 1973). Since magnesium is a coenzyme of a great many biological events, it is significant that lithium so closely resembles its chemical properties. The clinical interactions will be discussed later.

3.2. Lithium and Cell Membranes

As a general overview, there are two major types of cell membranes found in nature—nonexcitable and excitable. The latter category encompasses nerve and muscle cells, which in their resting state are more permeable to potassium than sodium, and when active, experience a massive sodium permeability change, so that they become much more permeable to sodium than potassium. This is accomplished primarily by altering sodium influx and efflux, while potassium exchange remains nearly constant (Hodgkin and Katz, 1949).

There are three possible mechanisms by which any substance can pass through the two types of membranes: (1) direct movement through a membrane; (2) passage through a pore; and (3) pinocytosis (possibly) (Swanson and Stahl, 1972). Membrane permeability to directly diffusing substances depends on hydrogen-binding groups, size of the molecule, and sometimes the number of bare methylene groups, and therefore applies only to nonelectrolytes (Swanson and Stahl, 1972).

Monovalent cations move across all cell membranes in a fashion that jumbles the order most often seen based on purely chemical properties mentioned earlier. There seems to be a selectivity, based on a mechanism to be discussed later, that does not relate to any basic physical property *per se* and is not even compatible with the naturally occurring abundance of the group IA cations in the body. Potassium most readily crosses any resting cell membrane, followed by rubidium, cesium, sodium, and finally lithium (Williams, 1973). This order becomes even more confusing when ionic permeability is considered in the action state of nerve and muscle fibers; sodium becomes most readily permeable, followed by lithium, potassium, rubidium, and then cesium (Williams, 1973). This order may account for the fact that lithium can almost completely substitute for sodium in generating an action potential (Hodgkin and Katz, 1949). It is apparent that it is most difficult to get lithium to pass through a resting membrane, and enter a cell, which may account for the large doses needed to effect lithium's action (Williams, 1973) and the clinically observed six- to ten-day lag period needed before lithium is effective (Gershon and Yuwiler, 1960; Tupin, 1970; Davis *et al.*, 1973a). In order to explain the differential permeability to cell membranes noted for the monovalent cations, the theory of ionic movement based on ion and pore size must be modified.

3.3. Lithium and Facilitated Diffusion

Singer and Rotenberg (1973) feel that many of the biologic characteristics of lithium are due to its physical and chemical similarities with sodium and potassium. However, they hasten to add that lithium "is not handled precisely like either" of the most abundant cations in the human body and suggest that lithium imperfectly substitutes for sodium or potassium, sharing a membrane "carrier" to facilitate entry into a cell, or interferes with the action of a "cation pump," thereby accounting for its intracellular accumulation (Singer and Rotenberg, 1973). The explanation for these mechanisms of influx and efflux rests with the concept of "facilitated diffusion" and "active transport" (Swanson and Stahl, 1972; Williams, 1973); also it is compatible with the mechanisms of a "semipermeable" membrane (Abood, 1972). Certain molecules pass through membranes faster than would be predicted based on purely a "pore-size" theory alone, and there seems to be a specific carrier system involved in this facilitated diffusion which does not involve any metabolic energy (Swanson and Stahl, 1972). This is a mechanism which may explain ionic entry into a cell, and it is significant that this system obeys Michaelis–Menten kinetics, which imparts to the membrane carrier the enzyme-like properties of saturation, specificity, and competition (Swanson and Stahl, 1972). Many transport systems have been suggested, but the group most intimately concerned with lithium transport is that of the macrocyclic compounds, which have a "dramatic ability to discriminate between monovalent cations" (Swanson and Stahl, 1972). Cyclic polyethers are especially selective, and there is an "excellent correlation between the ionic diameters of Li^+ (1.20 Å), Na (1.90 Å), K (2.66 Å), and the 'holes' of the cyclic polyethers. The 4-oxygen, 5-oxygen, and 6-oxygen polyethers have holes approximately 1.8, 2.7, and 4.0 Å in diameter to accommodate ions, which probably accounts for their indicated ion preferences. Complexes are not formed if the ion is too large to lie in the hole of the polyether ring" (Swanson and Stahl, 1972). This system can work in either an active or passive fashion, but for the moment, only the latter will be considered. The cyclic polyether carrier could stack together within the membrane, like a roll of Life Savers, providing a channel through which monovalent cations could pass (Swanson and Stahl, 1972). Regardless of which channel is open, i.e., sodium, potassium, or lithium, lithium can have an inhibitory effect "since it has a lower conductance than either sodium or potassium," as mentioned earlier (Williams, 1973). The direction of cation exchange is determined according to a Donnan equilibrium ratio.

Recently, Richelson (1977) reported that lithium enters excitable cell membranes (such as neurons) through the sodium channels or ionophores. In a well-designed experiment, he demonstrated increased lithium uptake into a neuronal cell by using veratridene, an alkaloid which selectively increases the permeability of electrically excitable membranes to sodium ions. Conversely, tetrodotoxin, which blocks the action potential of a nerve cell by blocking the "fast sodium channel, caused a 50% inhibition of the veratridene-stimulated lithium entry, while oubain, a (Na^+,K^+)ATPase inhibitor, had no effect on lithium entry by itself or in the presence of veratridene (Richelson, 1977). It would seem that Richelson has clearly demonstrated that, at therapeutic serum levels, lithium uses sodium channels as the major pathway into the cell; and cell membrane diffusion is less significant. To quote Richelson (1977), "this pathway of entry of lithium ions into a nerve cell may be the most important one with respect to lithium salt's therapeutic effects in the treatment of mania. For example, this Li^+ entry through the sodium channel may inhibit calcium entry during the action potential and thereby inhibit stimulus-coupled release of norepinephrine" (see Sections 4.3 and 4.4).

The second possible mechanism of facilitated diffusion employs a mobile carrier in lieu of a channel through the membrane (Swanson and Stahl, 1972). Ion specificity is based on the proposed formation of a mobile, lipid-soluble complex between cation and a selective active molecule, which would transport the cation from one interior surface of the membrane to the other (Swanson and Stahl, 1972). The facilitation or inhibition of this process at various critical points, i.e., the cation binding with the carrier, movement through the membrane, or release of the cation (permeant), can determine the degree and direction of transport (Swanson and Stahl, 1972).

3.4. Lithium and Active Transport

The active transport of sodium out of a cell, through a semipermeable membrane against an electrochemical gradient, is a well-accepted neurophysiological explanation for the low cellular concentration of sodium. This is an energy-dependent process that requires the presence of ATP and potassium in order to function (Swanson and Stahl, 1972). The generation of a nerve impulse temporarily inhibits the cation pump, allowing sodium to enter the cell; afterwards, the pump proceeds to remove sodium and restore the normal imbalance of sodium concentration across the cell membrane.

Cation pumping is thought to be dependent on the presence of an enzyme in the cell membrane which requires both sodium and potassium to function optimally. The sodium–potassium-activated-ATPase [(Na^+,K^+)ATPase] enzyme seems necessary for the active transport pump since it has several features which suggest its similarity to the active cation transport system (Swanson and Stahl, 1972):

1. It is located in the cell membrane.
2. Cation requirements are similar to those of the active transport system: There is a higher affinity for sodium on the intracellular side of a cell membrane and a higher affinity for potassium on the outside.
3. Substrate requirements coincide; both utilize ATP as an energy source for the movement of cations.
4. The enzyme system hydrolyzes ATP at a rate dependent on the intracellular sodium concentration.
5. The system is found in all cells with an active, sodium-linked transport of cations.

6. There is a good correlation between enzyme activity and rates of cation flux in different tissues.

The location of (Na^+,K^+)ATPase and its cation requirements for activity have major implications in elucidating the mechanism of action of lithium. The highest level of activity is found in tissues that have the property of electrical excitability, or a secretory function, i.e., brain, nerve, muscle, kidney, choroid plexus, and the ciliary body (Swanson and Stahl, 1972). Additionally, subcellular fractionation localizes (Na^+,K^+)ATPase in the fractions that contain cell membranes, while further subdivision of mammalian brain pinpoints the exact locale, not to the mitochondrial or synaptic vesicle, but to the external synaptosomal membranes (Swanson and Stahl, 1972).

The cations required for (Na^+,K^+)ATPase activity are obviously sodium and potassium, by definition. However, there are implications that rubidium can substitute for potassium without much of a decline in enzyme activity (Swanson and Stahl, 1972; Tobin et al., 1974). This is not true with lithium substitution for potassium. Lithium reduced the activity of (Na^+,K^+)ATPase by substituting for potassium at one-eighth the affinity and one-fourth the efficacy (Tobin et al., 1974; Ploeger, 1974). However, conflicting reports exist within the literature, and only by defining the term of lithium administration (acute vs. chronic), the setting (in vivo or in vitro), and the tissue studied, can the discrepancies be resolved.

One paper suggests that lithium activates the cation pump, by exchanging for potassium, and hyperpolarizes nerve cells in the brain of rats because of membrane stabilization (Tobin et al., 1974). The rationale for this proposal is based on the fact that lithium, in vitro, stimulates ATP hydrolysis, in the presence of magnesium, thereby increasing the dephosphorylation of (Na^+,K^+)ATPase (Tobin et al., 1974). Rubidium, on the other hand, had a biphasic effect on dephosphorylation, stimulating, then inhibiting it, in the presence of physiologic concentrations of potassium (Tobin et al., 1974). However, Ploeger (1974) administered lithium to rats for 14 days prior to conducting studies on peripheral nerve tissue (vagus) and found both (Na^+,K^+)ATPase activity, and (Mg^{2+})ATPase activity were reduced ($P \leq 0.05$, and $P \leq 0.01$, respectively). He proposes that the mechanism of action for lithium is a competitive inhibition of the carrier protein that normally transports potassium into the cell (Ploeger, 1974). Due to a postulated slow dissociation of lithium from the carrier complex, there is less carrier available for sodium and potassium transport and therefore an inhibition of the cation pump (Ploeger, 1974).

The effect of lithium on sodium sheds more light on its somewhat obscure mechanism of action. It has been well established that lithium can substitute for sodium in the mechanism generating either nerve or muscle action potential (Hodgkin and Katz, 1949; Keynes and Swan, 1959a,b; Carmeliet, 1964), but only to a limited extent (Small and Small, 1973), and the effect is short-lived (Huxley and Stampfli, 1951). Additionally, there is little change in the resting membrane potential, and lithium can passively diffuse through a membrane in a fashion similar to sodium (Keynes and Swan, 1959b; Carmeliet, 1964). However, once lithium is inside the cell, it is removed by the active cation pump at only one-eighth to one-twenty-fifth the rate of sodium (Keynes and Swan, 1959a; Giacobini, 1969), and the cell loses both sodium and potassium as a result of this (Carmeliet, 1964; Giacobini, 1969), although the potassium loss is more apparent (McKusick, 1954). Also, lithium cannot substitute for sodium in stimulating $(Na^+,K^+)ATPase$ (Schou et al., 1970). Thus lithium readily accumulates inside the cell, at the expense of other cations, and resides intracellularly at concentrations that can far exceed extracellular levels (Carmeliet, 1964).

In summary, the effect lithium has on action potentials differs from its effect on the activity of $(Na^+,K^+)ATPase$, an enzyme which is thought to be an integral part of the cation pump of cellular membranes. Lithium cannot substitute for the sodium-dependent functions of the enzyme, and inhibits its potassium-dependent functions, as it does for other potassium-dependent enzymes, such as pyruvate kinase, phosphatases, and diol-dehydratase (B_{12}) (Williams, 1973). The fact that some of these enzymes are also magnesium-dependent will be discussed later.

4. MECHANISM OF ACTION

4.1. Intracellular Concentration

Many authors conclude that for various reasons, some of which are mentioned above, lithium accumulates intracellularly (Giacobini, 1969; Vizi et al., 1972; Mendels and Frazer, 1973; Singer and Rotenberg, 1973). Significantly, it usually takes six to ten days for this intracellular accumulation to occur (an equilibrium between serum and intracellular concentration), which corresponds to the delay in the onset of its action observed clinically (Gershon and Yuwiler, 1960; Tupin, 1970; Davis et al., 1973a).

This fact has led Mendels and his co-workers (Mendels and Frazer, 1973, 1974; Mendels, 1973) to propose the red blood cell (RBC) as a model for the intracellular accumulation of lithium seen in the brain (CNS). Others share Mendels's view (Swanson and Stahl, 1972). In fact, in an elegantly designed experiment, Mendels' group fairly conclusively demonstrated that in acute and chronic lithium administration, in high and low doses, as much as a 96% correlation between RBC and CNS levels of lithium existed, while plasma levels had a far lower correlation in most cases (Frazer et al., 1973). By examining the decay curves presented in Frazer's paper, one sees that plasma levels in acute administration of lithium do not correlate very well with CNS levels for both high (4 mEq/kg) (46%) and low (2 mEq/kg) (64%) doses of lithium, but the RBC-to-CNS correlation for both acute doses is 95%

(Frazer *et al.*, 1973). Significantly, intracellular accumulation of lithium does not reach maximal levels until 8 hr after a single acute dose (Frazer *et al.*, 1973), and the lack of initial (0–1 hr) intracellular accumulation may account for the short-lived ability of lithium to replace sodium in generating an action potential (Huxley and Stampfli, 1951; Small and Small, 1973). Consequently, one must maintain a certain degree of skepticism when interpreting data from acute experiments, and a comparison between studies employing acute lithium administration vs. those using chronically pretreated subjects can be tenuous.

4.2. Lithium Adenylate Cyclase and Cyclic Adenosine 3',5'-Phosphate (cAMP)

The enzyme cAMP was first identified as the mediator of the hepatic glycogenolytic effect of norepinephrine and glucagon in 1960, and it is now recognized as the cellular regulatory agent for many hormones (Robison and Sutherland, 1971). Also, one cannot talk of cAMP without discussing adenylate cyclase, which is an integral part of the cell-surface receptor site for hormones (Robison and Sutherland, 1971; McEwen, 1975). It converts ATP into cAMP, which then proceeds to activate an intracellular receptor that stimulates phosphorylation of intracellular proteins (Singer and Rotenberg, 1973; McEwen, 1975). The phosphorylated intracellular proteins enter the cell nucleus and alter cell function through this mechanism. Significantly, this mechanism of cellular stimulation is found only for hormones that are amino acid derivatives (epinephrine) and polypeptides (glucagon and ACTH) (Sutherland, 1970), with the exception of triiodothyionine (T_3), which is a polypeptide but has a mechanism of action similar to steroids (McEwen, 1975).

The mechanism of cellular action of steroid hormones is different from that of amino acid and polypeptide hormones. Being more lipid soluble, they are able to pass through the cell membrane and bind to a specific steroid hormone receptor in the cell cytoplasm; the steroid/receptor complex enters the cell nucleus and in turn binds to specific sites on the DNA, thus activating the production of a new mRNA. The mRNA mediates intracellular protein synthesis, resulting in altered cellular functioning (McEwen, 1975). This concept differs from the earlier proposed hormonal action of steroids which utilized adenyl cyclase and cAMP (Cuthbert and Painter, 1969; Fanestil, 1969; Goodman *et al.*, 1969). The "permissive hormones" (steroids, thyroxine, and growth hormone) may influence the formation or action of cAMP, but the mechanism is obscure (Robison and Sutherland, 1971).

For the moment, this discussion will center on the effect of lithium on adenylate cyclase and cAMP. Clinical studies suggest that cAMP excretion in the urine is altered in depression and mania (Abdulla and Hamadah, 1970;

Paul *et al.*, 1970), but there is no certainty about the cause-and-effect relationship (Berg and Glinsman, 1970). Administration of lithium to manic patients with elevated urinary cAMP greatly reduced the excretion of cAMP, but this response was felt to be due to clinical improvement, rather than a direct inhibition, since the reverse was seen with depressed patients, with low cAMP, who were placed on lithium (Paul *et al.*, 1970). Later Paul and his associates (1971) found no elevation of cAMP in physically active subjects.

Studies on the effect of lithium on cAMP and adenylate cyclase in various organs demonstrated that CNS adenyl cyclase was unique, since it was much more sensitive to low concentrations of lithium than the vasopressin-sensitive adenyl cyclase of the renal medulla, the parathyroid-sensitive adenyl cyclase of the renal cortex, and the glucagon-sensitive adenyl cyclase of the liver (Dousa and Hechter, 1970*a*,*b*). Interestingly, it was demonstrated that the action of lithium can be differentiated, not only on the basis of organ specificity, but also on the site of action within like tissue. Singer and Franko (1973) were able to differentiate lithium-mediated blockage of ADH-induced cAMP on the mucosal surface of a toad's bladder, but not on the serosal surface.

One may also examine regional differences in the CNS. Brain tissue is rich in cAMP, which is located in the nuclear and mitochondrial fractions (Friedman, 1973). Adenyl cyclase is also concentrated in CNS tissue, in the membrane and synaptic portions of the cell; however, it is not clear whether it resides in the pre- or postsynaptic area (Friedman, 1973). Adenyl cyclase activity in homogenates of rat and rabbit cortex is inhibited by lithium (Forn and Valdecasas, 1971), but one is not certain if this is an artifact due to the effect of "cell breakage" on the activity of CNS adenyl cyclase, which is exquisitely sensitive to this process, in counterdistinction to platelet adenyl cyclase, which maintains its activity (Robison and Sutherland, 1971). The mechanism of inhibition is thought to be due to the loss of membrane calcium in the CNS tissue (Robison and Sutherland, 1971).

Forn and Valdecasas (1971) found that lithium inhibited histamine and norepinephrine-induced cAMP formation at a concentration of 2 mM, which approximates serum levels in manic patients, and postulate that this is possible due to adenyl cyclase inhibition. More importantly, they mention that adenyl cyclase needed magnesium or manganese for optimal epinephrine-stimulated activity, but only ACTH-stimulated adenyl cyclase activity was diminished by the absence of calcium, while epinephrine, glucagon, and fluoride stimulation were not (Forn and Valdecasas, 1971). Others concur with the idea that magnesium is needed for adenylate cyclase activation by prostroglandin E_1, and that lithium inhibits this interaction (Wang *et al.*, 1974).

Recently, investigators have begun to question exactly where lithium works in its blockade of the amino acid and polypeptide hormone-induced activation of adenyl cyclase. Since adenyl cyclase resides on the cell membrane (Robison and Sutherland, 1971; Singer and Rotenberg, 1973; Mc-

Ewen, 1975) and has its effect on the intracellular conversion of ATP to cAMP (Singer and Rotenberg, 1973; McEwen, 1975), one might assume both extracellular and intracellular lithium can inhibit hormone-induced activity. The major unanswered question is exactly where in this process lithium inhibition occurs. Four possibilities exist. Lithium could inhibit the binding of a hormone to the inactive adenyl cyclase, thus preventing its activation. This process would seem to be more dependent on extracellular lithium levels, therefore could occur in acute lithium administration, and continue throughout chronic administration. The other three possible sites of inhibition would occur intracellularly and therefore would be progressively inhibited over a six- to ten-day period of time, as internal lithium achieved equilibrium with extracellular concentrations. This intracellular lithium could (1) inhibit the dephosphorylation of ATP by adenyl cyclase, thus reducing cAMP formation; (2) inhibit cAMP coupling with the intracellular receptor resulting in protein phosphorylation (McEwen, 1975); or (3) interfere with the effect of the resulting protein/cAMP complex, possibly by altering the tertiary structure of DNA (Singer and Rotenberg, 1973).

Singer and his co-workers (1972) felt that lithium blocked the interaction of ADH and adenyl cyclase but did not interfere with the action of cAMP. They attribute the inhibition to a lithium/magnesium interaction that would alter the binding capacity of adenyl cyclase (Singer *et al.*, 1972). Earlier work suggests lithium competes with magnesium, with a reversal of adenyl cyclase inhibition being accomplished by increasing the magnesium concentration (Wolff *et al.*, 1970). A more recent work challenged this idea, since the administration of cAMP did not counteract lithium-induced diabetes insipidus, which is notoriously unresponsive to ADH administration (Forrest *et al.*, 1974). For this reason, the authors felt chronic lithium administration interferes with one of the intracellular steps distal to cAMP formation (Forrest *et al.*, 1974). Indeed, Forrest (1975) cautions readers to reject the "hypothesis that lithium may be a general inhibitor of hormones mediated via the adenylate cyclase–cyclic AMP system. . . ." The same distal site of action is proposed for the inhibition of TSH activity in rats receiving long-term lithium administration (Forrest, 1975). This conflict is resolved by Cox and Singer (1975), who feel that lithium can act both proximally and distally to cAMP.

4.3. Cellular Magnesium and Calcium

Some of the studies of lithium's effect on cAMP and adenyl cyclase suggest that the real mechanism of hormonal inhibition resides with the cationic competition involving magnesium and calcium. It has been reported that fat-cell adenyl cyclase has two binding sites for magnesium (a site altered by the action of ACTH and a catalytic site), and magnesium serves as a coenzyme in the adenyl cyclase-mediated conversion of ATP into cAMP

(Birnbaumer *et al.*, 1969). Lithium would be a likely candidate to interfere with the coenzyme activity of magnesium because of the remarkable similarities in both the atomic and crystal ionic radius (Birch, 1974). Indeed, many magnesium-dependent enzymes are inhibited by the presence of lithium (Kadis, 1974; Birch, 1974). Birch cautions that one must be observant of the concentration of lithium used, since it sometimes far exceeds tissue levels in patients, as it did in a report that demonstrated inhibition of DNA polymerase (Birch, 1974). However, there is fairly conclusive evidence that physiologic concentrations of lithium can inhibit magnesium-dependent enzymes such as hexokinase, alkaline phosphatase, pyruvate kinase (Birch, 1974), pyruvate decarboxylase, and L-alanine amino transferase (glutamic acid pyruvate transaminase), with inhibition of the last-mentioned enzyme resulting in reduced alanine formation (Kadis, 1974). Additionally, the expected and observed competition between lithium and magnesium and/or sodium (Williams, 1973) is more strikingly seen in Mg^{2+}-dependent ATPase than in (Na^+,K^+)ATPase in the vagus nerves of rats pretreated with lithium for 14 days (Ploeger, 1974). It is thought that Mg^{2+}-dependent ATPase is an integral part of the (Na^+,K^+)ATPase cation active transport, and even though two models exist for this transport system, both include magnesium as a coenzyme (Swanson and Stahl, 1972). The Mg^{2+}-dependent ATPase is thought to be the actual carrier molecule in one theory, while in the second, it provides the energy for the phosphorylation of (Na^+,K^+)ATPase, and magnesium catalyzes the cis/trans transformation, with the resulting enzyme being capable of binding either sodium or potassium depending on its allosteric configuration (Swanson and Stahl, 1972). Therefore, any inhibition of magnesium by lithium may account for an impaired cellular exchange of sodium or potassium.

Evidence for an antagonism between lithium and calcium is more obscure (Williams, 1973). In nonexcitable tissue, calcium is excreted by erythrocytes in the presence of ATP (Swanson and Stahl, 1972) and is thought to be antagonistic to cAMP in platelets and smooth muscle (Robison and Sutherland, 1971). In cardiac and striated muscle, calcium is needed for contracture (Lorkovic, 1972), can antagonize lithium-induced abnormalities (McKusick, 1954), and in turn can be inhibited by lithium or sodium nearly to the same degree (Lorkovic, 1972).

The role of calcium in nervous tissue is less conclusive, although the model for any excitatory membrane includes a Ca^{2+}–ATP phospholipid–protein complex (Abood, 1972). Replacement of external sodium with lithium reduced the efflux of calcium from a giant squid axon, while calcium uptake in brain slices is increased by the inhibition of active sodium and potassium transport (Swanson and Stahl, 1972), which is one of the actions of lithium.

It is critical to make a distinction, at this time, between axonal and synaptic activation. Thus far, neuronal excitability and various cationic influences have been reviewed. However, one cannot discuss lithium/calcium interaction without considering synaptic transmission. It has been suggested that calcium participates in the storage and release of neurosynaptic transmitters (Koelle, 1965; Abood, 1972). While calcium does not appear to be necessary for the activation of adenyl cyclase by the catecholamines (Robison and Sutherland, 1971), the synaptic junctions are very sensitive to magnesium/calcium ratios (Williams, 1973). In acetylcholine mediated ganglionic transmission, the calcium effects on synaptic transmission are inhibited by lithium (Giacobini, 1969), probably because lithium increases calcium influx (Vizi *et al.*, 1972). Calcium also appears to be involved in the excitation-coupled release of norepinephrine from neurons in the CNS (Schildkraut, 1973), but not in the peripheral sympathetic nervous system (Horst *et al.*, 1968). Centrally, lithium inhibits norepinephrine release, but lithium's action can be overcome by the addition of calcium (Katz and Kopin, 1968). Conversely, norepinephrine re-uptake is enhanced by the absence of calcium and inhibited by an overabundance of this cation (Horst *et al.*, 1968). Richelson (1977) demonstrated lithium enters CNS nerve cells via the sodium channel during the action potential, and this may block concurrent calcium entry, thereby inhibiting stimulus-coupled release of norepinephrine.

4.4. Synaptic Release and Synthesis of Catecholamines

Thus far, lithium's effect on cellular functioning has been examined in regards to active transport pumps, membrane alterations, carrier proteins, and competitive inhibition with other cations. The exploration of lithium's effect on catecholamines may provide clues to the biogenic amine hypothesis of manic-depressive disease (Schildkraut, 1965) and will combine two or more of the previously mentioned factors at any one time, thus unifying rather than fractionating ideas about the mechanism of action of lithium. The classic report in this field was published in 1966 (Schildkraut *et al.*, 1966) and demonstrated a 50% increase in deaminated catechols (intracellular MAO-mediated) after acute lithium administration, while there was a slight reduction in normetanephrine levels (12%) (extracellular COMT-mediated). The authors felt this indicated a shift in norepinephrine metabolism from synaptic cleft *O*-methylation to intracellular deamination (Schildkraut *et al.*, 1966), but their interpretation is difficult to accept based on possible artifacts as the result of their techniques, i.e., acute lithium administration, and the use of brain homogenates. Nonetheless, the thought that lithium may increase intracellular deamination was intriguing, and a more sophisticated study compared the effects of long-term lithium administration to acute (Schildkraut *et al.*, 1969). In both acute and chronically lithium-treated rat brains, there was an increase in deaminated norepinephrine, suggesting that lithium had an intracellular monoamine oxidase (MAO) stimulating effect (Schildkraut *et al.*, 1969). Short-term (4 hr) lithium administration showed that it reduced the amount of norepinephrine and normetanephrine

(COMT-mediated), while increasing deaminated catechol metabolites (MAO-mediated), which suggested that acute lithium administration resulted in an increased turnover and deamination of norepinephrine (Schildkraut *et al.*, 1969). However, after seven days of lithium, a slight, but nonsignificant, reduction of norepinephrine re-uptake (presynaptically) was noted, and norepinephrine levels were decreased by 35%, while normetanephrine was 25% lower than controls (Schildkraut *et al.*, 1969). Additionally, the turnover of norepinephrine was less, so Schildkraut and his co-workers (1969) felt that, on a percentage basis, there was really a net increase of deamination of norepinephrine in rats receiving long-term lithium administration. Other studies on rats receiving chronic lithium administration showed that the lithium pretreatment enhanced norepinephrine reuptake by the synaptosomal fraction (presynaptic membrane, synaptic vesicles, etc.) of brain homogenates by as much as 30% compared to controls (Colburn *et al.*, 1967). This same group found that the lithium concentration in synaptosomes was nearly three times that of myelin and more than six times greater than mitochondrial concentration (Colburn *et al.*, 1967).

Peripheral, acute studies in the perfused spleen indicate that lithium indeed facilitates the re-uptake of norepinephrine by 20–110% from control levels (Pomeroy and Rand, 1971), possibly due to the ability of lithium to inhibit calcium, thereby enhancing norepinephrine re-uptake (Katz and Kopin, 1968). Additionally, the acute perfusion of lithium reduced the amount of catechols released after splenic nerve stimulation (Bindler *et al.*, 1971), again possibly due to lithium's inhibition of calcium.

Perhaps here one should briefly review what is the accepted mechanism of norepinephrine's synaptic action. Norepinephrine is produced in a presynaptic vesicle and stored until stimulation. Prior to stimulation, vesicular norepinephrine exchanges with presynaptic (mobile) norepinephrine under the influence of magnesium-dependent ATPase (Iverson and Bloom, 1970) and is subject to degradation by MAO, resulting in the deaminated metabolite (Koelle, 1965). After norepinephrine release into the synapse, the action of the neurosynaptic transmitter is inhibited primarily by re-uptake by the presynaptic area. As much as 95% of the released norepinephrine is "inactivated" this way, and, with the exception of acetylcholine, which is enzymatically degraded, all known neurosynaptic transmitters use this "re-uptake" form of inactivation (Snyder, 1974). Any remaining norepinephrine in the synaptic cleft is inactivated to normetanephrine by COMT (Koelle, 1965).

Thus, chemicals that can facilitate the presynaptic re-uptake of norepinephrine reduce the amount available in the synaptic cleft for each nerve impulse, thus diminishing the noradrenergic effect. Conversely, blockage of presynaptic release also inhibits the noradrenergic effect. Based on this concept, it becomes difficult to interpret data that claim one function or the other. A study using rats that received a single dose of lithium found the effects of dexamphetamine [which causes the release of norepinephrine, and blocks its re-uptake (Snyder, 1974)] were not inhibited (U'Prichard and Steinberg, 1972). However, the third possible action of amphetamine, that of a partial, postsynaptic agonist of norepinephrine, was not considered and may explain the data.

Two groups found that fairly substantial acute doses of lithium increased the turnover of endogenous norepinephrine (Corrodi *et al.*, 1967; Stern *et al.*, 1969), while after chronic lithium administration in rats, norepinephrine was significantly lower in the CNS (Schildkraut *et al.*, 1969). Also, deaminated *O*-methylated metabolites (3-methoxy-4-hydroxyphenyglycol or MHPG, and 3-methoxy-11-hydroxymandelic acid or VMA) (Schildkraut, 1973) were found to be elevated on large chronic doses of lithium (3 mEq/kg for ten days), while there was a marked rate of disappearance of exogenously administered norepinephrine from the CNS, with a slight but nonsignificant lowering of endogenous norepinephrine (Greenspan *et al.*, 1970*a*).

Chronic lithium administration in rats has been shown not to effect endogenous levels of norepinephrine or dopamine (Corrodi *et al.*, 1969; Ho *et al.*, 1970; Bliss and Ailion, 1970) in the cerebral cortex, cerebellum, hypothalamus, brain stem, and diencephalon (Ho *et al.*, 1970), while some slight decrease in deaminate metabolites was found (Bliss and Ailion, 1970).

The effect of lithium on synaptic transmission and/or uptake has been discussed to some degree above, but it will be repeated here in a different context. One study found lithium inhibits norepinephrine release, and this action can be counteracted by calcium (Katz and Kopin, 1968). Colburn and his co-workers (1967), using chronic lithium pretreated rats, found the uptake of norepinephrine from synaptosomes was increased, as did Kuriyama and Speken (1970), while the absence of calcium enhanced norepinephrine re-uptake (Horst *et al.*, 1968). *In vivo* studies, with chronically lithium-treated rats, did not confirm the finding of increased norepinephrine uptake (Schildkraut *et al.*, 1969).

In summary, there seems to be a short-term lithium effect on norepinephrine which is manifested as an increase in the turnover rate of the catecholamine (Schildkraut, 1973). However, after at least two weeks of lithium administration, there is no increase in observed norepinephrine turnover (Schildkraut, 1973). This suggests that there is a temporally linked biphasic norepinephrine response to lithium, with a marked increase in its uptake and enzymatic degradation initially, which is followed several weeks later by a relatively steady state, with perhaps a lower "set-point" for all functions.

The evaluation of clinical studies is far more complicated than animal experimentation. Many works have been done on norepinephrine metabolites in the urine, but significantly, only one metabolite, normetanephrine, is solely dependent on COMT activity. The other commonly studied metabolites are deaminated and *O*-methylated VMA, which depend on both MAO and COMT. Only 3,4-hydroxymandelic acid depends on MAO alone, but, like normetanephrine, it is usually converted to VMA (Koelle, 1965).

In any event, early researchers noted a rise in VMA in the urine of nonpsychotic patients for two days after lithium administration; levels returned to normal after three to five days (Haskovec and Rysanek, 1969). In a manic patient, Schildkraut (1973) found a rise in urinary MHPG which lasted one week as a result of lithium administration. Greenspan and his co-workers (1970b) found that normetanephrine (the COMT-catalyzed metabolite of norepinephrine) and metanephrine (the COMT-catalyzed metabolite of epinephrine) decreased in the urine of patients after lithium administration, while lithium had no effect on norepinephrine, epinephrine, VMA, or MHPG levels, which seemed to correlate more with the clinical state of patients. The authors suggest that MHPG is the major metabolite of CNS norepinephrine and normetanephrine, both of which may not readily leave the CNS because of the blood–brain barrier (Katzman, 1972), and since as much as 50% of urinary MHPG is thought to be from the CNS (DeLeon-Jones et al., 1975), they feel that studies of MHPG will be the best indicator of CNS norepinephrine activity (Greenspan et al., 1970b). However, they recognize the shortcomings of such studies, since MHPG is also synthesized in the kidneys and liver, making interpretation of urinary data difficult (Greenspan et al., 1970b). Recently, studies of MHPG in the cerebrospinal fluid (CSF) have shown elevated MHPG in manics prior to lithium, and a reduction after lithium treatment (Wilk et al., 1972). Indeed, in the future, the method of metabolic investigation of the CSF may provide data that is far more representative of CNS functions of catecholamines than urine or blood studies, especially with the advent of the probenecid technique (Goodwin et al., 1973).

4.5. Indoleamines and Lithium

Alterations in serotonin metabolism have been implicated in affective disorders for a number of years (Mendels and Frazer, 1975), but the study of indoleamines has always taken a secondary role compared to catecholamines and is perhaps hampered by the various potential sources of error (Mendels and Frazer, 1975). The effects of lithium on indoleamine metabolism parallel catecholamine studies, and an early work by Katz and his co-workers (1968) showed that the addition of lithium to the perfusate of brain slices inhibited the stimulated release of both serotonin and norepinephrine, while it did not alter spontaneous efflux. Again, this study might be interpreted as showing that lithium facilitated the re-uptake of norepinephrine and serotonin, which has been reported elsewhere (Davis and Fann, 1971). Additionally, rats pretreated with lithium for 48 hr prior to the experiment (i.e., acutely) had a significantly reduced baseline content of both norepinephrine and serotonin

(Katz *et al.*, 1968). Other studies have examined both the acute and more prolonged effect of lithium on serotonin. Ho and co-workers (1970) examined five areas of the CNS of rats after 28 days of lithium administration. In the hypothalamus, brain stem, and diencephalon there was, respectively, a 46%, 26%, and 25% decline in synthesis of serotonin, while the cerebellum showed a 37% increase in turnover rates, and the brain stem, cortex, and hypothalamus showed decreased turnover rates of 30%, 15%, and 51%, respectively (Ho *et al.*, 1970). Additionally, in the same rats, only the hypothalamus had a significant reduction of norepinephrine turnover (29%) (Ho *et al.*, 1970).

Knapp and Mandell (1973) examined both short- and long-term effects of lithium on serotonin metabolism and found lithium increased the uptake of tryptophan, a precursor of serotonin, by striate-area synaptosomes. Also, tryptophan hydroxylase activity slowly decreased over time, while the conversion of tryptophan to serotonin increased with the additional uptake of tryptophan (Knapp and Mandell, 1973).

Clinical data suggest both catecholamines and indoleamines play a role in affective disorders, but one must be careful to distinguish between the subtypes, i.e., unipolar depressed, bipolar, and endogenous depressions with high or low MHPG in the urine. Ashcraft and co-workers (1972) found 5-hydroxindolacetic acid (5-HIAA), a metabolite of serotonin, and homovanillic acid (HVA), a deaminated, *O*-methylated metabolite of dopamine, both to be reduced in the CSF of unipolar depressed patients compared to controls. The group also reported a significant difference between the CSF levels of 5-HIAA in unipolar vs. bipolar depressed patients (Ashcroft *et al.*, 1972). After lithium treatment of manics, with elevated 5-HIAA and HVA, there was a nonsignificant reduction of CSF 5-HIAA (Ashcroft *et al.*, 1972). However, other studies show reduced 5-HIAA in the CSF of *both* depressed and manic patients, with a concomitant reduction of tryptophan in the same groups, and the authors note that lithium is effective in both disorders if properly selected (Mendels and Frazer, 1975). After a review of these studies, one may concur with the lament of both Schildkraut (1973) and Davis and co-workers (1973*b*). Further investigation is required before any firm conclusions may be drawn.

4.6. Effect of Lithium on Acetylcholine

An early work on mammalian sympathetic ganglion, in an acute preparation, claimed that nonphysiologic levels of lithium blocked postganglionic transmission, an acetylcholine-mediated synapse (Pappano and Volle, 1967), which led Giacobini (1969) to conclude that lithium was a postsynaptic inhibitor of cholinergic events. Moving up in date, but further down the phylogenetic scale, Waziri (1968) noted lithium reduced both inhibitory and excitatory postsynaptic potentials (IPSP and EPSP) in *Aplysia* neurons. Since this phenomenon could be explained either by blockage of presynaptic release or postsynaptic inhibition, acetylcholine was added to the lithium medium, and IPSP as well as EPSP returned to normal, thus suggesting presynaptic interference (Waziri, 1968). Later, Bjegovic and Randic (1971) found that when lithium was substituted for sodium it did not alter the spontaneous release of acetylcholine in a perfused cat cortex, but if synaptic firing was evoked by peripheral stimulation, there was less acetylcholine released. If one assumes that lithium indeed inhibits presynaptic acetylcholine release, the questions remaining to be answered are: (1) does lithium alter membrane qualities; or (2) does it interfere with the actual synthesis of acetylcholine. Williams (1973) mentions that lithium acts in a very different way from cholinergic drugs when one considers blockade of cation "channels." The tetraethylammonium ion $(NET_4)^+$, a cholinergic drug, utilizes or "blocks" the potassium pore in the cell membrane to almost the same degree as potassium itself, while lithium itself has the least, if any, effect of any monovalent cation (Williams, 1973). However, the reverse is true for sodium pores, where lithium approximates the action of sodium, while tetraethylammonium has practically no effect (Williams, 1973). Thus, it seems unlikely that lithium can inhibit acetylcholine release *per se.*

Vizi and his co-workers (1972) proceeded in a very logical and orderly fashion in their attempt to answer the questions posed above. Using the rationale that (1) lithium can replace sodium in generating an action potential; (2) the permeability of a nonmyelinated C fiber axon to lithium is almost that of sodium; (3) lithium is about as effective as sodium in maintaining a resting potential; (4) lithium is removed from a cell at one tenth the rate of sodium; (5) the intracellular concentration of lithium can exceed the extracellular concentration, while the intracellular concentration of sodium and potassium progressively diminish obviously in exchange for lithium; (6) as previously mentioned, lithium promotes presynaptic norepinephrine uptake, thereby diminishing the perceived norepinephrine "effect" on the postsynaptic receptor; and (7) lithium reduces the release of norepinephrine and serotonin, Vizi's group (1972) proceeded to examine the various effects of lithium on acetylcholine release and synthesis. Using an isomolar lithium chloride to replace sodium chloride, they found the lithium-containing perfusate initially (50 min) stimulated acetylcholine release from brain slices of rat cortex, but after 150 min no effects were observed (Vizi *et al.*, 1972). They postulate the initial release is due to the increase of calcium ion influx, which would cause acetylcholine release, but this was only the initial response at massively unphysiological doses of lithium (117.9 mM). The net long-term effect was a reduction in acetylcholine synthesis, which accounted for the lower levels of acetylcholine found presynaptically (Vizi *et al.*, 1972), and the blockade of ganglionic and cortical transmission (Waziri, 1968; Giacobini, 1969; Bjegovic and Randic, 1971).

4.7. Lithium and GABA

For the sake of completeness, one should consider a study of lithium's effect on the amino acid neurosynaptic transmitter GABA (gamma-aminobutyric acid). About 30% of the neurons in a rat's cortex utilize GABA as a neurosynaptic transmitter (Bloom and Iverson, 1971). Thus, it should be no surprise that lithium, when directly injected into the amygdala of awake monkeys, produced EEG changes which were mimicked by L-glutamate injections (Davis *et al.*, 1973*b*). Additionally, acute lithium administration decreases whole brain glutamate 20–60 min after injection (Delgado and DeFeudis, 1969). Obviously, whole brain studies can obscure regional changes (Davis *et al.*, 1973*b*), so a division of the response to lithium based on anatomical subdivisions of the CNS over time would be desirable. Gottesfeld and his group (1971) examined both glutamate and GABA in the hypothalamus and amygdala of rats receiving a single dose of lithium, as well as a five-day course of administration. Since GABA can block "attack behavior" evoked by glutamate stimulation of the hypothalamus (Gottesfeld *et al.*, 1971), lithium has been used to treat aggressive behavior (Sheard, 1971; Quitkin *et al.*, 1973; Demers, 1975). Furthermore since stimulation of both the hypothalamus (Smith *et al.*, 1970) and amygdala (Ursin, 1960) can result in aggressive behavior, chemical differentiation is desirable. A group of researchers in Hoebel's laboratory noted that crystalline carbacol application via chronic cannulae in the hypothalamus could produce aggressive behavior (Hendler, 1966) and that cholinergically induced "killing behavior" could be inhibited by norepinephrine (Smith *et al.*, 1970). Since there seems to be a similar antagonism between GABA and glutamate, as mentioned before, one might expect a concomitant response to lithium. Acute lithium administration resulted in a rise of both GABA and glutamate in both regions of the CNS, i.e., hypothalamus and amygdala (Gottesfeld *et al.*, 1971). These data may explain the lithium and L-glutamate effect on EEGs and the subsequent glutamate depletion (Delgado and DeFeudis, 1969). However, after five days of lithium administration, only glutamate levels were elevated in both CNS areas, while the concentration of GABA was unchanged in the amygdala and slightly elevated in the hypothalamus (Gottesfeld *et al.*, 1971). To date, no one has studied lithium's effect on the re-uptake of GABA, which one would suspect as another possible modality of GABA inhibition (Snyder, 1974).

4.8. Lithium and the Electrolyte/Membrane Theory of Affective Disorders

The effects that lithium has on active and passive membranes, enzymes, and cellular electrolytes have been discussed earlier (Section 3). However, there are practical considerations and applications for that material. Just as there has been a biogenic amine theory of affective disorders, there has existed, for some time, a body of literature supporting an electrolyte/ membrane theory. This seems most plausible, in view of the fact that the most specific and effective treatment to date of manic-depressive illness and some forms of depression is a simple electrolyte—lithium.

Electrolyte abnormalities have been frequently described in affective psychiatric disorders. Baker (1971) noted that the transfer rate of $^{22}Na^+$ from the plasma to the cerebrospinal fluid (CSF) in 18 patients with affective disease (psychotic depression, depressed manic-depressives, manic manic-depressives) was sigificantly lower than the rate for 28 neurotically depressed and schizophrenic patients, which confirmed earlier work by Coppen (1960). Carroll (1972), in his review of studies using this method, indicated that when the affective diseases were subdivided, manics have even a lower plasma/CSF transfer rate than depressed patients, and others noted that residual sodium (exchangeable sodium minus extracellular sodium) was increased in mania more than in depression (Coppen et al., 1966). Baer's group (1970a–c) noted that sodium retention occurred in depression and that residual sodium fell with recovery from depression. It was also reported that the CSF concentration of sodium in depressed patients is reduced (Baer et al., 1970a–c), probably secondary to the reduced transfer rate of sodium into the CSF (Baker, 1971). Others (Bunney et al., 1972; Mendels and Frazer, 1973, 1974) attempted to explain the abnormality of electrolyte metabolism in terms of altered membrane activity. Mendels and Frazer (1973) reported that depressed patients who had a higher lithium concentration in their red blood cells (RBC) demonstrated a good antidepressant response to lithium. The explanation offered for the altered lithium concentration in RBC was a postulated difference in the cell membrane of these two groups (Mendels and Frazer, 1973, 1974). However, Mendels and his co-workers (Mendels and Frazer, 1974; Mendels et al., 1974) cannot divorce the electrolyte/membrane theory of affective disorders from the biogenic amine theory, any more than the widely published and respected group of authors such as Bunney, Gershon, Murphy, and Goodwin (1972) can do the reverse. The marriage of the two theories is the best way to understand how lithium may work.

4.9. Integration of the Mechanisms of Action of Lithium and the Theories of Affective Disorders

Thus far, the action of lithium has been examined only from one particular point of view. Obviously, this approach is absurd, since every bodily function is the result of many processes interacting simultaneously. It is impossible to divorce cell membrane activity from neurosynaptic transmitter release and re-uptake, just as one cannot examine lithium's effect on a single cation. One cannot separate the cationic antagonisms of lithium from its enzymatic influences, which then again leads to examination of membrane activity and neurosynaptic transmitter synthesis, release, and re-uptake.

Bunney and his co-workers (1972) have updated the classic concepts regarding biogenic amine synthesis, release, re-uptake, and degradation. They suggest that lithium (a) acts at the presynaptic cell membrane, preventing biogenic amine release, (b) facilitates re-uptake of biogenic amines by the presynaptic membrane, thus counteracting the membrane deficiency in re-uptake postulated to be the process of the "switch into mania," and (c) increases the biogenic amine uptake by the synaptic vesicles (Bunney et al., 1972). This theory unifies the indoleamine and catecholamine theories of affective disorders and is in agreement with the research of others, which suggested biogenic amine uptake by synaptosomes proceeded by means of a saturable, sodium-dependent process obeying Michaelis–Menten kinetics (Bogdanski et al., 1970). It also encompasses the electrolyte/membrane theory of affective disorders, since the presynaptic membrane is identified as part of the mechanism of the pathological process of affective disease (Bunney et al., 1972). Significantly, there are three membrane processes to be identified; they are (1) biogenic amine release, (2) biogenic amine re-uptake, and (3) synaptic vesicle exchange of biogenic amines with the presynaptic mobile pool.

It has been reported that sodium is not needed for vesicular storage of norepinephrine, since there is no sodium–potassium-dependent ATPase in the synaptic vesicle (Horst et al., 1968; Swanson and Stahl, 1972). However, it seems that this process is determined by magnesium-dependent ATPase (Iverson and Bloom, 1970). Since Ploeger (1974) reported that both magnesium and sodium–potassium-dependent ATPase are inhibited by lithium, with more of an effect on the magnesium-dependent ATPase being observed, and others report that lithium blocks magnesium-dependent enzymes (Kadis, 1974; Birch, 1974), one may assume that lithium can inhibit the exchange of biogenic amines between the synaptic vesicle and the mobile presynaptic pool. Lithium also facilitates the re-uptake of biogenic amines into the mobile pool (Colburn et al., 1967; Davis and Fann, 1971), probably by inhibiting the action of calcium on the presynaptic membrane (Katz and Kopin, 1968; Horst et al., 1968; Abood, 1972). This, coupled with the fact that lithium may inhibit the release of biogenic amines, again possibly by blocking calcium (Abood, 1972; Schildkraut, 1973), may result in the accumulation of biogenic amines in the presynaptic mobile pool after lithium administration. For a biogenic amine, residence in the area is tenuous at best, since monoamine oxidase readily metabolizes any biogenic amine; this may explain, in a multifactorial fashion, the observation of Schildkraut et al. (1969) of increased deaminated norepinephrine after lithium administration and the hypothesis that reduced "apparent," i.e., usable by the synapse, levels of biogenic amines account for the salutory effect of lithium on affective disorders (Bunney et al., 1972). While one author suggests that the link between the "biogenic amine" and "electrolyte" hypothesis of affective disorders resides with lithium's ability to inhibit both the enzymatic and membrane transport effects of magnesium-dependent processes (Birch, 1974), another suggests that it is really lithium's action on the ratio of magnesium to calcium that determines its effect (Williams, 1973). Additionally, another group suggests that one should not examine absolute values of biogenic amines, but rather their ratio to one another, and attempts to demonstrate a correlation, not only between one biogenic amine and another, but the relationship of biogenic amines to electrolytes, over the course of studying a manic-depressive patient for 69 days (Mendels et al., 1974). They indeed did find that there were many correlations, namely, an increase in red blood cell (RBC) sodium and potassium, associated with a rise in 5-HIAA and VMA in the urine, respectively, as the patient's depression improved in response to lithium (Mendels et al., 1974). They also noted, as the depression improved with lithium treatment, a reduction in RBC magnesium associated with an increase of urinary 5-HIAA and RBC sodium (Mendels et al., 1974). Although only one patient was studied, the integration of the various theories of affective disorder, and the correlation of all components of lithium-produced effects, is a significant step towards developing a comprehensive understanding of lithium's mechanism of action. Hopefully, more studies of this breadth and depth will be forthcoming.

5. PHYSIOLOGY

5.1. Absorption

According to Schou (1957), lithium may be readily absorbed from the intestine, after oral ingestion, or from the subcutaneous, intramuscular, and intraperitoneal routes, after injection; it is detectable in tissue fluids and organs a few minutes after administration. However, serum levels do not peak until 1–4 hr after a single oral dose, with the majority of studies reporting 2 hr (Gershon and Yuwiler, 1960; Sugita et al., 1973; Baer, 1973; Smith-Kline Corp., 1974). This fluctuation in serum levels led to the convention that serum level determinations should be obtained 8–12 hr after the last dose of lithium (Baer, 1973). Some external factors may effect lithium absorption from intestinal tract, even though lithium is not protein bound (Schou et al., 1970). The type of anion combined with lithium, i.e., the type of salt, does not effect absorption (Amdisen and Schou, 1967), but possibly heavier patients need larger doses to achieve the same serum level as lighter people (Baer, 1973). While it is possible that ingesting large quantities of glucose or sodium-containing substances may alter jejunal absorption of lithium (Singer and Rotenberg, 1973), the most revealing evidence regarding altered absorption comes from other factors. Sugita and his co-workers (1973) demonstrated that the actual dosage form of lithium employed could dramatically influence serum levels. Comparing the brand-name lithium carbonate product from Smith, Kline and French laboratories against one from another pharmaceutical firm, they found that the former compound was 90% in solution after 15 min when using distilled water, synthetic intestinal fluid, or 0.10 N HCl, while the latter product was only 10% in solution at 15 min, and at 200 min, only 20% of it was dissolved in water, 28% in "intestinal fluid," and 43% in 0.10 N HCl (Sugita et al., 1973). Additionally, the same oral dose of medication resulted in serum levels of 0.91 mEq/liter for the Smith, Kline and French product and 0.40 mEq/liter for the other, with concomitant reductions in the urine (Sugita et al., 1973).

5.2. Distribution

Lithium rapidly distributes to the liver and kidney and is more slowly absorbed by muscle, bone, and brain (Schou et al., 1970). While Bakay (1956) reports it takes 8 hr for sodium to equilibrate across the blood–brain barrier, others report that 60 hr is needed for both sodium and potassium (Gershon and Yuwiler, 1960; Baker and Winokur, 1966). Lithium has been reported to take 22–26 hr to reach maximal levels in the brain (Baer, 1973), and the time course of absorption across the blood–brain barrier indicates a slow equilibrium, with the serum-to-CSF ratio being 24.6 : 1 at 2–4 hr, 5.7 : 1 at 7–8 hr, and 3.6 : 1 at 24 hr after acute administration (Platman and Fieve, 1969; Davis and Fann, 1971). Baker and Winokur (1966) did not find a significant difference in the serum-to-CSF lithium ratio between manic, depressed, and schizophrenic patients, with the CSF values usually being one-fourth those of serum values at 8 hr. This ratio is true for chronic lithium administration (Baer, 1973), and Baer (1973) also noted a similarly altered plasma-to- RBC ratio of lithium, i.e., 3 : 1. Others have reported differences between certain groups of patients, finding that manic patients retained lithium and that it entered cells faster than in a control group (Almy and Taylor, 1973), while a similar increased cellular uptake has been noted in depressed manic-depressive or unipolar depressed patients (Mendels and Frazer, 1973). These observations have been confirmed by research demonstrating that RBC lithium is a better predictor of CNS lithium than is serum (Frazer et al., 1973) and that the ratio of RBC/serum could serve as a predictor of patients who would respond to lithium (Mendels and Frazer, 1974) after seven days of lithium therapy (Mendels and Frazer, 1973). The fact that lithium resides intracellularly has been discussed earlier (Section 4.1) and accounts for the observation that lithium space exceeds calculated total body water (Baer, 1973).

There is also a possibility that a differential uptake of lithium exists between various areas of the CNS. Samoelov (1972) reported that lithium is selectively collected in hypophysical tissue, which may be explained using the concepts of the blood–brain barrier. Classically, the anatomical blood–brain barrier has been considered to be the perivascular end-feet of astrocytes (Fleishhauer, 1957, 1958, 1960). Later, a physiological barrier was suggested, consisting of an active transport process moving substances from the brain to the blood against a concentration gradient (Edstrom *et al.*, 1961; Steinwall, 1961). The anatomical barrier has been considered to be a lipid membrane, since the influx rate of most substances appears to vary with the lipid solubility of the molecule as it exists in the plasma (Brodie and Hogbon, 1957; Mayer *et al.*, 1959; Brodie *et al.*, 1960). Due to the physiological barrier, however, accumulation of a substance, unlike influx, is not necessarily related to lipid solubility (Barlow, 1964). Thus, when the central nervous system concentration of a substance is unequal to that of a plasma ultrafiltrate, it is possible that a steady-state equilibrium simply has not been reached or that an active transport process may have altered the steady-state equilibrium (Barlow, 1964). The latter explanation may account for the slow equilibrium of lithium mentioned earlier in this section.

Recently, Rapoport and his group (1972) have confirmed earlier theories which suggested that the blood–brain barrier acts like a layer of cells (probably capillaries of the brain) that respond to osmotic influences by shrinking or swelling, thereby opening up spaces between them. The state of the cells and therefore the spaces between them determines the presence or absence of a "blood–brain barrier" (Rapoport *et al.*, 1972) and certainly could be dramatically influenced by the intracellular accumulation of lithium.

An important factor which is often neglected in studies of the blood–brain barrier is its nonuniformity. Certain areas of the CNS, among them the adenohypophysis, neurohypophysis, area postrema, intercolumnar tubercle, pineal gland, subfornical organ, supraoptic crest, and parts of the tuber cinereum and median eminence have been shown to accumulate for greater amounts of dyes and tracers than do other parts of the central nervous system (Bakay, 1956; Wilson and Brodie, 1961). The lack of uniformity of the blood–brain barrier and the specific areas not protected may account for lithium's preferential influence on certain hormones.

5.3. Excretion

As mentioned in the introduction, patients with affective diseases metabolize lithium in a different fashion than control subjects (Trautner *et al.*, 1955), and animal studies really do not give a precise picture of the human physiology (Thomsen and Schou, 1968). Also, after chronic lithium administration the pharmacodynamics differ greatly from the "single-dose" dynamics. In general, the major route of lithium elimination is the kidney (Schou, 1957; Thomsen and Schou, 1968; Schou *et al.*, 1970), with 90–95% recovery in the urine being the figure usually quoted (Trautner *et al.*, 1955; Baer, 1973). However, there is some elimination in feces, sputum, sperm, and sweat (Trautner *et al.*, 1955). Lithium is freely filtered by the glomerulus, since it is not protein bound (Baer, 1973), and its renal clearance and excretion is independent of plasma concentration, water loading, furosemide, bendroflumethiazide, ethacrynic acid, ammonium chloride, spironolactone, or potassium chloride (Thomsen and Schou, 1968). These findings, coupled with the fact that osmotic diuresis, sodium bicarbonate, acetazolamide, and aminophylline increase lithium excretion, suggest that lithium is reabsorbed in the proximal tubule (Thomsen and Schou, 1968; Schou *et al.* 1970). Four fifths of lithium is reabsorbed by the proximal tubules (Schou *et al.*, 1970). Additionally, the one-fifth of the lithium that is excreted is concentrated in the loop of Henle by the countercurrent mechanism, much the same as with sodium (Thomsen and Schou, 1968). The distal tubule is not involved with lithium reabsorption, as suggested by the work of Baer (1973), since DOCA (a mineralocorticoid) does not enhance lithium reabsorption. Also, spirono-lactone (an inhibitory analog of the mineralocorticoid aldosterone), which blocks sodium reabsorption at the distal tubule, does not influence lithium reabsorption (Davis and Fann, 1971; Baer, 1973). However, the actual cation, sodium, does influence lithium reabsorption and excretion. Dietary sodium restriction can lead to the accumulation of lithium (Baer, 1973), presumably because the kidney will reabsorb more lithium at the proximal tubule in the absence of sodium (Thomsen and Schou, 1968).

Studies done on normal subjects, using a single oral dose of lithium (600 mg Li_2CO_3 = 16.2 mEq of lithium), demonstrated lithium clearance to be 19.25 cc/min with C_{Li}/C_{Cr} = 0.17–0.23 with a standard deviation of 0.02 (Thomsen and Schou, 1968). Other studies compare lithium excretion and retention between manic patients and normal controls. In an early work (Gershon and Yuwiler, 1960), lithium (19–50 mEq) was given to control subjects in a single dose, and after 15 min, began to appear in the urine, with a peak of urinary elimination occurring at 1–2 hr. Over the next 6–7 hr there was a slow decline, with 30–70% being eliminated in 8 hr after ingestion (Gershon and Yuwiler, 1960). This single dose resulted in increased urinary pH, a transient diuresis, and a marked increase of sodium chloride as well as some increase in potassium chloride in the urine (Gershon and Yuwiler, 1960). After repeated lithium administration, and urinary measurement, urinary lithium excretion rose sharply, and then leveled off after five to six days, with sodium and potassium alterations stopping after six days (Gershon and Yuwiler, 1960). Measurement of lithium excretion over an 8-hr period of time in both normal and manic patients showed that the former excreted 30% of 27 mEq of lithium given in one dose, while the latter excreted 27% (Epstein *et al.*, 1965). Epstein and his co-workers (1965) did not find any variation in 24-hr excretion of lithium between manics and controls, but others have found manics do retain lithium (Trautner *et al.*, 1955; Greenspan *et al.*, 1968; Almy and Taylor, 1973). In one study, normal controls would excrete 45–75% of an initial single dose in 24 hr, while active manic patients excrete only 12–20% in the same period (Gershon and Yuwiler, 1960). Almy and Taylor (1973) found after a single test dose of lithium (24.75 mEq), manics retained 16 mEq of the dose in 36 hr (65%), while controls retained only 10 mEq (44%). They also found that the half-life of lithium was 18 hr in controls and greater than 36 hr in manics, and ascribe this to a rapid intracellular accumulation of lithium in manics (Almy and Taylor, 1973). Greenspan and his group (1968), using a manic patient as his own control, demonstrated that lithium retention occurred until day 12, i.e., the oral dose of lithium exceeded urinary excretion by 5–20 mEq/day. After 12–14 days, lithium equilibrated and lithium intake equaled its output (Greenspan et al., 1968). Once equilibrium is established, i.e., lithium intake equals urinary output, one may calculate the maintenance dosage in mEq/24 hr by multiplying renal lithium clearance (cc/min, determined by a single dose of lithium) by average serum concentration of lithium times 1.44 (Schou et al., 1970). This is useful in older patients, children, and patients with impaired renal functions (Schou et al., 1970).

In summary, one may say that manics retain lithium, as do certain depressed patients (Mendels and Frazer, 1973), and that it takes 6–14 days for lithium to equilibrate in the body. Thus, the reportedly higher doses of lithium needed early in manic episodes in order to achieve therapeutic blood levels may be explained by the previously mentioned research which demonstrates an increased ability to absorb and intracellularly retain lithium in severe affective disorders.

5.4. Interactions with Other Cations

Lithium has been shown to influence both monovalent and divalent cations, and for the sake of simplicity, each will be examined in turn. Many authors have reported a biphasic effect of lithium on the sodium ion (Trautner et al., 1955; Baer et al., 1970a, 1971; Davis and Fann, 1971), which indicates a natriuresis lasting 1–2 days, after the onset of continuous lithium administration; this is followed by a period of sodium retention, lasting 2–5 days, with a return to normal sodium balance by 6–10 days. Baer and his group (1970a, 1971) also reported that potassium follows roughly the same pattern of excretion and retention, but to a lesser degree. Exogenously administered sodium can only slightly lower the serum lithium levels (Demers and Heninger, 1971), but a reduction of sodium intake results in significantly elevated serum lithium levels (Baer, 1973). The interrelationship between sodium and lithium is well outlined in a paper by Baer and co-workers (1970b). By measuring "sodium space" using [24]Na, they found manic and hypomanic patients who responded to lithium had more exchangeable sodium space and less intracellular or residual sodium space (Baer et al., 1970b), and this may be due to a lithium-induced change in sodium distribution (Baer, 1973).

The role of the renin–angiotensin–aldosterone system in sodium/lithium interactions, and in affective disorders in general, has been explored by several groups of investigators. Animal studies reveal that chronic lithium administration results in sodium depletion, which is greater in the CNS than the rest of the body (Baer *et al.*, 1970c). Concomitantly, there was potassium loss as well, but not to the same degree as sodium. Depletion of these cations over a 14-day period of lithium administration does not parallel what is noted in human studies, nor can it be explained solely on the basis of aldosterone inhibition (Baer *et al.*, 1970c). Smith and Thompsen (1973) noted that relative renal lithium clearance was related to sodium intake in both adrenalectomized and control rats, but the reduced absolute lithium clearance noted in adrenalectomized rats was not related to creatinine clearance, urine flow, or to sodium and potassium excretion. Baer and his co-workers (1973) gave DOCA to rats receiving lithium and a control group. They noted a reduced ability to retain sodium in the lithium-treated rats and concluded that lithium blocked the mineralocorticoid effect of DOCA (Baer *et al.*, 1973), which is certainly feasible, based on the mechanism of action of aldosterone and lithium (Fanestil, 1969). In humans, the acute response to lithium administration is a natriuresis with a concomitant rise in renin noted by some researchers (Demers *et al.*, 1971; Baer, 1973). Others have felt lithium does not increase renin, and note, instead, a reduced pressor response to angiotensin II (Fleischer *et al.*, 1971). However, the authors do suggest there is a temporary rise in aldosterone, which they feel is related to a direct lithium effect on the zona glomerulosa of the adrenal (Fleischer *et al.*, 1971). The transient rise in aldosterone has been noted by others, and usually lasts 2–10 days (Murphy *et al.*, 1969; Hendler *et al.* 1976), which coincides with the transient rise seen in renin secretion, probably in response to the lithium-induced natriuresis and not as a result of direct stimulation (Baer, 1973). Several authors have reported elevated aldosterone in the untreated manic phase of manic-depressive disease (Allsopp *et al.*, 1972; Akesode *et al.*, 1976; Hendler, 1975), which returns to normal levels after 14 days of lithium administration (Hendler, 1975, Hendler *et al.*, 1976). Whether or not these findings are related to the pathogenesis of affective disease remains to be seen.

The influence of lithium on divalent cations is related to its previously discussed enzymatic effects. The only comprehensive study attempting to relate the various cationic effects of lithium was done longitudinally on one patient by Mendels and his group (1974). They found a reduction in RBC magnesium as the patient's urinary 5-HIAA increased and as the concentration of lithium in the RBC increased (Mendels *et al.*, 1974). However, even though RBC potassium and sodium rose with increased RBC lithium, there was no correlation with magnesium (Mendels *et al.*, 1974). Again, in one patient studied longitudinally, Bunney and his group (1968) noted a correlation of improvement of mania associated with increased serum levels of lithium and magnesium. The fact that serum and RBC levels of magnesium may not coincide was demonstrated by Nielsen (1964a), who reported an elevated serum magnesium in manic patients treated with lithium compared to a control group, while no differences were found in RBC magnesium between the manic and control group. The effect may be related to the duration or dosage of lithium, since both Nielsen (1964b) and Andreoli and co-workers (1972) found increases in serum magnesium from days 4–14 at high lithium doses in rabbit and rat, respectively. Serum calcium has been found to rise in response to lithium in rats (Andreoli *et al.*, 1972), and this has been found to have clinical significance. Depressed patients, who met the criteria for primary affective disorder, were given lithium, and serum levels of both magnesium and calcium were determined for five days following the institution of lithium therapy (Carmen *et al.*, 1974). The best predictor of an antidepressant response to lithium was found when patients demonstrated a rise in both calcium and magnesium, with 15/16 patients improving (Carmen *et al.*, 1974). Additionally, 13/17 patients, who experienced a fall in either magnesium and calcium or both within five days of instituting lithium therapy, did not respond to the antidepressant effects of lithium, while the best predictor of a nonresponder was a decrease in magnesium in response to lithium, with 10/11 failures (Carmen *et al.*, 1974). In light of the previously discussed effect of lithium on magnesium- and calcium-dependent enzymes, this work could be of great clinical significance.

6. INTERACTIONS WITH PHARMACEUTICALS

6.1. Concurrent Use of Diuretics

As was mentioned earlier, lithium toxicity is enhanced by reduced sodium intake (Baer, 1973). The earliest reported toxicities with lithium were reported in patients using diuretics that cause sodium loss, but despite this longstanding *caveat*, patients still are placed on natriuretic agents with lithium, and serious consequences have resulted. Even after the discontinuance of lithium, one may experience toxicity induced by the addition of diuretics (Hurtig and Dyson, 1974). The safest rule of thumb is offered by Singer (1974), who categorically states one should not use diuretic agents with lithium, unless they do not cause concurrent potassium loss (e.g., triamterene or amiloride).

6.2. Lithium and Haloperidol

No less an authority than Schou (1968) recommends the concomitant use of lithium and haloperidol. However, a recent study reported irreversible brain damage in patients receiving this combination (Cohen and Cohen, 1974), but one must examine the data carefully. The subjects were given high doses of haloperidol, and two of the four reported cases developed persistent dyskinesias (Cohen and Cohen, 1974), a well-established side effect of haloperidol. In a well-designed and -controlled study, Leonard and co-workers (1974) report a beneficial synergistic effect of lithium and haloperidol on Huntington's chorea patients, with no indications of any CNS impairment. Furthermore a report suggesting the use of lithium to treat tardive dyskinesia (Reda *et al.*, 1975), the very effect that Cohen and Cohen (1974) report it causes, lends credence to the acceptance of the combined use of lithium and haloperidol.

6.3. Lithium and Insulin

Lithium seems to increase serum insulin after two weeks of therapy, with or without weight gain (Mellerup *et al.*, 1972). Additionally, glucose tolerance increases after long-term lithium administration, i.e., lower blood glucose levels were observed after a glucose load (van der Velde and Gordon, 1969; Heninger and Mueller, 1970). Singer and Rotenberg (1973) suggest the mechanism of this action is the similarity of both lithium and insulin in decreasing cAMP levels, inhibiting adenyl cyclase, and blocking glucose and fat release. Therefore, one may have to reduce insulin dosage slightly in a diabetic patient receiving lithium, assuming the renal status is not impaired.

6.4. Lithium and Tricyclic Antidepressants

Shopsin and Gershon (1973) indicate that "there have been no controlled studies carried out expressly for the purpose of assessing the toxic liability or interaction between lithium and other psychoactive drugs or ECT." However, Lingjaerde and others (1974) noted a synergism between lithium and imipramine-H-oxide in combination, given to endogenously depressed patients, when compared to tricyclics alone or other tricyclics with lithium; they attribute this response to lithium's inhibition of tricyclic degradation. Another report indicates that lithium and imipramine have antagonistic effects on platelets, with the latter inhibiting biogenic amine transport, while lithium was found to enhance serotonin and metaraminol transport and uptake by the platelets (Murphy *et al.*, 1970). The only nonclinical synergism with tricyclic antidepressants reported is lithium's ability to serve as a reversible, competitive inhibitor of butyrylcholine esterase (Davis *et al.*, 1973*b*).

6.5. Lithium and the MAOI-Tranylcypromine

The classic, if not only, paper in this area suggests that since the sedative side effects of tricyclic antidepressants add to anergy, retardation, and hypersomnia, a trial on MAOI was warranted (Himmelhock *et al.*, 1972). Twenty-one depressed unipolar or bipolar patients were given tranylcypromine, while 20 were concomitantly on lithium, and 11 had no previous response with tricyclic antidepressants (Himmelhock *et al.*, 1972). Of the 21 patients, 11 had a complete remission, another five improved substantially, and the remaining five improved, then in four or five days began to show paranoid ideation, foreshadowing a manic episode (Himmelhock *et al.*, 1972). This was attributed to the amphetamine-like structure of tranylcypromine (Himmelhock *et al.*, 1972), and the remarkable recovery in 16 of the 21 patients far outweighs the precipitated manic-like episodes.

6.6. Lithium and Diphenylhydantoin

Erwin and his co-workers (1973) reported the administration of lithium to 15 epileptic patients already receiving diphenylhydantoin and still averaging 4.4 seizures a month. No status epilepticus was noted after the addition of lithium, and six had 50% fewer seizures, while ten had 25% fewer seizures, and nine demonstrated a reduced (greater than 25%) number of epileptiform discharges on EEG (Erwin *et al.*, 1973). On a purely neurophysiological basis, one might expect a synergism between diphenylhydantoin and lithium, and one cannot forget the early reports of its success in epilepsy. However, one of the 15 patients cited above did have increased (166%) seizure activity (Erwin *et al.*, 1973) and one of 62 patients did have a grand mal seizure as the result of lithium administration (Baldessarini and Stephens, 1970), so one must be careful not to become overly enthusiastic as yet.

7. EFFECTS ON CLINICAL TESTS

7.1. ECG (EKG)

As early as 1957, Schou (1957) reported T-wave abnormalities as the result of lithium administration in one-fifth of patients receiving the drug. Recently, using a very thorough recording of ECG, employing a 12-lead technique, Demers and Heninger (1970) found all nine manic-depressive patients on lithium had some T-wave depression, even though all were on high-sodium diets. While patients with substantial T-wave depression developed U waves, there was no consistent P or QRS change, nor were rhythm abnormalities noted (Demers and Heninger, 1970). A follow-up study by the same authors (Demers and Heninger, 1971a) noted that the T-wave depression starts within five days after lithium administration and returns to normal three to five days after discontinuing lithium. They also reported the T-wave alterations were variable on a day by day basis, did not correlate with a high-

or low-sodium diet, and enzyme levels were not elevated (Demers and Heninger, 1971a). The conclusion drawn by the authors was that ECG changes needed to be determined on a serial basis in order to demonstrate T-wave changes and to counteract the variability (Demers and Heninger, 1971a). A single case report indicates lithium could cause ectopic foci, PVCs, and irregularly irregular beats, and the authors (Tangedahl and Gau, 1972) suggest discontinuing lithium and replacing potassium slowly to counteract the intracellular hypokalemia.

7.2. EEG

In an encouraging paper by Erwin and his co-workers (1973), they report 9 of 15 seizure patients had greater than a 25% reduction of epileptiform discharges, with clinical improvement in ten. A less optimistic account is given by others who reported diffuse slowing and widening of the frequency spectrum in all nine patients (Mayfield and Brown, 1966), but their subjects were either manic at the time of the study, or had a history of mania, and the EEGs were recorded 2 hr after lithium administration. In a well-controlled study, Platman and Fieve (1969) demonstrated more EEG changes in 45 manic-depressed patients on lithium than on placebo, with slowing (3–7 cps) being the most common abnormality. In another study over a one-year time span, using each patient as his own control, James and Reilly (1971) noted that lithium had a normalizing effect on frequency and could convert delta and beta rhythm to alpha during the course of one year. This is in counterdistinction to the toxic effect of lithium noted by Schou and his group (1968) in which EEG alpha activity was reduced and theta and delta rhythm increased. Based on the above, it is apparent that lithium's effect on EEGs varies with the clinical state of the subject, the time course, and degree of lithium administration.

7.3. WBC

Lithium has been noted to cause a leukocytosis, with neutrophilia and lymphopenia, in counterdistinction to chlorpromazine, which caused a leuko-penia (Shopsin *et al.*, 1971). However, the leukocytosis is felt to be reversible and innocuous (Shopsin *et al.*, 1971) and may be related to a steroid effect on bone marrow (Watanabe *et al.*, 1974a). It was also reported that the neutrophilia is due to a shift in segmented neutrophils (51–67%), but no correlation was noted between serum lithium levels and leukocytosis (Watanabe *et al.*, 1974a,b).

7.4. Serum Sodium and Potassium

Much has already been said about the effect of lithium on intracellular, urinary, and RBC concentrations of sodium and potassium, but little regarding serum levels. This should be expected, because every effort is made by the body to maintain homeostasis, which for sodium and potassium is a proper serum level. Regardless of the wild swings in sodium and potassium in all other body spaces in response to lithium, *serum* levels of these cations (not *blood* levels which would include about 45% of its value from the RBCs) remain remarkably constant (Trautner *et al.*, 1955).

7.5. Serum Magnesium and Calcium

The reader is referred to Section 5.4 of this chapter.

8. CONCLUSION

Despite its erratic entry into the field of medicine, lithium has now become firmly entrenched as an indispensable therapeutic tool in psychiatry. Understanding the mechanism of action of lithium will do much for understanding the pathology of endogenous affective disorders and other syndromes responsive to lithium therapy. While lithium may not survive in psychiatry, as more specific treatments for various disorders evolve, it nonetheless has and will probably continue to serve psychiatry and mankind as new and sometimes surprising uses are found for it.

9. REFERENCES

ABDULLA, Y. H., and HAMADAH, K., 1970, 3′,5′-Cyclic adenosine monophosphate in depression and mania, *Lancet* **1:**378–381.

ABOOD, L. G., 1972, Excitation and conduction in the neuron, in: *Basic Neurochemistry* (W. Albers, G. Seigel, R. Katzman, and B. Agranoff, eds.), pp. 41–65, published for the American Society for Neurochemistry (first edition), Churchill/Livingstone, Edinburgh.

AKESODE, A., HENDLER, N., and KOWARSKI, A., 1976, A 24-hr monitoring of the integrated plasma concentration of aldosterone and cortisol in manic patients, *Psychoneuroendocrinology* **1:**419–426.

ALLSOPP, M. N. E., LEVEL, M. J., STITCH, S. R., and HULLIN, R. P., 1972, Aldosterone production rates in manic depressive psychosis, *Br. J. Psychiatry* **120:**399–404.

ALMY, G. L., and TAYLOR, M. A., 1973, Lithium retention in mania, *Arch. Gen. Psychiatry* **29:**232–234.

AMDISEN, A., and SCHOU, M., 1967, Biochemistry of depression, *Lancet* **1:**507–538.

ANDREOLI, V. M., LILLANI, F., and BRAMBILLA, G., 1972, Increased calcium and magnesium excretion induced by lithium carbonate, *Psychopharmacologia* **25**:77–85.

ANGST, J., WEIS, P., GROF, P., BAASTRUP, P. C., and SCHOU, M., 1970, Lithium prophylaxis in recurrent affective disorders, *Br. J. Psychiatry* **116**:604–614.

ASHCROFT, G. W., ECCLESTON, D., MURRAY, L. G., GLEN, A. I. M., CRAWFORD, T. B. B., and PULLAR, I. A., 1972, Modified amine hypothesis for the etiology of affective illness, *Lancet* **2**:573–577.

BAER, L., 1973, Pharmacology—lithium absorption, distribution, renal handling and effect on body electrolytes, in: *Lithium* (S. Gershon and B. Shopsin, eds.), pp. 33–50, Plenum Press, New York.

BAER, L., PLATMAN, S. R., and FIEVE, R., 1970*a*, The role of electrolytes in affective disorders, *Arch. Gen. Psychiatry* **22**:108–113.

BAER, L., DURELL, J., BUNNEY, W., JR., LEVY, B., MURPHY, D., GREENSPAN, K., and CARDON, P., 1970*b*, Na$^+$ balance and distribution in LiCO$_4$ therapy, *Arch. Gen. Psychiatry* **22**:40–44.

BAER, L., KASSIR, S., and FIEVE, R. R., 1970*c*, Lithium-induced changes in electrolyte balance and tissue electrolyte concentration, *Psychopharmacologia (Berlin)* **17**:216–224.

BAER, L., PLATMAN, S. R., KASSIR, S., and FIEVE, R. R., 1971, Mechanisms of renal lithium handling and their relationship to mineralo-corticoids: A dissociation between sodium and lithium ions, *J. Psychiatr. Res.* **8**:91–105.

BAER, L., GLASSMAN, A., and KASSIR, S., 1973, Negative sodium balance in lithium carbonate toxicity, *Arch. Gen. Psychiatry* **29**:823–827.

BAKAY, L., 1956, *The Blood Brain Barrier With Special Regard to the Use of Radioactive Isotopes,* Charles C. Thomas, Springfield, Illinois.

BAKER, E. F. W., 1971, Sodium transfer to cerebrospinal fluid in functional psychiatric illness, *Can. Psychiatr. Assoc. J.* **16**:167–170.

BAKER, M. A., and WINOKUR, G., 1966, Cerebrospinal fluid lithium in manic illnesses, *Br. J. Psychiatry* **112**:163–165.

BALDESSARINI, R., and STEPHENS, J., 1970, LiCO$_4$ for affective disorders, *Arch. Gen. Psychiatry* **22**:72–77.

BARLOW, D. F., 1964, Clinical aspects of the blood–brain barrier, *Am. Rev. Med.* **15**:187–202.

BERG, G., and GLINSMANN, W. A., 1970, Cyclic A.M.P. in depression and mania, *Lancet* **1**:834.

BINDLER, E. H., WALLACH, M. B., and GERSHON, S., 1971, Effect of lithium ion on the release of ^{14}C-norepinephrine by nerve stimulation from the perfused cat spleen, *Arch. Int. Pharmacol. Ther.* **190**:150–154.

BIRCH, N. J., 1974, Letter: Lithium and magnesium dependent enzymes, *Lancet* **2**(7886):965–967.

BIRNBAUMER, L., POHL, S. L., and RODBELL, M., (July) 1969, Adenyl cyclase in fat cells, *J. Biol. Chem.* **244**(13):3468–3476.

BJEGOVIC, M., and RANDIC, M., 1971, Effect of lithium ions on the release of acetylcholine from the cerebral cortex, *Nature* **230**:587–588.

BLISS, E. L., and AILION, J., 1970, The effect of lithium upon brain neuroamines, *Brain Res.* **24**:305–310.

BLOOM, F. E., and IVERSON, L. L., 1971, Localizing [^{3}H]GABA in nerve terminals of rat cerebral cortex by electron-microscopic autoradiography, *Nature* **229**:628–630.

BOGDANSKI, D. F., GLASZKOWSKI, T. P., and TISSARI, A. A., 1970, Mechanisms of biogenic amine transport and storage, *Biochem. Biophys. Acta* **211**:521–532.

BRODIE, B. R., and HOGBON, C. A., 1957, Some physico-chemical factors in drug action, *J. Pharm. Pharmacol.* **9**:345–380.

BRODIE, B. R., KURZ, H., and SCHENKER, L. A., 1960, The importance of dissociation constant and lipid solubility, *J. Pharmacol. Exp. Ther.* **130**:20–25.

BUNNEY, W. E., JR., GOODWIN, F. K., DAVIS, J. M., and FAWCETT, J. A., 1968, A behavior-biochemical study of lithium treatment, *Am. J. Psychiatry* **125**:499–512.

BUNNEY, W. E., JR., GERSHON, E. S., MURPHY, D. L., and GOODWIN, F. K., 1972, Psychobiological and pharmacological studies of manic-depressive illness, *J. Psychiatr. Res.* **9**:207–226.

CADE, J. F. J., 1949, Lithium salts in the treatment of psychotic excitement, *Med. J. Aust.* **36**:349–358.

CADE, J. F. J., 1970, The story of lithium, in: *Discoveries in Biological Psychiatry* (F. Ayd, Jr., and B. Blackwell, eds.), pp. 218–229, J. B. Lippincott, Philadelphia.

CARMAN, J. S., POST, R. M., TEPLITZ, T. A., and GOODWIN, F. K., 1974, Letter: Divalent cations in predicting antidepressant response to lithium, *Lancet* **2**(7894):1454.

CARMELIET, E. E., 1964, Influence of lithium ions on the transient wave potential and cation content of cardiac cells, *J. Gen. Physiol.* **47**:501–530.

CARROLL, B., 1972, Sodium and potassium transfer to cerebrospinal fluid in severe depression, in: *Depressive Illness: Some Research Studies* (B. Davies, B. Carroll, and R. Mowbray, eds.), pp. 247–257, Charles C. Thomas, Springfield, Illinois.

COHEN, W. J., and COHEN, N. A., 1974, Lithium carbonate, haloperidol, and irreversible brain damage, *J. Am. Med. Assoc.* **230**(9):1283–1287.

COLBURN, R. W., GOODWIN, F. K., BUNNEY, W. E., JR., and DAVIS, J. M., 1967, Effect of lithium on the uptake of norepinephrine by synaptosomes, *Nature* **215**:1395–1397.

COPPEN, A. J., 1960, Abnormality of the blood–cerebrospinal fluid barrier of patients suffering from a depressive illness, *J. Neurol. Neurosurg. Psychiatry* **23**:156–161.

COPPEN, A. J., SHAW, D. M., MALLESON, A., and COSTAIN, R., 1966, Mineral metabolism in mania, *Br. Med. J.* **1**:71–75.

CORRODI, H., FUXE, K., HOKFELT, T., and SCHOU, M., 1967, Effect of lithium on cerebral monoamine neurons, *Psychopharmacologia* **11**:345–353.

CORRODI, H., FUXE, K., and SCHOU, M., 1969, The effect of prolonged lithium administration on cerebral monoamine neurons in the rat, *Life Sci.* **8**:643–651.

COX, M., and SINGER, I., 1975, Lithium and the adenylate cyclase–cAMP system, *N. Engl. J. Med.* **293**(1):46.

CUTHBERT, A. W., and PAINTER, E., 1969, Mechanism of action of aldosterone, *Nature* **222**:280–281.

DAVIS, J. M., and FANN, W. E., 1971, Lithium, *Annu. Rev. Pharmacol.* **11**:285–302.

DAVIS, J. M., JANOWSKY, D., and EL-YOUSEF, M. K., 1973*a*, The use of lithium in clinical psychiatry, *Psychiatr. Ann.* **3**:78–99.

DAVIS, J. M., JANOWSKY, D. S., and EL-YOUSEF, M. K., 1973*b*, Pharmacology—the biology of lithium, in: *Lithium* (S. Gershon and B. Shopsin, eds.), pp. 167–189, Plenum Press, New York.

DeLEON-JONES, F., MAAS, J. W., DEKIRMENJIAN, H., and SANCHEZ, J., 1975, Diagnostic subgroups of affective disorders and their urinary excretion of catecholamine metabolites, *Am. J. Psychiatry* **132**:1141–1148.

DELGADO, J. M., and DeFEUDIS, F. V., 1969, Effects of lithium injections into the amygdala and hippcampus of awake monkeys, *Exp. Neurol.* **25**:255–267.

DEMERS, R. G., 1975, Personal communication.

DEMERS, R. G., and HENINGER, G., 1970, Electrocardiographic changes during lithium treatment, *Dis. Nerv. Syst.* **31**:674–679.

DEMERS, R. G., and HENINGER, G., 1971*a*, Sodium intake and lithium treatment in mania, *Am. J. Psychiatry* **128**(1):132–136.

DEMERS, R. G., and HENINGER, G., (October) 1971*b*, Electrocardiographic T-wave changes during lithium carbonate treatment, *J. Am. Med. Assoc.* **218**:381–386.

DEMERS, R. G., HENDLER, R., ALLEN, R. P., and BOYD, J., 1971, Edema and increased plasma renin activity in lithium treated patients, *Physicians' Drug Manual* **3**(1–2):2–5, 24.

DOUSA, T., and HECHTER, O., 1970*a*, Lithium and brain adenyl cyclase, *Lancet* **1**:834–835.

DOUSA, T., and HECHTER, O., 1970*b*, The effect of NaCl and LiCl on vasopressin-sensitive adenyl cyclase, *Life Sci.* **9**(1):765–770.

Dyson, W., and Mendels, J., 1968, Lithium and depression, *Curr. Ther. Res.* **10**:601–608.

Edstrom, E., Ricardo, P., and Steinwall, P., 1961, The blood–brain barrier phenomenon, *Acta Neurol. Scand.* **37**:1–21.

Epstein, R., Grant, L., Herjanic, M., and Winokur, G., 1965, Urinary excretion of lithium in mania, *J. Am. Med. Assoc.* **192**:409–410.

Erwin, C. W., Gerber, C. J., Morrison, S. D., and James, J. F., 1973, Lithium carbonate and convulsive disorders, *Arch. Gen. Psychiatry* **28**:646–648.

Fanestil, D., 1969, Mechanism of action of aldosterone, *Annu. Rev. Med.* **20**:223–231.

Fieve, R. R., Platman, S. R., and Plutchik, R. R., 1968, The use of lithium in affective disorders: I. Acute endogenous depression, *Am. J. Psychiatry* **125**:487–491.

Fleischer, K., Binick, E., Klaus, D., and Tolle, R., 1971, Effects of lithium on plasma renin and the pressor responsiveness to angiotensin in man, *Arzneim. Forsch.* **21**:1363–1364.

Fleishhauer, K., 1957, Untersuchungen am Ependym des Zwischenand Mettelhirns der Landschildkrote, *Z. Zellforsch.* **46**:729–767.

Fleishhauer, K., 1958, Uber die Feinstruktur der Faserglia, *Z. Zellforsch.* **47**:548–556.

Fleishhauer, K., 1960, Fluorescenzmikroskopische Untersuchungenan der Faserglia, *Z. Zellforsch.* **51**:467–496.

Forn, J., and Valdecasas, F. G., 1971, Effects of lithium on brain adenyl cyclase activity, *Biochem. Pharmacol.* **20**:2773–2779.

Forrest, J. N., 1975, Lithium inhibition of cAMP mediated hormones: A caution, *N. Engl. J. Med.* **292**(8):423–424.

Forrest, J. N., Cohen, A. D., Torretti, J., Himmelhock, J. M., and Epstein, F. H., 1974, On the mechanism of lithium-induced diabetes insipidus in man and rat, *J. Clin. Invest.* **53**:1115–1123.

Frazer, A., Mendels, J., Secunda, S. K., Cochrane, C. M., and Bianchi, C. P., 1973, The prediction of brain lithium concentrations from plasma or erythrocyte measures, *J. Psychiatr. Res.* **10**:1–7.

Friedman, E., 1973, Pharmacology—lithium's effect on cyclic AMP, membrane transport, and cholinergic mechanisms, in: *Lithium* (S. Gershon and B. Shopsin, eds.), p. 75–82, Plenum Press, New York.

Garrison, F. A., 1929, *History of Medicine*, 4th ed., pp. 93, 111–112, 118, 123, 125, 198, W. B. Saunders, Philadelphia.

Geldard, F., 1953, *The Human Senses*, p. 296, John Wiley and Sons, New York.

Gershon, S., and Yuwiler, A., 1960, Lithium ion: A specific psychopharmacological approach to the treatment of mania, *J. Neurol. Psychiatry* **1**:229–241.

Giacobini, E., 1969, The effect of lithium on the nerve cell, *Acta Neurol. Scand.* **207**:85–91.

Gjessing, L. R., 1967, Lithium citrate loading of a patient with periodic catatonia, *Acta Psychiatr. Scand.* **43**(4):372–375.

Goodman, P. B., Allen, R., and Rasmussen, D., 1969, On the mechanism of action of aldosterone, *Proc. Natl. Acad. Sci. U.S.A.* **64**:330–337.

Goodwin, F. R., Post, R. M., Dunner, D. L., and Gordon, E. K., 1973, Cerebrospinal fluid amine metabolites in affective illness—the probenecid technique, *Am. J. Psychiatry* **130**:73–79.

Gottesfeld, Z., Epstein, B. S., and Samuel, D., 1971, Effect of lithium on concentration of glutamate and GABA levels in amygdala and hypothalamus of rat, *Nature (London), New Biol.* **234**:124–125.

Greenspan, K., Green, R., and Durell, J., 1968, Retention and distribution patterns of lithium, a pharmacological tool in studying the pathophysiology of manic-depressive psychosis, *Am. J. Psychiatry* **125**(4):512–519.

Greenspan, K., Aronoff, M. S., and Bogdanski, D. F., 1970*a*, Effects of lithium carbonate on turnover and metabolism of norepinephrine in rat brain—correlation to gross behavioral effects, *Pharmacology* **3**:129–138.

Greenspan, K., Schildkraut, J. J., Gordon, E., Baer, L., Arnoff, M., and Durell, J.,

1970*b*, Catecholamine metabolism in affective disorders—III *J. Psychiatr. Res.* **7**:171–183.

HASKOVEC, L., and RYSANEK, K., 1969, Die wirkung von lithium auf den metabolismus der katecholamine und indolalkylamine bein menschen, *Arzneim. Forsch.* **19**:426–435.

HENDLER, N., 1966, The Effects of Hypothalamic Application of Crystalline Norepinephrine and Carbachol on Food Intake and Activity, Senior thesis, Psychology Department, Princeton University.

HENDLER, N., 1975, Lithium-responsive hyperaldosteronism in manic patients, *J. Nerv. Ment. Dis.* **161**(1):49–54.

HENDLER, N., UEMATSU, S., LONG, D., and ALLEN, G., 1976, Letter to the editor: Problems with lithium as treatment for inappropriate ADA secretion, *N. Engl. J. Med.* **294**(8):446.

HENINGER, G. R., and MUELLER, P. S., 1970, Carbohydrate metabolism in mania, *Arch. Gen. Psychiatry* **23**:310–319.

HIMMELHOCK, J. M., DETRE, T., KUPFER, D. J., and BYCK, R., 1972, Treatment of previously intractable depressions with tranylcypromine and lithium, *J. Nerv. Ment. Dis.* **155**:216–220.

HO, A. K. S., LOH, H. H., CRAVES, R. J., HITZEMANN, R. J., and GERSHON, S., 1970, The effect of prolonged lithium treatment on the synthesis rate and turnover of monoamines in brain regions of rats, *Eur. J. Pharmacol.* **10**:72–78.

HODGKIN, A. L., and KATZ, B., 1949, The effect of Na$^+$ ions on the electrical activity of the giant axon of the squid, *J. Physiol.* **108**:37–77.

HORST, W. D., KOPIN, I. J., and RAMEY, E. R., 1968, Influence of sodium and calcium on norepinephrine uptake by isolated perfused rat hearts, *Am. J. Physiol.* **215**(4):817–822.

HURTIG, H. I., and DYSON, W. L., 1974, Lithium toxicity enhanced by diuresis, *N. Engl. J. Med.* **290**(13):748–749.

HUXLEY, A. F., and STAMPFLI, R., 1951, Direct determination of membrane resting potential and action potential in single myelinated nerve fibers, *J. Physiol. (London)* **112**:476–495.

IVERSEN, L. L., and BLOOM, F. E., 1970, Transmitter release mechanisms, *Neurosci. Res. Prog. Bull.* **8**:407–415.

JAMES, J. F., and REILLY, E., 1971, The electroencephalographic recording of short- and long-term lithium effect, *South Med. J.* **64**:1722–1727.

KADIS, B., 1974, Letter: Lithium and magnesium-dependent enzymes, *Lancet* **2**(7890):1209.

KATZ, R. I., and KOPIN, S. J., 1968, Release of norepinephrine-^{3}H and serotonin-^{3}H evoked from brain slices by electrical field stimulation—calcium dependency and the effects of lithium, onabain, and tetrodotoxin, *Biochem. Pharmacol.* **18**:1835–1839.

KATZ, R. I., CHASE, T. N., and KOPIN, I. J., 1968, Evoked release of norepinephrine and serotonin from brain slices: Inhibition by lithium, *Science* **162**:466–467.

KATZMAN, R., 1972, Blood–brain–CSF barriers, in: *Basic Neurochemistry* (R. W. Albers, G. J. Siegal, R. Katzman, and B. W. Agranoff, eds.), pp. 327–339, published for the American Society for Neurochemistry, Churchill/Livingston, Edinburgh.

KEYNES, R. D., and SWAN, R. C., 1959*a*, The permeability of frog muscle fibers to lithium ions, *J. Physiol. (London)* **147**:626–638.

KEYNES, R. D., and SWAN, R. C., 1959*b*, The effect of external sodium concentration on the sodium fluxes in frog skeletal muscle, *J. Physiol. (London)* **147**:591–625.

KLINE, N. S., 1969, Lithium: The history of its use in psychiatry, in: *Modern Problems of Pharmacopsychiatry*, Vol. 3 (F. A. Freyhan, N. Petrilowitsch, and P. Pichot, eds.), pp. 3–21, S. Karger, Basel.

KLINE, N. S., 1973, A narrative account of lithium usage in psychiatry, in: *Lithium* (S. Gershon and B. Shopsin, eds.), pp. 5–13, Plenum Press, New York.

KLINE, N. S., WREN, J., COOPER, T. B., VARGA, E., and CAROL, O., 1974, Evaluation of lithium therapy in chronic and periodic alcoholism, *Am. J. Med. Sci.* **268**(1):13–22.

KNAPP, S., and MANDELL, A., 1973, Short- and long-term lithium administration: Effects on the brain's serotonergic biosynthetic systems, *Science* **180**(4086):645–647.

KOELLE, G., 1965, Drugs acting at synaptic and neuroeffector junctional sites, in: *The*

Pharmacological Basis of Therapeutics, 3rd ed. (L. S. Goodman, and A. Gilman, ed.), pp. 399–440, Macmillan, New York.

KURIYAMA, K., and SPEKEN, R., 1970, Effect of lithium on content and uptake of norepinephrine and 5-hydroxythyptamine in mouse brain synaptosomes and mitochondria, *Life Sci.* **9:**1213–1220.

LEONARD, D. P., KIDSON, M. A., SHAUNON, P. J., and BROWN, J., 1974, Double-blind trial of lithium carbonate and haloperidol in Huntington's chorea, *Lancet* **2**(7890):1208–1209.

LINGJAERDE, O., EDLUND, A. H., GORMSEN, C. A., GOTTFRIES, C. G., HAUGSTAD, A., HERMANN, I. L., HOLLNAGEL, P., MAKIMATTILLA, A., RASMUSSEN, K. E., REMVIG, J., and ROBAK, O. H., 1974, The effects of lithium carbonate in combination with tricyclic antidepressants in endogenous depression: A double-blind, multicenter trial, *Acta Psychiatr. (Scand.)* **50:**233–242.

LORKOVIC, H., 1972, Antagonism between calcium and monovalent cations in depolarized denervated muscles, *Am. J. Physiol.* **222:**1427–1434.

MAYER, S., MARCKEL, R. P., and BRODIE, B. R., 1959, Kinetics of penetration of drugs and other foreign compounds into cerebrospinal fluid and brain, *J. Pharmacol. Exp. Ther.* **127:**205–211.

MAYFIELD, D., and BROWN, R., 1966, The clinical laboratory and electroencephalographic effects of lithium, *J. Psychiatr. Res.* **4:**207–219.

MCEWEN, B. S., 1975, The brain as a target organ of endocrine hormones, *Hosp. Pract.* **10**(5):95–104.

MCKUSICK, V. A., 1954, The effects of lithium on the electrocardiogram of animals and the relation of this effect to the ratio of the intracellular and extracellular concentration of potassium, *J. Clin. Invest.* **33:**598–610.

MELLERUP, E. T., GRONLUND, R., THOMSEN, H., BJORUM, H., and RAFAELSON, O. J., 1972, Lithium, weight gain, and serum insulin in manic-depressive patients—untreated manic-depressives, *Acta Psychiatr. Scand.* **48**(4):332–336.

MENDELS, J., 1973, Lithium and depression, in: *Lithium* (S. Gershon and B. Shopsin, eds.), pp. 253–269, Plenum Press, New York.

MENDELS, J., and FRAZER, A., 1973, Intracellular lithium concentration and clinical response: Towards a membrane theory of depression, *J. Psychiatr. Res.* **10:**9–18.

MENDELS, J., and FRAZER, A., (November) 1974, Alterations in cell membrane activity in depression, *Am. J. Psychiatry* **131**(11):1240–1246.

MENDELS, J., and FRAZER, A., 1975, Reduced central serotonergic activity in mania: Implications for the relationship between depression and mania, *Br. J. Psychiatry* **126:**241–248.

MENDELS, J., SECUNDA, S. K., and DYSON, W. L. A., 1972, A controlled study of the antidepressant effects of lithium carbonate, *Arch. Gen. Psychiatry* **26:**154–157.

MENDELS, J., FRAZER, A., SECUNDA, S. K., and STOKES, J. W., 1974, A study of electrolyte and biogenic amine metabolism in manic-depressive disease, *Int. Pharmacopsychiatry* **9:**206–217.

MURPHY, D. L., GOODWIN, F. K., and BUNNEY, W. E., JR., 1969, Aldosterone and sodium response to lithium administration in man, *Lancet* **2:**458–461.

MURPHY, D. L., COLBURN, R. W., DAVIS, J. M., and BUNNEY, W. E., JR., 1970, Imipramine and lithium effects on biogenic amine transport in depressed and manic depressed patients, *Am. J. Psychiatry* **127:**339–345.

NIELSEN, J., 1964*a*, Magnesium–lithium studies 1: Serum and erythrocyte magnesium in patients with manic states during lithium treatment, *Acta Psychiatr. Scand.* **40:**190–196.

NIELSEN, J., 1964*b*, Magnesium–Li$^+$ studies 2: Effect of Li$^+$ on serum Mg^{++} in rabbits, *Acta Psychiatr. Scand.* **40:**197–202.

PAPPANO, A. J., and VOLLE, R. L., 1967, Action of lithium ions in mammalian sympathetic ganglia, *J. Pharmacol. Exp. Ther.* **157:**346–355.

PAUL, M. I., CRAMER, H., and GOODWIN, F. K., 1970, Urinary cyclic AMP in affective illness, *Lancet* **1:**996.

PAUL, M. I., CRAMER, H., and BUNNEY, W. E., JR., 1971, Urinary adenosine 3',5'-monophosphate in the switch process from depression to mania, *Science* **171**:300–303.

PLATMAN, S. R., and FIEVE, R. R., 1969, The effects of lithium carbonate on the electroencephalogram of patients with affective disorders, *Br. J. Psychiatry* **115**:1185.

PLOEGER, E. J., 1974, The effects of lithium on excitable cell membranes, the influence of ATPase of homogenates of the non-myelinated nerve fibers of the rat, *Arch. Int. Pharmacodyn. Ther.* **210**(2):374–382.

POMEROY, A., and RAND, M. J., 1971, Facilitation of noradrenaline uptake by lithium, *Aust. N.Z. J. Psychiatry* **5**:280–285.

QUITKIN, F. M., RIFKIN, A., and KLEIN, D., 1973, Lithium in other psychiatric disorders, in: *Lithium* (S. Gershon and B. Shopsin, eds.), pp. 295–316, Plenum Press, New York.

RAPOPORT, S. I., HORI, M., and KLATZO, I., 1972, Testing of a hypothesis for osmotic opening of the blood–brain barrier, *Am. J. Physiol.* **223**:323–331.

REDA, F. A., ESCOBAR, J. I., and SCANLAN, J. M., 1975, Lithium carbonate in the treatment of tardive dyskinesia, *Am. J. Psychiatry* **132**(5):560–562.

RICHELSON, E., 1977, Lithium ion entry through the sodium channel of cultured mouse neuroblastoma cells: A biochemical study, *Science* (in press).

ROBERTS, E. L., 1950, A case of chronic mania treated with lithium citrate and terminating fatally, *Med. J. Aust.* **37**:261.

ROBISON, G. A., and SUTHERLAND, E. W., 1971, Cyclic AMP and the function of eukaryotic cells: An introduction, in: *Cyclic AMP and Cell Function* G. A. Robison, G. G. Nahas, and L. Triner, eds.), pp. 5–9, Vol. 185, Annals of the New York Academy of Science, New York.

SAMOELOV, N. N., 1972, Lithium distribution in rabbits, *Med. Radiol.* **17**(9):61–66.

SCHILDKRAUT, J. J., 1965, The catecholamine hypothesis of affective disorders: A review of supporting evidence, *Am. J. Psychiatry* **122**:509–522.

SCHILDKRAUT, J. J., 1973, Pharmacology—the effects of lithium on biogenic amines, in: *Lithium* (S. Gershon and B. Shopsin, eds.), pp. 51–75, Plenum Press, New York.

SCHILDKRAUT, J. J., SCHANBERG, S. M., and KOPIN, I. J., 1966, The effects of lithium ions on H³-norepinephrine metabolism in brain, *Life Sci.* **5**:1479–1483.

SCHILDKRAUT, J. J., LONGUE, M. A., and DODGE, G. A., 1969, The effects of lithium salts on the turnover and metabolism of norepinephrine in rat brain, *Psychopharmacologia (Berlin)* **14**:135–141.

SCHOU, M., 1957, Biology and pharmacology of the lithium ion, *Pharmacol. Rev.* **9**:17–58.

SCHOU, M., 1968, Lithium in psychiatric therapy and prophylaxis, *J. Psychiatr. Res.* **6**:67–95.

SCHOU, M., AMDISEN, A., and TRAP-JENSEN, J., 1968, Lithium poisoning, *Am. J. Psychiatry* **125**(4):520–527.

SCHOU, M., BAASTRUP, P. C., GROF, P., WEIS, P., and ANGST, J., 1970, Pharmacological and clinical problems of lithium prophylaxis, *Br. J. Psychiatry* **116**:615–619.

SHEARD, M. H., 1971, Effect of lithium on human aggression, *Nature* **230**:113–114.

SHOPSIN, B., and GERSHON, S., 1973, Pharmacology-toxicology of the lithium ion, in: *Lithium* (S. Gershon and B. Shopsin, eds.), pp. 107–146, Plenum Press, New York.

SHOPSIN, B., FRIEDMANN, R., and GERSHON, S., 1971, Lithium and leukocytosis, *Clin. Pharmacol. Ther.* **12**:923–928.

SINGER, I., 1974, Reply to letter to the editor, *N. Engl. J. Med.* **290**(13):749.

SINGER, I., and FRANKO, E. A., 1973, Lithium-induced A.D.H. resistance in toad urinary bladder, *Kidney Int.* **3**:151–159.

SINGER, I., and ROTENBERG, D., 1973, Mechanisms of lithium action, *N. Engl. J. Med.* **289**(5):254–260.

SINGER, I., ROTENBERG, D., PUSCHETT, J., and FRANKO, E., 1972, Lithium-induced nephrogenic diabetes insipidus—*in vivo* and *in vitro*, *J. Clin. Invest.* **51**:1081–1091.

SKOU, J. C., 1960, Further investigation on a Mg^{++} ion and Na^+ ion, *Biochem. Biophys. Acta* **42**:6–23.

SMALL, J. G., and SMALL, I. F., 1973, Pharmacology–neurophysiology of lithium, in: *Lithium* (S. Gershon and B. Shopsin, eds.), pp. 83–107, Plenum Press, New York.

SMITH, D. F., and THOMSEN, K., 1973, Renal lithium clearance in adrenalectomized rats, *Am. J. Physiol.* **225**(1):159–161.

SMITH, D. F., KING, M. B., and HOEBEL, B. G., 1970, Lateral hypothalamic control of killing: Evidence for a cholinoceptive mechanism, *Science* **167**:900–901.

SMITH-KLINE CORP., 1974, Eskalith in Psychiatry, Company publication.

SNYDER, S., 1974, *Madness and the Brain*, pp. 235–247, McGraw-Hill, New York.

STEINWALL, P., 1961, Transport mechanisms in certain blood–brain barrier phenomena—a hypothesis, *Acta Psychiatr. Neurol. Scand. Suppl.* **1950:3**14–318.

STERN, D. N., FIEVE, R. R., NEFF, N. H., and COSTA, E., 1969, The effect of lithium chloride administration on brain and heart norepinephrine turnover rates, *Psychopharmacologia* **14**:315–322.

SUGITA, E. T., STOKES, J. W., FRAZER, A., GROF, P., MENDELS, J., GOLDSTEIN, F. J., and NIEBERGALL, P. J., 1973, Lithium carbonate absorption in humans, *J. Clin. Pharmacol.* **13**(7):264–270.

SUTHERLAND, E. W., 1970, On the biological role of cyclic AMP, *J. Am. Med. Assoc.* **214**:1281–1288.

SWANSON, P. D., and STAHL, W. L., 1972, Ion transport, in: *Basic Neurochemistry* (W. Albers, G. Siegel, R. Katzman, and B. Agranoff, eds.), pp. 21–40, published for the American Society for Neurochemistry (first edition), Churchill/Livingstone, Edinburgh.

TANGEDAHL, T. N., GAU, G. T., 1972, Mycardial irritability associated with lithium carbonate therapy, *N. Engl. J. Med.* **287**:867–869.

THOMSEN, K., and SCHOU, M., 1968, Renal lithium excretion in man, *Am. J. Physiol.* **215**:823–827.

TOBIN, T., AKERA, T., HAN, C. S., and BRODY, T. H., 1974, Lithium and rubidium interactions with sodium- and potassium-dependent adenosine triphosphatase: A molecular basis for the pharmacological action of these ions, *Mol. Pharmacol.* **10**:501–508.

TRAUTNER, E. M., MORRIS, R., NOACK, C. H., and GERSHON, S., 1955, The excretion and retention of ingested lithium and its effect on the ionic balance of man, *Med. J. Aust.* **2**:280–291.

TUPIN, J., 1970, The use of lithium in manic-depressive psychosis, **21**:17–24.

U'PRICHARD, D. C., and STEINBERG, H., 1972, Selective effects of lithium on two forms of spontaneous activity, *Br. J. Pharmacol.* **44**:349–350.

URSIN, H., 1960, The temporal lobe substrate of fear and anger, *Acta Psychiatr. Neurol. Scand.* **35**:378–396.

VAN DER VELDE, C. D., and GORDON, M. W., 1969, Manic-depressive illness, diabetes mellitus and lithium carbonate, *Arch. Gen. Psychiatry* **21**:478–485.

VIZI, E. S., ILLES, P., RONAI, A., and KNOLL, J., 1972, Effect of lithium on acetylcholine release and synthesis, *Neuropharmacology* **11**:521–530.

WANG, Y. C., PANDY, G. N., MENDELS, J., and FRAZER, A., 1974, Effect of lithium on prostaglandin E-stimulated adenylate cyclase activity of human platelets, *Biochem. Pharmacol.* **23**:845–855.

WATANABE, S., TAGUCHI, K., NAKASHIMA, Y., EBARA, T., and IGUCHI, K., 1974a, Leukocytosis during lithium treatment and its correlation to serum lithium levels, *Folia Psychiatr. Neurol. Jpn.* **28**:161–165.

WATANABE, S., ISHINO, H., FUJIWARA, J., and OTSUKI, S., 1974b, Relationship between serum lithium level and clinical response to depression treated with lithium carbonate, *Folia Psychiatr. Neurol. Jpn.* **28**:167–177.

WAZIRI, R., 1968, Presynaptic effects of lithium on cholinergic synaptic transmission in *Aplysia* neurons, *Life Sci.* **7**:865.

WHITE, M. G., and FETNER, C. D., 1975, Treatment of the syndrome of inappropriate secretion of antidiuretic hormone with lithium carbonate, *N. Engl. J. Med.* **292**(18):390–392.

WILK, S., SHOPSIN, B., GERSHON, S., and SUHL, M., 1972, Cerebrospinal fluid levels of MHPG in affective disorders, *Nature* **235:**440–441.

WILLIAMS, R. J. P., 1973, The chemistry and biochemistry of lithium, in: *Lithium* (S. Gershon and B. Shopsin, eds.), pp. 15–31, Plenum Press, New York.

WILSON, C. M., and BRODIE, B. R., 1961, The absence of blood–brain barrier from certain areas of the central nervous system, *J. Pharmacol. Exp. Ther.* **133:**332–334.

WOLFF, J., BERENS, S. C., and JONES, A. B., 1970, Inhibition of thyrotropi-stimulated adenyl cyclase activity of beef thyroid membrane by low concentrations of lithium ion, *Biochem. Biophys. Res. Commun.* **39:**77–82.

7

LITHIUM: CLINICAL CONSIDERATIONS

Baron Shopsin and Samuel Gershon

1. INTRODUCTION

Lithium is available in the United States in the carbonate form and is marketed in the form of capsules or tablets containing 300 mg. Lithium carbonate is a white, light alkaline powder with the molecular formula Li_2CO_3 and molecular weight 73.89. This ion is an element of the alkali-metal group with atomic number 3, atomic weight 6.94, and an emission line at 671 nm on the flame photometer.

1.1. Indications

"Lithium carbonate is indicated in the treatment of manic episodes of manic depressive illness. Maintenance therapy prevents or diminishes the intensity of subsequent episodes in those manic depressive patients with a history of mania."*

At the time of writing, there are no provisions in the FDA-approved package insert for its use in acute depressive episodes, nor is it officially recognized as a maintenance therapy in staving off or modifying subsequent episodes in manic-depressives who suffer only recurrences of depression.

Lithium has moved across the therapeutic spectrum from poison to

* FDA-approved package inserts.

Baron Shopsin and Samuel Gershon • Neuropsychopharmacology Research Unit, New York University–Bellevue Hospital Center, New York, New York.

panacea. In the present chapter we will review and critically evaluate various clinical studies in attempting to delineate a therapeutic profile for the use of lithium in psychiatry. As a practicum we cover the various lithium preparations as well as dosage requirements in the control of mania and as maintenance therapy against manic-depressive recurrences. The toxicology of the lithium ion is intended as a guideline for evaluating the possibilities for its safe use in the narrow range of psychiatric patients for which this drug is primarily intended.

2. LITHIUM IN MANIA

We will review some of the major open and single-blind studies and then focus on controlled studies comparing lithium to chlorpromazine and haloperidol in the treatment of mania. In addition to their obvious practical significance, the more recent studies comparing lithium to other neuroleptics are of special importance because they bear on the question of the *specificity* of lithium against the manic syndrome—a question that has theoretical implications for the underlying pathophysiology of mania.

2.1. Uncontrolled and Single-Blind Studies

Table 1 summarizes the major uncontrolled and single-blind studies* of lithium's effectiveness in acute mania. In general, these open studies represent the early clinical trials of lithium, and they do not utilize a double-blind design or placebo-group comparison. The great majority of these studies do not use rating scales for the evaluation of clinical response, nor do they define their diagnostic criteria for mania, particularly in relation to the borderline between manic and schizoaffective states. However, many of the studies report the clinical observation that the patient most likely to respond to lithium is the "typical" manic, with the drug being less effective as more patients with schizoaffective states are included in the sample. An assessment of all the uncontrolled studies conducted by many different groups over a number of years consistently demonstrates a high incidence of response within about a week of starting lithium. When these studies are globally tabulated (Table 1), 334 out of 413 patients (or 81%) showed improvement in mania during acute lithium treatment.

Nonblind studies in psychopharmacology are frequently dismissed as uninterpretable. However, clinical experience suggests that mania, a major

---

* This review was confined to studies in the English-language literature.

TABLE 1
Lithium in Mania—Uncontrolled and Single-Blind Studies[a]

Study	Number of manic patients	Results		Comments
		Im-proved	Unim-proved	
Cade (1949)	6	6	0	Individual case reports presented.
Noack and Trautner (1951a,b)	30	25	5	Two cases reported.
Glessinger (1954)	21	15	6	No case reports. Lithium citrate used.
Schou et al. (1954)	30	27	3	12 responders were "definite" and 15 were "possible." Ratings used and diagnostic criteria specified.
Schou (1959)	119	91	28	Includes "typical" and "mixed" manic syndromes.
Kingstone (1960)	17	16	1	3 case reports presented.
Wharton and Fieve (1966)[b]	25	17		Single-blind ratings; diagnostic criteria specified.
Schlagenhauf et al. (1966)	68	61	7	Some patients were continued on other medication.
Blinder (1968)	22	21	1	Patients described as "hypomanic."
Van der Velde (1970)	75	55	20	Diagnostic criteria specified.
Totals	413	334 (81%)	71 (17%)	

[a] Prepared by F. K. Goodwin and M. H. Ebert (1973).
[b] The data from this study are reported as number of episodes of mania. There were 19 patients in the trial.

psychotic illness, is not particularly responsive to the subtle environmental and interpersonal factors which contribute to high placebo response rates. A greater difficulty in the interpretation of these open trials derives from the fact that mania is a cyclic phenomenon which, in the absence of intervention, will generally remit spontaneously. However, it is unusual for this to occur over a time period of several days to several weeks, i.e., the time period within which most of the antimanic responses to lithium occurred. Thus, it is quite unlikely that the rapid disappearance of manic symptoms during the first week of lithium therapy in the large majority of patients would be due to chance or to a placebo effect.

2.2. Controlled Studies

Lithium carbonate is now an established treatment modality for manic phase, manic-depressive illness (Gershon and Shopsin, 1973). With few exceptions, the published studies, both open and controlled, support the claim for lithium carbonate's efficacy in this disorder.

To date, only 11 studies have used control groups (Schou *et al.*, 1954; Maggs, 1963; Bunney *et al.*, 1968, Goodwin *et al.*, 1969; Johnson *et al.*, 1968, 1971; Spring *et al.*, 1970; Platman, 1970; Prien *et al.*, 1971; Shopsin *et al.*, 1975; Takahashi *et al.*, 1975); four used placebo (Schou *et al.*, 1954; Maggs, 1963; Bunney *et al.*, 1968; Goodwin *et al.*, 1969), seven chlorpromazine hydrochloride (Johnson *et al.*, 1968, 1971; Spring *et al.*, 1970; Platman, 1970; Prien *et al.*, 1971; Takahashi *et al.*, 1975; Shopsin *et al.*, 1975) and one compared lithium to haloperidol (Shopsin *et al.*, 1975). An assessment of these 11 controlled studies does not permit any direct comparisons inasmuch as the experimental designs and study methods varied. In summarizing these studies, it can be stated that all those comparing lithium carbonate with placebo show clear treatment superiority with lithium carbonate. However, the controlled studies comparing lithium carbonate and neuroleptics cannot *unequivocally* establish the superiority of lithium carbonate conclusively, based on statistical (biometric) significance.

Four double-blind controlled studies failed to show statistically significant differences between lithium carbonate and chlorpromazine (Spring *et al.*, 1970; Platman, 1970; Johnson *et al.*, 1971; Shopsin *et al.*, 1975); in one investigation (Prien, *et al.*, 1971) results with these two drugs are different depending on division of manic patients into "highly active" and "mildly active," and lithium carbonate appeared to be the "better" treatment in only mildly active patients.

Although inherent differences in study design and methodology in studies comparing lithium carbonate and chlorpromazine do not permit direct comparison of results, an additional look at the studies is important in order to assess this problem of differential drug effects more clearly. In 1968 (Johnson *et al.*, 1968), a controlled study comparing lithium carbonate with chlorpromazine indicated superiority for lithium carbonate over chlorpromazine; the two drugs differed in quality of action on clinical description, with lithium carbonate superior in normalizing ideation and mood while chlorpromazine acted more quickly in controlling motor activity. A follow-up study (Johnson *et al.*, 1971) appeared to bear out these preliminary findings, although statistically significant differences among different rating devices were not consistently seen and chlorpromazine did produce significant improvement in manic patients. These discrepancies may be accounted for on the basis of a lack of specific and relevant rating devices with which to delineate changes in manic psychopathology. Rate of discharge in these investigations clearly testified to differences in treatment outcome. In later studies by Spring *et al.* (1970) and Platman (1970), the advantage of lithium carbonate over chlorpromazine in the treatment of mania also surfaces. Although Spring *et al.* (1970) were unable to disclose any significant difference between the two treatments on a statistical basis, of the 14 patients studied by these investigators, eight of nine responded to lithium carbonate while only three of six responded to chlorpromazine (including the crossover trial). In addition, the specific "target" symptoms that are most characteristic of mania showed considerably more change with lithium carbonate than chlorpromazine. In the study by Platman (1970), a three-week double-blind comparison between lithium carbonate and chlorpromazine showed no statistically significant difference between the two treatments. Platman believed, however, that lithium carbonate was superior to chlorpromazine by the end of the third week and that the advantage was reflected in the fact that the majority of the lithium carbonate group were able to be discharged while no patient receiving chlorpromazine was discharged. Again, a disparity surfaces between clear-cut differences on discharge rate and failure to confirm this on the rating scales.

The VA-NIMH collaborative studies differ from the preceding studies in several respects. The possible study method disparities in the VA-NIMH project deserve comment because they likely relate to the differences in treatment outcome. Also, these methodological issues should be highlighted because the large number of patients used will make it impossible for investigators to duplicate for some time to come. First, the VA-NIMH project was a large, multihospital, cooperative study. While this provides the advantage of a large sample size, the disadvantages include the distinct possibility of both diagnostic and treatment heterogeneity, variation in clinical settings and professional staff, and less intensive clinical evaluation of individual patients. The diagnostic dilemma surrounding manic-depressive illness, manic phase, and schizophrenic illness, schizoaffective excited phase, has perplexed even *soi-disant* experts in the field. It becomes obvious that, in the VA-NIMH studies, diagnostic heterogeneity comes critically into question due to the many physicians involved in such a large number of hospitals (Shopsin *et al.*, 1975), all different both on an administrative (private, general, and VA) and geographical level. This issue is highlighted in their study, in that the "highly active" patients were noted to be more disturbed and disorganized than the mildly active patients, an observation that raises the question of whether some patients in the highly active group might be considered as schizoaffective or atypical by others. The literature suggests that typical patients clearly do less well with lithium carbonate and, in fact, such patients can show an aggravation of psychopathology or predisposition to neurotoxic symptoms. This point may be highly relevant for the highly active group in the VA study, in which the majority of patients receiving lithium carbonate were eliminated because of inability to complete the three weeks of treatment. This latter lithium carbonate group had a higher incidence of severe toxic reactions, which may indicate diagnostic nonspecificity. The high rate of 40% dropouts in lithium carbonate patients in the VA-

NIMH study is clearly at variance with findings reported by others. Inexperience with lithium carbonate and lack of knowledge concerning the pharmacology of this ion, as well as individual (heterogeneous) treatment styles, could certainly account for this high dropout rate. This has not been the case in most other studies that have compared the use of lithium carbonate with chlorpromazine in controlled fashion. Even if the highly active manic patients became somewhat toxic with lithium carbonate in the VA-NIMH study, one questions why the patients would be eliminated rather than have their dosage adjusted, which in most instances would rectify the situation.

The varying orientations and levels of experience of patient raters and treating physicians in the large variety of hospitals in the collaborative study appear to represent a critical variable. The conclusion by Prien *et al.*, 1971) that chlorpromazine is more effective than lithium carbonate in treating highly active patients should therefore be viewed with caution. The criticisms above may in fact account for the disparity between the results in this latter study and those of extensive clinical observations by Schou (1968) and others (Goodman and Ebert, 1973) that the *effect of lithium carbonate and neuroleptics on mania is qualitatively quite different, i.e., that the neuroleptics are generally observed to suppress the hyperactivity without altering the underlying manic thoughts or mood, while lithium carbonate, although slower to show an initial effect, eventually has a more specific therapeutic effect on the manic symptoms.*

A multi-institutional cooperative study comparing lithium carbonate with chlorpromazine was conducted in Japan, using a controlled double-blind design in a series of 80 manic patients, to evaluate the drugs' clinical utility and efficacy, characteristics of therapeutic effect, and side effects. Physicians' overall ratings showed lithium carbonate as significantly superior to chlorpromazine in efficacy for manic psychosis. Improvements of basic mood and of disturbance in speech and voice were prominent with lithium carbonate. Onset of the therapeutic effect of lithium carbonate was within 10 days of medication in 65% of the patients, significantly faster than with chlorpromazine. Side effects encountered with lithium carbonate therapy at dose levels not higher than 1800 mg/day were milder and less frequent compared with those seen with chlorpromazine.

This study suffers from many methodological problems which render overall assessment of comparable drug efficacy most difficult. The multihospital nature of this study is subject to the same criticisms as that of the VA-NIMH collaborative venture reported by Prien *et al.* (1971). The rating scale used is unknown outside Japan and was not given, so that we do not know the criteria used for improvement. Those few symptoms given would not appear to be the most relevant symptoms of mania by any means. The highest dosage given of chlorpromazine was 450 mg; even acknowledging that Japanese patients with mania appear to require less chlorpromazine than their U.S. counterparts (Ishida *et al.*, 1972), we are not given the average dose per patient or even the number of patients requiring maximum dosage. Considering the poor treatment response in those manics treated with chlorpromazine, dosage was likely critical. Of greatest cause for scepticism, the Japanese report indicates that lithium acted more rapidly than chlorpromazine, a finding that goes contrary to every piece of data, both open and controlled, in the world literature. Then too, the therapeutic effect of lithium carbonate failed to show any significant correlation with the dose or serum concentrations of lithium. The mean serum level of lithium was ± 0.56 mEq/liter, which is quite modest to alleviate the symptoms of acute mania.

Thus, although this large-scale Japanese study reports statistically superior treatment efficacy for lithium over chlorpromazine, the data are sufficiently questionable on methodological grounds, as well as possible cross-cultural differences, as to preclude closure on the outcome.

The butyrophenone haloperidol has been widely used in the treatment of acute mania; to date, there has been only one double-blind controlled study comparing its efficacy with that of lithium carbonate or chlorpromazine. Several investigators propose a particular efficacy for haloperidol in the treatment of manic disorder (Shopsin and Gershon, 1971a); the *British Textbook of Clinical Psychiatry* highly endorses the use of haloperidol intravenously in dramatically reducing manic excitement. Such pioneers and advocates of lithium carbonate as Schou (1968) and Baastrup (1968) indicate in separate communications that an acute manic state is treated effectively and more rapidly with haloperidol and electric convulsive therapy (ECT) than with lithium carbonate. The drug is in fact considered by some (Ban, 1969) to be one of the most effective drugs in the therapy for mania.

Despite the commercial availability of this drug since April 1967, it had not been used in controlled studies with manic patients until very recently. A study was finally undertaken to compare, in a controlled double-blind fashion, the effects of lithium carbonate, chlorpromazine, and haloperidol in moderate to severely disturbed hospitalized manic patients (Shopsin et al., 1975). It is the only double-blind controlled study in which lithium carbonate has been compared with a butyrophenone and the only double-blind evaluation between chlorpromazine and haloperidol in this psychiatric disorder.

In synthesizing the results of this investigation, lithium carbonate and haloperidol emerge as the superior treatments in our group of manic patients. Although there was generally no statistically significant difference across different rating scales from baseline to termination among the three drug groups as measured by analysis of variance, repeated measures model, both qualitative and quantitative differences surface with overall cross-comparisons between drug groups. In the case of chlorpromazine, and irrespective of this drug's overall treatment efficacy at treatment termination, it had an insignificant effect on manic ideation or behavior. Qualitative differences between lithium carbonate and either neuroleptic are clearly reflected in discharge rate. Haloperidol more rapidly subdued hyperactivity as well as some affect and ideational psychopathology, without untoward side effects of sedation. However, these effects were not complete; only one of the patients receiving haloperidol met criteria for discharge at the end of study. Lithium carbonate appeared to act more evenly on all symptoms of mania, showing a more total normalization of affect, ideation, and behavior by study termination that permitted most patients to be discharged; a full recovery was most frequently seen with lithium carbonate treatment. Similar findings have been reported in an open study by Russian investigators (Nuller and Rabinovich, 1971). Also, chlorpromazine tended to sedate patients and was not effective in controlling the manic state. Thus, under conditions o both haloperidol and chlorpromazine treatment, the manic state, however improved compared with baseline values, was not totally normalized. Increasing dosage of either neuroleptic beyond the fixed study dosage did not resolve this situation.

Implications are that the rating scales employed across different studies under standard interview conditions cannot pick up the total manic psychopathology. In fact, the key words in defining the neuroleptic effect in manic patients are "modification" and "control" without qualitatively altering the underlying mania. While receiving the neuroleptic compounds, some patients are controlled to the point at which mania is sufficiently suppressed to show significant improvement on rating scales such as the BPRS, CGI, and other ward-behavior ratings. However, normalization is not usually complete; despite the substantial neuroleptic impact on items depicting mania, such as excitement, euphoria, grandiosity, mannerisms, and cooperativeness, the underlying mania is not qualitatively modified to the point at which patients could be discharged at study termination. These manic patients continue to show, however modified, some flight of ideas, grandiosity, overspending, enhanced interests, involvement with others, and enhanced overzealous business interests. Many continue to show an air of self-assurance, some breezy affability, self-satisfaction, and increased assertiveness. While less demanding and more compliant, some remain uninhibited, childishly proud, intolerant (although sometimes controllably so) of criticism, still glib of tongue, and witty. Thus, the rating scale results belie the true clinical (manic) state in that: (1) their crude and sweeping symptom items show noticeable change scores largely by virtue of the behavioral control in patients receiving neuroleptics; and (2) they are too insensitive to elicit true manic psychopathology. Apropos of these issues, it is important to mention that the neuroleptics may permit patients to control their behavior exceedingly well in the interview situation, such that only their comportment under other conditions not subject to clinical scrutiny would reflect that the manic ideation is not substantially ameliorated. This is most readily apparent in patients receiving haloperidol, in whom the antimanic effect, including behavioral control, can be more pronounced than with chlorpromazine and is not accompanied by sedation.

New scales must be devised to measure manic ideation and behavior more clearly; existing scales are clearly inadequate and do not take into account social adjustment measurements. Merely subduing manifest belligerence, hostility, anger, irritability, quarrelsomeness, grandiosity, jocularity, unconventional speech, and intolerance does not signify sufficient or acceptable control of the manic state; factors such as sleep, a more discreet appreciation of social participation and interaction, general performance, and flow of items are necessary considerations. These latter areas become critically important when considering drug specificity in mildly manic patients who may not require hospitalization or when comparing drug treatment in mildly active hospitalized patients. This may indeed account for the failure of the VA-NIMH collaborative study (Prien *et al.*, 1971) to report any significant differences between treatment outcomes in mildly active patients receiving either chlorpromazine or lithium carbonate. It is precisely this lack of sensitivity in any of the rating scales that accounts for the apparent disparity between the objective scales and dischargeability of patients under different drug treatments as reported by us (Johnson *et al.*, 1968, 1971; Klein and Davis, 1969) and others (Spring *et al.*, 1970; Platman, 1970).

2.2.1. Closing Remarks

The many open and controlled trials of lithium in mania show a remarkable degree of consistency in concluding that this simple salt has definite therapeutic properties in the great majority of manic patients. There are, however, two major questions concerning the efficacy of lithium as an acute treatment for mania which are still open. First, what is the *relative* efficacy of lithium as compared to phenothiazines or haloperidol in the management of acute mania; and, second, what clinical or diagnostic features might be used to define the potential lithium responder?

A critical review of the evidence makes it clear that definite "answers" to these two questions are not yet possible. Nevertheless, the bulk of the available evidence does suggest that lithium occupies a unique position in the chemical treatment of mania, in that it exerts diagnostically related psychopharmacological specificity which does not resemble the preclinical or clinical pharmacological profiles of the neuroleptic compounds used in manic disorder. Lithium's effect in mania differs distinctly from that of the neuroleptics (such as chlorpromazine and haloperidol) on three points. First, they have different time courses. Chlorpromazine and haloperidol usually act more rapidly than lithium, whose full effect cannot be expected for 7–10 days of treatment. This is of considerable importance when the acute and unusually violent cases of mania are treated. Second, while the sedative action of conventional neuroleptics is largely independent of the illness causing agitation, lithium acts more specifically against mania, its best results being obtained in patients with clinical pictures dominated by mood elevation, irritability, restlessness, talkativeness, and jocularity. Third, and perhaps most important, the responses to lithium and neuroleptic treatments differ in quality. Neuroleptics, while producing an effective suppression of the manic overactivity and restlessness, are accompanied by a drugged effect of sedation and drowsiness. Thus, the phenothiazines and butyrophenones merely place a lid over the manic state; the patients usually retain, below the surface, their characteristic symptoms of mania. Lithium, on the other hand, seems to remove the manic symptoms in a more specific manner, dissolving the elevated mood, hyperactivity, restlessness, talkativeness, sleeplessness, etc., with sedation or the feeling of being drugged. The patient is "normalized," and brought into a state that cannot be distinguished subjectively or objectively (Schou, 1968) from his normal, premorbid condition.

2.2.2. Factors Affecting Response: Diagnostic Precision

In order to appreciate the specific therapeutic effects of lithium, it should be prescribed for patients showing a clear diagnostic indication for this drug. The manic phase of manic-depressive illness is the prime indication for lithium treatment. The ambiguities surrounding the diagnosis of manic illness, and especially that shadowy interface between manic phase, manic-depressive disorder, and schizophrenia, schizoaffective type and excited phase, present a diagnostic dilemma in that both illnesses share large components of both affective as well as behavioral disturbance. The resolution of this problem of differential diagnosis is critical, however, since several studies have indicated that patients do less well on lithium when the manic picture is clouded with "atypical" features (Schou, 1954; Hartigan, 1963; Fries, 1969). This "atypical" group includes subjects with schizophrenic symptoms, and the significance of such differential drug responsiveness has been underlined in several recent studies (Johnson et al., 1968; Aronoff and Epstein, 1969; Shopsin et al., 1971b). In discussing their trial on lithium, Aronoff and Epstein noted that some of their schizoaffective cases, which they acknowledged might well have been designated "atypical manic-depressive illness" by others, showed only moderate response or symptom aggravation under lithium treatment. It is on this sort of explicitness about diagnostic ambiguities that progress in delineating lithium's therapeutic usefulness depends. The studies by Johnson et al. (1968) and Shopsin et al. (1971b) underscore lithium's specificity of action; both investigations indicate strongly that lithium has no apparent sedative or neuroleptic properties and that it can, in fact, precipitate or contribute to futher decompensation of schizophrenic symptomatology. The affective, psychomotor, or paranoid components of this psychiatric illness, like the core process itself, fail to show any selective symptom amelioration during treatment with lithium. *If there are those patients with schizophrenic features who do respond to lithium, and it appears that there are such individuals, we cannot at this time define the clinical profile with which to predict response. Lithium should be considered for such cases only under investigational circumstances; the availability of specialized treatment facilities and the potential hazards of lithium dictate a conservative treatment posture for the practicing psychiatrist.*

3. LITHIUM IN ACUTE ENDOGENOUS DEPRESSION

There are no FDA provisions for lithium's use in acute depressive disorders or as a prophylaxis against recurrent unipolar depressions (i.e., individuals experiencing only recurrences of acute depression). There are, nevertheless, data to suggest that lithium may exert therapeutic efficacy in some endogenously depressed patients. (Endogenous depression is a term commonly used to define an autonomous, chemically related illness as distinct from neurotic or exogenous depressions that are triggered by external/situational events.) There are several very legitimate reasons for the general reluctance to accept a possible role for lithium in depression. The use of an "antimanic" drug against acute depression requires careful scrutiny of the published reports, inasmuch as these effects are seemingly paradoxical. Much of the current psychopharmacological and biological research into the affective illnesses has emphasized an apparent bipolar relationship between depression and mania; changes in these two states are largely viewed to be in opposite directions, as the biochemical–pharmacological studies also view these as polar opposites. Then too, as is the case in other areas of psychopharmacology research, the evaluation of lithium's efficacy in acute depression is complicated by a variety of issues that critically center about differences in research design and methodology across different studies. These discrepancies contribute to the lack of consistency in reported findings and include diagnostic consideration, treatment duration, dosage, and criteria for improvement. It is against this background, and not surprisingly, that any suggestion that lithium carbonate may be effective in the treatment of depression has been received with reservation.

As with the use of lithium in mania, the diagnostic issues attending the application of lithium in depression are perhaps strategic. The emergence of differentially effective forms of pharmacotherapy has led to a renaissance of interest in the phenomena and clinical classification of the affective disorders (Lehman, 1968), and this literature has been reviewed recently (Beck, 1967; Mendels and Cochrane, 1970; Winokur, 1973; Klerman, 1973). Since the early studies of Grinker and his co-workers, numerous investigators have attempted to classify and subdivide the depressive disorders according to presenting signs, symptoms, and history. Many workers have focused on the distinctions between endogenous (or endogenomorphic or autonomous or vital) and nonendogenous (or reactive or "neurotic" or chronic characterological) depressive syndromes (Hamilton and White, 1959; Kiloh and Garside, 1963; VanPraag *et al.*, 1965; Rosenthal and Klerman, 1966). The distinction between bipolar (manic-depressive) and unipolar depressive disorders has also been emphasized in recent years (Angst, 1966; Perris, 1966; Winokur *et al.*, 1969); a number of biological correlates of this clinical distinction have been reported. These findings have been reviewed recently (Klerman, 1973). The distinction between primary and secondary affective disorders has been stressed by one group of investigators (Robins and Guze, 1972); specific diagnostic criteria for identifying these disorders have been proposed (Feighner *et al.*, 1972).

Then too, for a number of years, investigators have recognized the possibility that different subgroups of patients with depressive disorders might exhibit different specific biochemical alterations that might ultimately contribute to the development of a more meaningful biochemical classification of the affective disorders and a more rational approach to treatment with greater prediction of treatment response.

Early uncontrolled studies by Australian investigators in 1949 (Cade, 1949) and 1951 (Noack and Trautner, 1951*a,b*) noted an absence of any therapeutic response to lithium in depressed patients. After an interval of some years, several European investigators reported on the successful use of lithium in small numbers of depressed patients (Vojtechovsky, 1957; Andreani *et al.*, 1958; Hartigan, 1963). In more recent years, different groups of American investigators have published findings from further studies, some of them controlled comparisons, in attempts to define more clearly lithium's role in depression. Fieve *et al.* (1968) compared lithium and imipramine and concluded that any antidepressant effect of lithium was mild; imipramine was vastly superior. Zall *et al.* (1968) and Van der Velde (1970) were both unable to show an antidepressant effect for lithium. Dyson and Mendels, first in an open study (1968) and later in a controlled trial comparing lithium with desimipramine, concluded that lithium showed marked antidepressant properties—equivalent to desimipramine's—in the latter study. In the open study by Dyson and Mendels the population is difficult to define. They had both inpatients and outpatients. Diagnoses included bipolar patients, neurotic/reactive depressives, cyclothymic personalities with depression, and unipolar endogenous depressives. Although more patients who improved with lithium were bipolar, this is not at all surprising since an equal number of the patients who did not respond had a neurotic/reactive depression and would not be expected to even with other, more standard, antidepressants. It is also curious that 10 patients that responded had cyclothymic personality disorders with a history of depression; 2 of these patients did have a history of unipolar depression, but the diagnosis in the remaining 8 is really undetermined. Thus, all unipolar patients responded (the 2 unipolar patients described both responded). In the double-blind study by Mendels *et al.* (1972) there was no statistically significant difference in the rate of improvement among bipolar and unipolar patients. The NIMH group has suggested, on the other hand, that it may be the bipolar patient who appreciates a more favorable response to lithium carbonate. Johnson's study is difficult to evaluate, and efficacy for lithium is difficult to assess inasmuch as he had a mixed population including neurotic, unipolar, and bipolar patients. If lithium showed any type of therapeutic response in that population, it was in the unipolar patients, and again it was suggested that a subgroup of depressed patients could respond to lithium. Thus, the existing data are not at all clear. In fact they are somewhat confusing, and the numbers are certainly too small in each study to make clear the exact therapeutic effect that lithium may have in depression or the particular subgroup of depressives that would show the best response.

Studies in more recent years, especially those using plasma–red blood cell lithium as possible predictors of antidepressant response, have certainly lent sophistication to the work but, as in other areas of psychobiology, have only tended to greatly confound the issues. Mendels, Frazer, Secunda and their group have carried out several studies exploring intracellular lithium concentration and clinical antidepressant response to lithium in forwarding a membrane theory of depression. Mendels' group has (basically) shown that patients who respond to lithium appear to have a higher intracellular lithium concentration for a given plasma level than patients who do not improve. Furthermore, they feel that it is the bipolar manic-depressive patients in depressed phase who are more likely to respond to lithium treatment than are the recurrent unipolar depressives, suggesting that the diagnostic difference may be associated with some difference in cell membrane properties. Mendels has also shown that depressed patients treated with lithium who show an increase in RBC sodium are more likely to improve than patients who do not show any increase in RBC sodium. Thus, patients who show a clinical response to lithium, with regard to antidepressant properties for this drug, have higher red blood cell lithium concentrations and show an increased red blood cell sodium; these patients are largely or all bipolar. Finally, they found that the lithium ratio was higher in patients with a higher baseline red blood cell sodium concentration. A critical evaluation of some of the work by Mendels and his group is required. As stated, their bipolars tended to improve with lithium whereas the unipolars did not. However, clinical response was noted in a unipolar patient who had lower red blood cell lithium, and red blood cell lithium was also lower in another patient albeit he was bipolar and did show a clinical response. Another bipolar patient showed no response and also had lower red blood cell lithium. Thus of the 14 patients reported on by Mendels, only 11 patients may be said to supply the data for the proposed membrane theory of depression. The numbers are obviously small, constituting only 4 patients in the unipolar group and 6 patients in the bipolar group with which to make clinical–chemical comparisons for lithium's antidepressant response.

In a recent communication delivered by Carroll (APA Meeting, Anaheim, California; First Pacific Congress of Psychiatry, Melbourne, Australia, 1975), a larger number of depressed patients were given lithium in an open trial. It was found that an almost equal number of patients showed some antidepressant response compared with those who did not show any response. More importantly, Carroll showed that of those patients who responded, and despite changed scores in the Hamilton Rating Scale which did indicate significance, no fundamental change in depressive pathology surfaced, and in fact these patients were unable to return to a functioning capacity or be discharged from hospital. Although there was a tendency for more of the "responders" to be bipolar, there was no difference in the red blood cell lithium between this group (0.44 mEq/liter) and the nonresponders (0.41 mEq/liter). Thus Carroll could not show any difference between intracellular–extracellular lithium and specifically intracellular lithium with regard to responders and nonresponders, and the term responders must be used very guardedly inasmuch as Carroll reported no remarkable alteration in the basic depressive illness which would warrant discharge from hospital or return to a normal functioning capacity. Again, as in previous studies, the unipolar–bipolar type of distinction could not always be made. Carroll was able to confirm our findings (Elizur et al., 1972) that intracellular red blood cell lithium could be used as both a marker and harbinger for lithium toxicity in that lithium appears to flood (or is unable to extrude from) cells during neurotoxic changes.

Adding further problems to eventual data interpretation is a report by Lyttkens et al. (1976), who report an important variable of sex, disease, and age for RBC to plasma lithium ratio, which is significantly higher in female subjects with manic-depressive disease. This difference persists even during long-term lithium therapy. Older female schizophrenics also have higher RBC lithium than age matched males. The findings emphasize the importance of endocrine investigations in this area and support the view that plasma lithium in humans does not always reflect the intracellular levels. The report by Lyttkens et al. must be regarded with caution also, in that the data themselves are subject to criticism. The groups are subdivided into normal subjects, schizophrenic subjects, and manic-depressive individuals; all are subdivided into male and female populations. However, some individuals were inpatients, others were outpatients; different dosages were given during subacute treatment, others had prolonged chronic treatment, the duration of treatment extending from weeks to years. In addition and to really confound the issues, schizophrenic patients also received other "antipsychotic medication" during the trial period with lithium. Thus, without any type of clarification or subdivision, the differences among males and females, healthy individuals and patients, may reflect, because of the inherent methodological difficulty in this study (without any breakdown of data), differences related to variables of hospitalization, diet, activity, acute illness vs. illness interphase, the influence of other medications, and length of lithium therapy (days, weeks vs. months, years).

In addition to RBC lithium, other variables have been reported to be associated with the antidepressant effect of lithium:

1. Manic-depressive or bipolar illness (Dyson and Mendels, 1968; Goodwin et al., 1972).
2. Family history of bipolar illness (Dyson and Mendels, 1968).
3. "Endogenous" symptom pattern (Dyson and Mendels, 1968).
4. Increased average evoked responses (Baron et al., 1975).

5. "High" baseline plasma calcium/magnesium ratio (Carmen *et al.*, 1974).
6. Initial increase in plasma magnesium (and calcium) concentration with lithium treatment (Carmen *et al.*, 1974).
7. Reduced accumulation of 5-hydroxyindoleacetic acid in lumbar spinal fluid (Goodwin and Post, 1974).

None of these claims have met with any reasonable degree of duplication or critical evaluation. They are recorded here for their academic interest.

Thus we may well ask ourselves, "where are we with regard to lithium's antidepressant effect?" The answer is hard to come by. It is obviously of theoretical importance that this ion may be effective in select cases of depression, since such an effect is difficult to reconcile with the catecholamine hypothesis of affective illness if one also considers that lithium is highly specific against mania and shows prophylactic efficacy against both recurrent mania and depression. Therefore the data, despite their provocative nature and because the numbers in each study have been far too small to come away with any type of real appreciation for lithium's efficacy in depression, do not really permit us to state that any clinical or chemical index exists with which to consistently predict treatment outcome with lithium in depressed patients. The work does, however, warrant further investigational effort for critical evaluation and eventual delineation of lithium's possible efficacy in select cases of depression.

Until further data are forthcoming, lithium should not be used or approved as a standard psychoactive drug treatment of acute depression.

4. USE OF LITHIUM IN PSYCHIATRIC DISORDERS OTHER THAN MANIA OR DEPRESSION

The evidence for a therapeutic value of lithium in illnesses other than manic-depressive psychosis has been extensively reviewed (Quitkin *et al.*, 1973). A review of the vast literature indicates that although lithium has been tried in a myriad of illnesses related and unrelated to manic-depressive illness, the only reasonably well-controlled studies published have been on the treatment of schizoaffective schizophrenics (excited phase), a mixed group of schizophrenics experiencing an exacerbation of psychosis, emotionally unstable character disorders (EUCD), the prophylaxis of schizoaffective illness, and obsessive-compulsive neurosis.

Johnson *et al.* (1971), comparing a small number of schizoaffectives (manic) treated with lithium or chlorpromazine, found the latter treatment superior. As previously indicated in a foregoing section on mania, legitimate questions arise about the conclusions drawn from the statistical computations presented.

Prien *et al.* (1971*b*) found that in highly active schizoaffective patients chlorpromazine was definitely superior to lithium; in less active patients there was no difference. Similarly, in extremely active manic-depressive manic patients Prien *et al.* (1971*a*) found chlorpromazine superior to lithium, but in the less active patients both drugs were equally effective. The VA-NIMH group document the schizoaffectives' improvement in cognitive as well as affective spheres. This finding is contrary to earlier thinking about lithium-sensitive areas of psychopathology and must be considered in any theoretical formulation of the distinctions between the two illnesses, as well as in theories concerning lithium specificity.

Shopsin *et al.* (1971*a*) found chlorpromazine vastly superior to lithium in a mixed group of schizophrenics experiencing exacerbation of their illness. Strikingly, neurotoxicity occurred in 6 of 11 patients at usually nontoxic blood levels. Neurotoxicity included toxic confusional states and behavioral deterioration.

Review of the literature reveals that to date there is no clear-cut evidence that lithium has any beneficial effect on the schizophrenic process. In fact, the only two controlled studies (Johnson *et al.*, 1968; Shopsin *et al.*, 1971) carried out in schizophrenic patients to compare the efficacy of lithium to an established neuroleptic compound both indicate that lithium appears to be without any sedative or neuroleptic properties, and in fact can precipitate or contribute to further decompensation of schizophrenic symptomatology. These findings hold irrespective of the schizophrenic reaction or diagnostic subtype. The affective, psychomotor or paranoid components of this psychiatric illness, like the core process itself, fail to show any selective symptom amelioration during treatment with lithium. Furthermore, and perhaps of greatest significance, our studies suggest that schizophrenic patients as a population have a decreased threshold tolerance or sensitivity for the lithium ion, which exposes them to central nervous system toxicity at moderate to low levels of serum lithium (Shopsin *et al.*, 1971*b*).

It appears that the lithium effect is perhaps disease-specific, with its only clear-cut therapeutic use in the manic phase of manic-depressive illness.

At the time of writing, Small *et al.* (1975) have reported their findings of a placebo-controlled study of lithium combined with neuroleptics in 22 hospitalized chronic schizophrenic patients. Minimal neurotoxicity or other side effects occurred. Ten of the patients benefited significantly with lithium as compared to placebo in terms of blind psychiatric and nursing ratings and nonblind clinical judgments of outcome. These results contrast with previous negative reports in the literature and the generally poor prognosis in chronic schizophrenic patients. The authors suggest that a trial combining lithium with psychotropic drugs is warranted in carefully selected schizophrenic patients who do not respond satisfactorily to conventional treatment.

Angst *et al.* (1970), utilizing a design of successive control and study periods, found in schizoaffective states that the period on lithium was characterized by fewer psychotic exacerbations and hospital admissions. The methodology of the study has been criticized because the drug effect is confounded with order and sequence, and the therapists and patients were not "blind." Angst counters these arguments with evidence that the duration of cycles (time from beginning of one episode to the next) in manic-depressive illness decreases, and therefore, during the second treatment period (with lithium) the natural history of the illness would seem to predict greater morbidity. He also invokes controversial ethical arguments against long-term placebo-controlled studies.

Geisler and Schou (1969) studied obsessive-compulsive neurotics using a repeated measure design consisting of multiple 2-week periods during which lithium and placebo were alternated. A blind rater was unable to differentiate between treatments.

In a pilot study testing the usefulness of lithium in the control of violence and aggression, Tupin (1970) has suggested potential efficacy for this ion, and in another pilot study by Sheard (1971) on the use of lithium in explosive personalities, encouraging results were presented. These investigations appear to have important implications in light of the growing social–political concern in the control of violence and aggression. Efficacy for lithium in the control of unmanageable antisocial behavior, as well as in cyclothymic personalities, has been mentioned in reports by other investigators over the years.

Because of its obvious affective component and inherent periodicity, it would seem logical to explore the use of lithium in the premenstrual syndrome. Separate open studies by Sletten and Gershon (1966) and Fries (1969), however anecdotal, indicated promising results with lithium in this disorder. Currently in the United States, research centers are actively engaged in comparing lithium in double-blind fashion with other drugs more conventionally used in the treatment of premenstrual tension (PMT), such as hydrochlorthiazide. It should be stated that the use of hydrochlorthiazide in symptoms of premenstrual tension is largely empirical, inasmuch as there is a paucity of data to substantiate the routine use of such diuretics in this disorder.

In a long-term double-blind controlled comparison, lithium has been compared to hydrochlorthiazide and placebo in women suffering from PMT. The data would clearly suggest that lithium is the drug of choice for most women over time (Shopsin *et al.*, 1976). The drug is more typically started 7–10 days before bleed (menses) and increased gradually to the optimum dosage–blood level for each patient up to day of bleed, at which time lithium is discontinued and restarted again 7–10 days prior to the subsequent menses. Variations in this treatment schema depend upon factors such as individual tolerance and appearance and symptoms with regard to ovulation–bleed, etc. Data reveal that the premorbid history and clinical character of the syndrome are crucial in appreciating a therapeutic response to lithium.

Those patients suffering from a more characteristically cyclic flare-up during the premenstrual period with remission at bleed and normal interphases between may be said to more typically respond. Those women who experience an exacerbation (however intense) of perpetual-personality–neurotic conflicts are seen to do less well or not respond at all to lithium treatment over time. Placebo effects and a variable course are factors which confound data interpretation; they require control in long-term studies in this area of psychobiological research.

In a study carried out by the Veterans Administration Hospital in Togus, Maine, patients were randomized into a group receiving lithium and another group receiving identical-appearing placebo during the abstinence phase of their illness following hospitalization for excessive drinking (Kline *et al.*, 1974; Wren *et al.*, 1974). Patients were selected who had a history of chronic alcoholism and nonpsychotic depression. The investigators chose one objective criterion of change in drinking habits: whether the patient had an episode of drinking that led to hospitalization for detoxification. They did not try to measure the amount or frequency of drinking, just the number of episodes which required hospitalization.

As expected, the patient population was unreliable. Of the 73 patients selected, 43 failed to complete the first follow-up period of 44 weeks. Of the remaining 30 who completed the 48 weeks of continuous treatment, 14 were from the placebo group and 16 from the lithium group. When the readmission rate of the two groups was compared, lithium appeared to modify the patients' drinking; the lithium group did not appear to repeat as frequently as did the control. Although both groups were less depressed at the end of one year, when compared with depression ratings at the beginning of the project, there was no significant difference between groups when analyzed using analysis of covariance. This finding was in contrast to the original assumption of these investigators that lithium might control alcoholism by controlling depression.

The data suggest an exciting avenue for future research. It should be emphasized, however, that such studies need be undertaken with caution, since lithium and alcohol are not always compatible; there may be a risk of severe toxicity (including neurotoxic manifestations) when alcohol, especially in large quantities, is consumed under conditions of lithium ingestion.

4.1. Lithium in Tardive Dyskinesia

During recent years, various investigators have reported on the usefulness of lithium in tardive dyskinesia as well as Huntington's chorea (Prange *et al.*, 1973; Dalen, 1973; Mattsson, 1973; Manyam and Bravo-Fernandez, 1973; Reda *et al.*, 1975). Two of the most recent double-blind trials have appeared in the literature: one of these claimed "slight" improvement in tardive symptoms with lithium (Gerlach *et al.*, 1975) and the other reported "essentially negative" results (Simpson *et al.*, 1976).

As with other reports of lithium efficacy in disorders other than mania, the data are far from confirmatory and await critical evaluation and the results of further controlled trials.

Thus, at the time of writing, and the interesting findings from some anecdotal and/or controlled studies notwithstanding, lithium has not (yet) proven itself as a therapeutic treatment modality in illnesses other than manic-depressive disorder. It may be said that even in the affective illnesses, the more atypical (e.g., schizoaffective, cyclothymic personality disorders) the disorder, the less likely it is that lithium will be efficacious. The data are, however, sufficiently encouraging and investigationally intriguing in the areas of premenstrual tension, emotionally unstable character disorders, schizoaffective illness (whatever these entities may prove to be), and tardive dyskinesia to warrant further research.

5. USE OF LITHIUM IN DISORDERS OF CHILDHOOD AND ADOLESCENCE

The authors recognize the many issues, both sociological and professional surrounding the use of the term "hyperactive child." A discussion of the relative merits of this term, or the definitional dilemmas surrounding its use, would far exceed the scope of this chapter. If, as many of us feel, the term denotes a behavioral syndrome without implication as to (variable) etiology, the specificity of psychoactive drugs in this group of disorders becomes difficult to evaluate except on an individual (patient) basis.

Likewise, we are sensitive to the fact that a diagnosis of depression, especially manic-depressive illness in children, highlights the constitutional, clinical, and psychodynamic bewilderment surrounding the entire problem of "classification" in child psychiatry.

5.1. Hyperactive Children

In a study carried out by Greenhill and Reider (1973) at the NIMH, nine severely hyperactive children, unresponsive to drugs and psychotherapy, were placed on a 3-month modified double-blind trial of lithium carbonate alternating with dextroamphetamine or placebo. The results of this study indicate that, while lithium carbonate appears to be a safe drug for investigation in children, this ion is inadequate for treating hyperactive children unresponsive to stimulant medication. In another study involving a controlled crossover between lithium and chlorpromazine in hyperactive severely disturbed young psychotic and nonpsychotic preschool-aged children, more symptoms diminished on chlorpromazine than on lithium (Campbell *et al.*, 1972). However, blind ratings indicated no statistically significant difference between the two drugs and an absence of any statistically significant change in behavior or psychopathology with either drug. The authors suggest that some of the observed effects by lithium on behavior warrant further studies to explore the effects of this ion in certain subdiagnostic categories with a cluster of symptoms, such as hyperactivity, aggressivity, and explosive affect. Gram and Rafaelsen (1972) also reported a decrease in hyperactivity, aggressiveness, stereotyped behavior, and psychotic speech in their controlled trial with lithium in psychotic children. Whitehead and Clark (1970), however, were unable to find any difference between lithium and placebo on hyperactivity in children. Wender (1972) has also failed to observe any drug effect with lithium in a group of hyperactive children unresponsive to, or responsive only to high doses of, amphetamines.

5.2. Mood Disorders

Annell (1969*a*) reported very effective results against manic symptoms in young Swedish children treated with lithium carbonate. She also believes that maintenance lithium therapy is good in preventing recurrences of mania, and particularly successful in averting depressions. This author reports the clinical impression that lithium also yields good results in children whose illnesses are not basically mood disorders (Annell, 1969*b*). An assessment of lithium's effect in these children is complicated by many issues. The dilemma of whether a diagnosis of manic-depressive illness is ever applicable in young children is further complicated by the fact that many of the patients described by this author would be acknowledged by many clinicians as schizophrenic. Perhaps the most critical issue in questioning the validity of overall results is that, for Annell, lithium would appear useful in any child, regardless of presenting symptoms. She described favorable effects in children with periodic stupor, schizophrenia, and/or organic brain damage. Such broad applicability for any one drug deserves serious critical scrutiny. Frommer (1968) also found lithium useful for emotionally disturbed children. Among them were children who showed behavior that, in an adult, would suggest hypomania. Lithium was also given a trial in other children who were described as periodically falling into moods marked by depressive features and temper outbursts of serious magnitude. Lithium therapy was considered successful in such cases. Other reports also suggest favorable results in children with affective disorder.

Rifkin *et al.* (1972) have done the only double-blind controlled study of lithium in this patient group. In their study, 21 inpatients, predominantly adolescent girls diagnosed as having emotionally unstable character disorder (EUCD), were included. EUCD was defined as including patients with chronic maladaptive behavior patterns, such as excessive dependency, disobe-dience, truancy, drug abuse, and lack of responsibility toward vocational or scholastic tasks, who in addition have the distinguishing psychopathologic phenomenon of mood swings. These mood swings last hours to days and are usually characteristically manifested by sadness, hostility, social withdrawal, and diminished spontaneous speech; the hypomanic periods by overactivity, over-talkativeness, poor social judgment, and a subjective mood of either great happiness or an uncomfortable sense of drivenness. In the study by Rifkin *et al.* (1972), using lithium in EUCD, lithium or placebo was administered in an initially random manner for six weeks followed by a crossover to the other drug. The serum level of lithium was maintained between 0.8 and 1.5 mEq/liter. During the last week of each drug period, the 21 patients were evaluated daily by "blind" raters. The hypothesis that lithium would dampen affective fluctuation was confirmed. Lithium was significantly better than placebo in two measures of mood fluctuation: global judgment and a rating of the daily range of mood.

The fact that both lithium and chlorpromazine diminish the mood fluctuations of EUCD is analogous to the relationship between the two drugs in manic-depressive and schizoaffective mania: both drugs are at times effective, but lithium may have fewer side effects. The side-effect issue is of particular importance in EUCD, for many of these patients object to the sedating effects of chlorpromazine; none objected to lithium.

6. PREPARATIONS, DOSAGE, AND CONTROL

6.1. Preparations

About 30 lithium preparations have been or will shortly be marketed. They are listed in Table 2 which also shows the type of preparation, the lithium content per tablet or capsule, the lithium salt used, the amount of salt per tablet or capsule, and the source of the preparation. In some instances the same preparation is sold in different countries under different names.

There are two types of lithium preparation, the ordinary and the sustained or slow release. In the latter, which is not commercially available in the United States, the lithium salt is embedded in some sort of matrix (of which there are several different types), so that it is released gradually in the intestine. Absorption of the lithium ion is thereby prolonged, and one avoids the sharp absorption peaks in the serum lithium concentration, often associated with side effects, that are seen with ordinary preparations.

A number of different lithium salts have been used, but no solid evidence is available to show that one salt is clearly better than the others.

As shown in the table, the lithium content of the tablets or capsules ranges from 3.9 to 12.2 mmol. It has been proposed that to clarify matters

TABLE 2

Lithium Preparations on the Market or Shortly to Be Marketed

Name	Type	Lithium content per tablet or capsule (mmol)	Lithium salt used	Amount of salt per tablet or capsule (mg)	Source
Camcolit	Conventional	6.8	Carbonate	250	Norgine, England
Carbolith	Conventional	8.1	Carbonate	300	Winley-Morris, Canada
Carbolitium	Conventional	8.1	Carbonate	300	Lab. Campinas, Brazil
Carbopax	Conventional	8.1	Carbonate	300	Lafi, Brazil
Carbopax A.P.	Sustained release	8.1	Carbonate	300	Lafi, Brazil
Cetoglution	Conventional	8.1	Carbonate	300	Ariston, Argentine
Demalit	Conventional	4.0	Carbonate	150	Mullda, Turkey
Eskalith	Conventional	8.1	Carbonate	300	Smith, Kline & French, U.S.A.
Hypnorex	Sustained release	10.8	Carbonate	400	Chodel, West Germany
Licarb	Conventional	8.1	Carbonate	300	Gilcross, Canada
Limas	Conventional	5.4	Carbonate	200	Taisho, Japan
Litarex	Sustained release	6.0	Citrate	564	Dumex, Denmark
Lithane	Conventional	8.1	Carbonate	300	Roerig, U.S.A.
Litheum	Conventional	8.1	Carbonate	300	Valdecasas, Mexico
Lithicarb	Conventional	6.8	Carbonate	250	Protea, Australia
Lithionit Duretter	Sustained release	6.0	Sulfate	330	Hässle, Sweden
Lithiofor	Sustained release	12.0	Sulfate	660	Vifor S.A., Switzerland
Lithium-Aspartat	Conventional	3.2	Aspartate	500	Köhler Chemie, West Germany
Lithium Carbonas	Conventional	5.4	Carbonate	200	Brocades, Holland
Lithium Carbonate Polfa	Conventional	6.8	Carbonate	250	Polfa, Poland
Lithium Carbonicum	Conventional	6.8	Carbonate	250	Vifor S.A., Switzerland

Name	Type	Li content	Compound	Dose (mg)	Manufacturer
Lithium Carbonicum Spofa	Conventional	8.1	Carbonate	300	Spofa, Czechoslovakia
Lithium Duriles	Sustained release	6.0	Sulfate	330	Astra, West Germany
Lithium Gammasol	Solution	0.04 in 2 ml	Gluconate	407 in 100 ml	Labcatal, Benelux
Lithium Mikroplex	Solution	0.04 in 2 ml	Gluconate	407 in 100 ml	Labcatal, West Germany
Lithium Negroni	Conventional	3.9	Glutamate (mono)	600	Negroni, Italy
Lithium Oligosol	Solution	0.04 in 2 ml	Gluconate	407 in 100 ml	Labcatal, France
Lithium Phasal	Sustained release	8.1	Carbonate	300	Pharmax, England
Lithium Scharffenberg	Conventional	8.1	Carbonate	300	Scharffenberg, East Germany
Lithizine	Conventional	4.0 and 8.1	Carbonate	150 and 300	Paul Maney, Canada
Lithocarb	Conventional	4.0	Carbonate	150	E. Merck, India
Litho-Carb	Conventional	4.0 and 8.1	Carbonate	150 and 300	Noco, Canada
Lithonate	Conventional	8.1	Carbonate	300	Rowell, U.S.A.
Lithotabs	Conventional	8.1	Carbonate	300	Rowell, U.S.A.
Litin Capsule	Conventional	8.1	Carbonate	300	Yurtöglu, Turkey
Litoduron	Sustained release	10.8	Carbonate	400	Orion, Finland
Mamialith	Conventional	6.8	Carbonate	250	Muir & Neil, Australia
Neurolepsin	Conventional	8.1	Carbonate	300	Kwizda, Austria
Neurolithium	Solution	5.0 in 5 ml	Gluconate	1000 in 5 ml	Labcatal, France
Plenur	Sustained release	10.8	Carbonate	400	Lasa, Spain
Priadel	Sustained release	10.8	Carbonate	400	Delandale, England
Quilonorm	Conventional	8.1	Acetate (anhydrous)	536	Penicillin-Ges. Dauelsberg, West Germany
Quilonorm retard	Sustained release	12.2	Carbonate	450	Penicillin-Ges. Dauelsberg, West Germany
Tabl. lithii carbonatis DAK	Conventional	8.1	Carbonate	300	DAK, Denmark
Tabl. lithii citratis Ph.N.	Conventional	5.3	Citrate	500	Pharmacop. Nord. 1963 Scandinavia
Théralite	Conventional	6.8	Carbonate	250	Théraplix, France

and guard against mistakes physicians give lithium doses in millimoles (or milliequivalents) of lithium rather than in milligrams of the salt used. It would serve the same purpose if the drug companies indicated clearly on the label of the bottles the lithium content, expressed in millimoles (or milliequivalents) of each tablet or capsule. This could be instead of, or in addition to, information about the amount of the salt; this latter information is required by legislation in some countries.

Lithium is monovalent and one millimole of lithium is therefore the same as one milliequivalent (in German, Millivalente). One millimole of lithium is equal to 6.9 mg of lithium and is contained in 66 mg of lithium acetate (anhydrous salt), 154 mg of lithium adipate, 37 mg of lithium carbonate, 94 mg of lithium citrate, 200 mg of lithium gluconate, 154 mg of lithium glutamate (mono salt), or 55 mg of lithium sulfate. It is the amount of active agent, the lithium ion, that is of importance.

In the following, lithium doses will be given in millimoles (mmol) and lithium concentrations in millimoles per liter (mmol/liter).

6.2. Stabilization of a Manic Episode

Once the diagnosis is established, stabilization of a patient on lithium medication is essentially a procedure similar to that of controlling a diabetic patient with insulin. Stabilization of a manic episode does not by necessity require hospitalization, although this is sometimes desirable. Any of the lithium salts may be used, but the most readily available and best tolerated is lithium carbonate, commercially available in the United States in the form of 300-mg tablets or capsules. It is advisable to start the patient on 3–4 capsules daily in divided dosages. We have found that in the more attenuated or hypomanic patients starting off with 1 capsule on day 1, 2 capsules on days 2 or 3, and 3 capsules in divided doses thereafter is helpful in avoiding intolerance and/or other inconvenient side effects. The more frequent initial side effects often coincide with the absorptive rise of lithium and likely correlate with the steepness of the rise rather than the actual peak of blood–tissue levels. Plasma levels should be monitored thereafter while the lithium dosage is increased; the dosage will vary, sometimes considerably, from one patient to another and will depend on illness severity and degree of motor activity, body weight, age, and rate of renal lithium clearance. Dosages of 1.5–3.5 g are often required, sometimes more, and care should be taken to keep lithium blood levels *below* 1.8 mEq/liter to avoid more serious side effects. In hospital, plasma levels should be determined every 3–4 days; outpatients may have blood drawn weekly or even biweekly in the more attenuated forms where frequent contact with the doctor and patient–family compliance are optimum. Careful clinical observation is often required in the more severe cases where dosage is more energetically increased. *Monitoring lithium blood levels is no substitute for good clinical observation*; lithium

maintenance is always a matter of clinical evaluation and blood-level surveil-
lance. When blood levels alone are used as a gauge for monitoring lithium
treatment, serious as well as hapless and needless suffering can result (Cohen
and Cohen, 1974).

Therapeutic response is usually achieved in the manic state, with plasma
lithium levels in the range of 0.8–1.5 mEq/liter. This remission more typically
occurs in 6–10 days.

The serum concentration of lithium may be determined through flame
emission photometry or atomic absorption spectrometry. Descriptions of
serum lithium determinations for clinical use may be found elsewhere
(Amdisen, 1967; Doerr and Stamm, 1968; Hansen, 1968). *Blood samples for
lithium should be drawn 8–12 hr after the last ingested dose.*

Determination of the serum lithium concentration with flame emission
photometry or atomic absorption photometry is rapid and accurate. It is
important that the blood samples for lithium determination are drawn at a
proper time in relation to the intake of lithium. Figure 1 shows that the
lithium concentration in serum varies considerably throughout the day.
During the absorptive peaks it may rise 100% over the postabsorptive level.
Accordingly, quite different results are obtained with blood samples drawn
just before, a short time after, and a long time after the intake of the last
lithium dose. Amdisen (1975) has shown that the postabsorptive serum
lithium concentration, determined at a standard interval after the last intake
of lithium, varies much less than does the concentration in blood samples

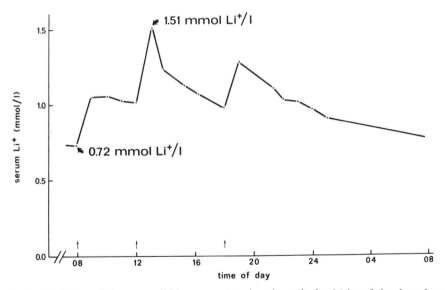

FIG. 1. Variation of the serum lithium concentration through the 24 hr of the day when
lithium is administered in three daily doses (↑) of 12 mmol each, given as ordinary tablets at
mealtimes (Amdisen, 1975).

drawn during the period of absorption. He therefore suggests that this postabsorptive or standard serum lithium concentration be used for monitoring the treatment. The period of absorption lasts about 3–6 hr with ordinary lithium preparations and about 8–10 hr with sustained-release preparations. The time interval chosen for the standard serum lithium must therefore be longer than 10 hr. It is, however, of no great consequence which time interval longer than 10 hr one chooses. Intervals of 12 or 18 hr are practical. The 12-hr interval is used for the patients who are able to come to the laboratory in the morning and the 18-hr interval for those who prefer to come in the afternoon. Since lithium is eliminated continuously through the kidneys, 18-hr serum values will be about 0.1–0.2 mEq/liter lower than 12-hr values.

In view of the large variation of the serum lithium concentration throughout the day, it is unfortunate that the literature (including some of our own previous publications) so often fails to give information about the time interval between the last lithium intake and the drawing of the blood sample.

A manic attack may be treated with a combination of lithium and a neuroleptic (i.e., chlorpromazine, haloperidol, etc.) The neuroleptic and lithium can be started simultaneously. We have often found it advisable to *gradually* increase lithium to 3–4 tablets or capsules daily over the first few days when initiating combined treatment with a neuroleptic in efforts to minimize any toxic synergism. When the behavioral manifestations are controlled, lithium can be further increased and the neuroleptic tapered down and gradually discontinued. The neuroleptic is thus given for greater degrees of behavioral control in the more difficult cases while awaiting the more specific, but delayed, normalizing effects of the lithium. Sometimes, under hospital conditions a more vigorous approach using higher doses of both lithium and neuroleptic is preferable; lithium is increased following the same guidelines described for giving lithium alone (i.e., gradually increased until toxic side effects develop, blood levels of 1.8 mEq/liter are reached, or clinical remission occurs, whichever occurs first). Careful clinical monitoring is the rule under such conditions of combined therapy.

Whether the initial treatment consists of lithium in high doses given alone or lithium in lower doses given with a neuroleptic, the administration is usually continued as a therapeutic maintenance treatment for as long as the manic episode would have lasted had it remained untreated, usually 1–2 months, and is then discontinued. This is the procedure one would follow in patients with a first episode or with episodes occurring at long intervals. In patients with frequent episodes, the treatment is often continued beyond the supposed end of the current episode in order to prevent further manic and depressive recurrences; one is then dealing with prophylactic maintenance treatment. Whether given therapeutically or prophylactically, the maintenance dosage must be based on serum lithium determinations; this is described in the following section.

There is no cookbook recipe for treating manic patients with lithium. The above are intended to serve as guidelines. Treatment carried out without a thorough knowledge of the principles involved can be hazardous.

6.3. Maintenance Treatment

Once the manic episode dissolves, the dosage of lithium must be lowered or toxicity will develop. The patient no longer is able to tolerate such high dosage; this seems to be a characteristic of the manic phase of manic-depressive illness and is likely related to renal lithium handling (see Shopsin *et al.*, 1975, for a review).

During maintenance treatment the intake of lithium must equal the elimination, and since lithium is excreted almost exclusively through the kidneys, it is primarily the renal lithium clearance which determines the maintenance dosage. The renal lithium clearance is ordinarily one-fifth the creatinine clearance. Like the latter, it varies a good deal between individuals and also falls with advancing years. The optimum maintenance dosage, that which gives maximum therapeutic and prophylactic effect with fewest side effects, accordingly varies a good deal from person to person. There are some patients, particularly among the young, who require and tolerate daily maintenance doses of 2000–3000 mg lithium carbonate/day and some, especially among the elderly, who only need and tolerate doses of 600 mg of lithium carbonate per day. Individual adjustment of maintenance doses is essential.

Determinations of the serum lithium concentration are of value in this connection. Experience has shown that most patients derive maximum benefit with a minimum of side effects if the lithium concentration in serum is between approx. 0.6–1.2 mEq/liter; this range refers to blood samples drawn 12 hr after the last intake of lithium. It is therefore advantageous to aim primarily for a serum lithium concentration within this range. In a few patients, relapses or troublesome side effects may necessitate after-adjustment to a higher or lower level. Once the optimum 12-hr serum level has been found for the individual patient, it should be maintained through regular serum lithium determinations and appropriate dosage corrections. Schou (1973) has suggested that many patients can be adequately treated by two daily doses of lithium, the smaller in the morning and the larger at bedtime. When maintenance dosage has been thoroughly established, it may be possible to give the total dose at bedtime; this can more often be done with sustained-release than with ordinary preparations, although this form of lithium is not presently available in the U.S.A.*

Control may be carried out at longer intervals, but at least every third month. Control should, however, take place at shorter intervals in patients

* Currently under investigational use in the United States.

suffering from kidney disease, during treatment with diuretic drugs, in patients on a low-salt diet (Thomsen and Schou, 1968) or a slimming diet (Schou *et al.*, 1975), and during the last six months of pregnancy and around delivery; lithium should be avoided during the first three months of pregnancy (Weinstein and Goldfield, 1973). It is often advisable to determine the serum lithium concentration at intervals of a few days during intercurrent disease, as well as during convalescence after such disease (Schou *et al.*, 1975).

If a limited, unexpected change in the control concentration occurs, the control should be repeated on the following two days in order to check the reliability of the observation. A consistent rise in the serum concentration should lead to a reduction in dosage; at the same time, the patient's kidney function should be examined.

If the 12-hr serum lithium concentration is found higher than 1.6 mEq/liter of lithium, or if there are symptoms of intoxication, lithium treatment should be discontinued immediately and the patient evaluated for hospitalization/observation.

Monitoring of lithium treatment through determinations of the lithium concentration should not replace clinical observation. It is sometimes advisable to inform the family and patient about the symptoms of moderate lithium intoxication. This should be done in order to be certain that the patient will call the doctor without delay at the slightest suspicion of this syndrome. Attention must, however, be drawn to the fact that the syndrome of lithium poisoning varies considerably among individuals (Schou *et al.*, 1975); one cannot necessarily rely on the layman's ability to recognize such a variable and complex medical syndrome.

Other considerations for lithium treatment are given in the section on toxicology.

It is only natural that patients who remain well day after day and month after month should sometimes forget their past episodes of ill-health. It is therefore not surprising that some patients become forgetful or negligent and that others ask to discontinue treatment. Nevertheless experience shows without any doubt that after discontinuation of treatment recurrences of mania or depression are just as likely to occur as before the treatment started; this is so no matter how long lithium may have been given (Baastrup *et al.*, 1970; Schou *et al.*, 1970*b*).

7. TOXICOLOGY OF THE LITHIUM ION

The lithium ion is unique among the available psychopharmaceutical drugs in that it exerts therapeutic activity without producing any undesirable side effects on emotional–intellectual functioning. However, there are unwanted somatic side effects that occur during lithium treatment. Although there are several classifications possible, we have divided these unwanted effects into three main types (Shopsin and Gershon, 1973). The first is represented by mild to moderate toxic effects and may be seen at low serum lithium concentrations; the second is the lithium intoxication or poisoning associated with accumulation of lithium to serum levels above 2.0 mEq/liter. This borderline is not absolute; patients occasionally have serum concentrations between 2 and 3 mEq/liter without being intoxicated (Schou, 1968), while symptoms of intoxication have been noted at serum lithium levels in the range of 0.75 mEq/liter (Shopsin *et al.*, 1970). The third type of side effect coincident with administration of lithium includes a variety of endocrine and metabolic effects; it may be more appropriate to view some of these effects as complications of treatment with this medication.

The various toxic manifestations are summarized in Table 3; there is no obligatory sequence of occurrence.

7.1. Mild–Moderate Toxic Side Effects: Minor Lithium Intolerance

Although the prepared list of side effects appears formidable, those effects most frequently observed are transient nausea, abdominal discomfort, loosening of stools, thirst, increased frequency of urination, muscular weakness, fine tremor of the hands, fatigue, and lethargy. The tremor produced by lithium does not yield to antiparkinsonian medication but may be responsive to the beta-adrenergic blocker, propranolol (Kirk *et al.*, 1972). Sometimes vomiting and diarrhea occur. These side effects often coincide with the absorptive rise of lithium and may be seen even when serum lithium peak values remain below 1.0 mEq/liter; certain observations indicate that their appearance may be correlated with the steepness of the rise rather than the height of the peak. These common toxic symptoms are usually transient in nature and spontaneously subside during the first few weeks of treatment with continued lithium medication. When symptoms persist, the temporary reduction of dosage or discontinuance of lithium is usually followed by cessation of symptoms. Some investigators have observed that some patients not responding to a temporary interruption of lithium ingestion will often tolerate a change to another lithium preparation.

Some of these side effects may persist or reappear at a later stage of treatment; they are also fully reversible. Occasionally they continue for months or years in patients continually maintained on lithium medication. Table 4 indicates the frequency of side effects appearing during the first week in 30 Scandinavian patients starting lithium treatment and in 100 patients given lithium continuously for periods of 1–2 years. This table was prepared by Schou *et al.* (1970) and does not necessarily reflect comparable findings by other investigators.

The various side effects cited above may thus be troublesome in nature

TABLE 3
Lithium Toxicity Checklist (LTCL)[a]

Gastrointestinal symptoms
   1. Anorexia
   2. Nausea
   3. Vomiting
   4. Diarrhea
   5. Constipation
   6. Dryness of the mouth
   7. Metallic taste

Neuromuscular symptoms and signs
   1. General muscle weakness
   2. Ataxia
   3. Tremor
   4. Muscle hyperirritability
     a. Fasciculation (increased by tapping muscle)
     b. Twitching (especially of facial muscles)
     c. Clonic movements of whole limbs
   5. Choreoathetotic movements
   6. Hyperactive deep tendon reflexes

Central nervous system
   1. Anesthesia of skin
   2. Incontinence of urine and feces
   3. Slurred speech
   4. Blurring of vision
   5. Dizziness
   6. Vertigo
   7. Epileptiform seizures
   8. Electroencephalographic (EEG) changes

Mental symptoms
   1. Difficulty concentrating
   2. Slowing of thought
   3. Confusion
   3, Somnolence
   5. Restlessness, disturbed behavior
   6. Stupor
   7. Coma

Cardiovascular system
   1. Pulse irregularities
   2. Fall in blood pressure
   3. Electrocardiographic (ECG) changes
   4. Peripheral circulatory failure
   5. Circulatory collapse

Miscellaneous
   1. Polyuria
   2. Polydypsia
   3. Glycosuria
   4. General fatigue
   5. Lethargy and a tendency to sleep (drowsiness)
   6. Dehydration
   7. Skin rash-dermatitic lesions
   8. Weight loss
   9. Weight gain
  10. Alopecia
  11. Quincke's edema

[a] Prepared by B. Shopsin and S. Gershon (1973).

but represent only minor symptoms to which patients acclimate quite readily. These mild signs of intolerance are an inconvenience rather than a hazard to the patient.

7.2. Lithium Poisoning

When serum lithium rises to values above 2 mEq/liter, poisoning with this ion may develop (Corcoran *et al.*, 1949; Hanlon *et al.*, 1949; Coats *et al.*, 1957; Verbov *et al.* 1965; Buhl and Hansen, 1968; Schou *et al.*, 1968*b*; Allgen, 1969). The onset is usually (but not necessarily) gradual, preceded by prodromal symptoms during several days. These include sluggishness, lassitude, drowsiness, confusion, slurred speech, ataxia, fine and coarse tremor or muscle twitching, anorexia, vomiting, and diarrhea. Severe lithium poisoning primarily affects the central nervous system. Consciousness is

TABLE 4
Initial and Late Side Effects During Prophylactic Lithium Treatment[a]

Side effects	Number of patients showing side effects	
	Initially $(N = 30)^b$	Late $(N = 100)$
None	4	65
Gastrointestinal irritation	10	0
Tremor	16	4
Muscular weakness	12	0
Thirst and polyuria	18	23
Weight gain 5 kg	0	11

[a] From Schou *et al.* (1970*a*).
[b] N = number of patients studied.

severely impaired and coma may develop. The muscles may be hypertonic or rigid with hyperactive deep tendon reflexes, and muscle tremor throughout or fasciculation can be seen. Toxic symptoms such as tremor, ataxia, rombergism, slurred speech, dysdiadochokinesia, and nystagmus imply cerebellar disturbance.

7.3. Treatment of Lithium Poisoning

The severity of symptoms and state of the patient, as well as serum lithium levels, will determine the specific treatment measures in cases of more severe lithium intoxication. Merely discontinuing the drug promotes a drop in levels and may be the only action required. Elimination experiments indicate that serum levels drop by 50% every 1–2 days after lithium has been discontinued (Melia, 1970). Allgen (1969) has demonstrated that levels up to 2.6 mEq/liter drop to zero within 10 days, while the levels of 3.0 mEq/liter totally disappear within 12 days. Gershon and Yuwiler (1960) have previously reported that single-dose lithium loads of 19–50 mEq/liter were detectable in the urine of normal individuals 15 min after ingestion, and excretion reached a peak in 1–2 hr. This was followed by a slow decline for the next 6–7 hr and, finally, a leveling off which continued for a considerable time. Between 30 and 70% of the initial dose is eliminated during the 8 hr following ingestion, and about 95% could be recovered within 10–14 days.

There is no specific antidote for lithium intoxication. Since lithium is the cause of the poisoning, the first and foremost goal of treatment should consist of eliminating this ion from the organism. In severe cases adjunctive treatment measures are aimed at averting the complications accompanying protracted states of unconsciousness and infection. Treatment is basically the same as that used in barbiturate poisoning: (1) elimination by lavage if there is likely to be significant amount of lithium in the stomach; (2) correction of fluid and electrolyte imbalance; and (3) regulation of kidney function. Infection prophylaxis, regular roentgenograms of the lungs, frequent determination of blood pressure, and preservation of adequate respiration are essential; pulmonary complications are implicated as the cause of death in those infrequent cases recorded (Schou, 1968). Obviously, blood and urine lithium determinations require continuous monitoring of the elimination of the ion. Some initial measures to be taken after admission to hospital are outlined here:(1) discontinue lithium; (2) stat lithium blood level, then daily or bidaily as required; (3) serum and potassium estimations (follow as required); (4) electrocardiograph (ECG) stat and periodically thereafter; (5) temperature and blood pressure every 4 hr; (6) infection prophylaxis (rotate patient, etc.); (7) optional measures include spinal tap and electroencephalogram (EEG): (8) if a question of infection exists, blood culture and viral studies of blood and cerebrospinal fluid are indicated.

The administration of sodium chloride was previously advocated in the treatment of lithium poisoning (Schou, 1959). More recent work by Thomsen and Schou (1968) confirm that such a procedure leads to a rise in lithium excretion, but the effect sets in slowly, and clinical experience has shown the procedure to be of only limited practical value (Schou et al., 1968b). More vigorous and rapid lithium excretion is obtained by infusion of sufficient quantities of saline, but caution is urged since in severely poisoned patients this procedure entails the risk of developing lung and brain edema. Osmotic diuresis, alkalinization of the urine, and administration of aminophylline together exert a rapid action on lithium excretion and may be used individually or together. The Scandinavians report that a combination of the first two has proven safe and reliable as a standard procedure for the treatment of barbiturate poisoning (Myschetzky and Lassen, 1963), and more recent experience with cases of lithium poisoning has shown that infusion of urea and sodium lactate can raise lithium excretion by 100–200% (Myschetzky et al., unpublished data, reported by Thomsen and Schou, 1968). Mannitol is also useful in this regard (Shopsin and Gershon, 1971a). Although Hawkins and Dorken (1969) describe a case of lithium poisoning which ended fatally despite hemodialysis, other reports clearly indicate the usefulness of this procedure (Amdisen and Skjoldborg, 1969).

Replacement of sodium, potassium, and water restores not only plasma ions, pH, and water balance, but also the vital functions of blood pressure, respiration, and excretion which are dependent on such vital balances. The specific regimen employed will obviously vary with each case. Mention is made that potassium replacement is often facilitated by the administration of glucose; glucose provides caloric intake, counteracts ketosis, and promotes intracellular transport of the potassium. Insulin may be added to facilitate glucose utilization.

Patients who recover from states of lithium poisoning, even those who

TABLE 5

Management of severe lithium poisoning[a]
  A. Discontinue lithium
  B. Stat blood lithium level—then daily or bidaily levels as required.
  C. Stat serum sodium and potassium estimations (follow as required).
  D. ECG stat and periodically thereafter.
  E. Temperature and blood pressure every 4 hr.
  F. Infection prophylaxis (rotate patient, etc.).
  G. Optional—spinal tap and EEG.
  H. If the question of infection exists: blood culture and viral studies of blood and CSF are
      indicated.

Treatment methods recommended
  1. Replace water and electrolytes as needed (sodium, potassium, calcium, magnesium).
      Total daily fluid should be at least 5–6 liters/day. Do not over-salinize, and avoid
      abrupt changes in electrolyte intake. Monitor if changes made.
  2. Forced lithium diuresis via urea—20 g i.v. 2–5 times daily (urea contraindicated if
      severe renal impairment antedates toxicity), or mannitol 50–100 g i.v. as total daily
      dose.
  3. Increase lithium clearance with aminophylline (which also suppresses tubular reab-
      sorption and increases blood flow). Dosage 0.5 g by slow i.v. administration (may cause
      sharp but transitory hypotension).
  4. Alkalinization of urine with i.v. sodium lactate has been recommended as an adjunc-
      tive measure.
  5. If poisoning is severe, the patient should be dialyzed (peritoneal dialysis or artificial
      kidney).

[a] Primarily via renal excretion: 4/5 of filtered lithium is reabsorbed in the proximal tuble (normal half-life
of lithium is 24 hr).

were previously comatose, show no permanent sequelae. It is usually possible
to resume lithium therapy provided the original cause of toxicity has been
removed.

7.4. General Considerations

As previously indicated (Schou, 1968), prevention of lithium intoxication
must be based on three essential points: (1) exclusion from therapy of
unsuitable individuals; (2) proper dosage; and (3) dosage/blood level control
during stabilization and maintenance. The contraindications to lithium
include kidney disease and cardiovascular illness. These may be considered
relative rather than absolute, however, inasmuch as there are patients for
whom lithium may be considered of critical importance in staving off manic
bouts potentially deleterious to their physical health. The central factor in the
safe use of lithium is avoidance of toxic tissue accumulation, and this
depends upon effective elimination via the kidneys. Patients with abnormal
kidney function (or those on a salt-restricted diet) constitute a definite

treatment risk. However, it is the stability of renal function, rather than any impairment, which is thought to be the key factor (Schou, 1968). It is thus that patients with polycystic kidney disease (McKnelly *et al.* 1970); bilateral glomerulonephritis (Gold and Kline, unpublished data); loss of one kidney (Warick, 1966); severe congenital and cardiac disease, generalized arteriosclerosis with congestive failure, coronary insufficiency (in a 76-year-old male), and immediate postcoronary infarction (Warick, 1966; McKnelly *et al.*, 1970) have been successfully treated with lithium carbonate. In each case the personal, social, and physical complications of recurrent manic episodes were weighed against the physical disabilities; lithium was used under these hazardous situations due to exceptional justifications. The different investigators demonstrated that with extreme caution and careful monitoring of the lithium and patients' physical state, lithium can be administered successfully and the medical illness controlled. We hasten to add, however, that these cases are exceptional; treatment of such individuals is not routinely recommended. Stabilization in these exceptional circumstances should be undertaken in hospital by experienced investigators with the aid of a competent medical team.

When an intercurrent illness develops in a patient receiving a stable dose of lithium, toxic symptoms can occur. It is advisable to have the patient stop medication when a physical illness develops and to be wary of physical illnesses if signs of toxicity develop in a patient on an otherwise stable regimen. Viral infections and elevated temperatures due to any cause often require a reduction or temporary cessation of medication. Illnesses leading to dehydration (e.g., vomiting and postoperative states) should also be an indication for temporary cessation of medication because of possible electrolyte imbalance. Likewise, a reduction of lithium dosage may be required during excessively hot weather.

Other factors that tend to mitigate against instituting lithium treatment are organic brain disorders and possibly age; organic change due to any cause may lead to diminished threshold tolerance for the lithium ion and predispose to toxicity. Although good kidney functioning in the elderly patient should guide the decision to treat, care should be used in older patients. We do not advocate the use of diuretics or oral/intramuscular steroid preparations (estrogen, cortisone, prednisone, etc.) during lithium treatment. Patients with a history of thyroid disease or dysfunction should be carefully evaluated before starting lithium treatment as should patients with any history of endocrine or metabolic disturbance (e.g., diabetes mellitus, low serum potassium, etc.). As indicated above, diagnosis may be a crucial factor in the predisposition of certain individuals to central nervous system toxicity (Shopsin *et al.*, 1970). Finally, it is advisable not to give lithium in the first trimester of pregnancy; this area is discussed elsewhere in this book.

Although there are a host of published reports and probably thousands of open trials where lithium has been used safely with other psychoactive drugs (e.g., tricyclic antidepressants, phenothiazines), there have been no controlled studies carried out expressly for the purpose of assessing the toxic liability or interaction between lithium and other psychoactive drugs or ECT. In fact, it has been our observation that lithium, by virtue of toxicity or other physical properties, does appear capable of modifying brain tissue, bringing about decreased threshold tolerance or sensitivity to other drugs (e.g., phenothiazines or tricyclic compounds), even those previously tolerated prior to lithium ingestion.

Why some patients become toxic, whether apparently accumulating the lithium ion on constant dose regimens or with lithium levels well within the normal therapeutic range (not usually associated with toxicity), can only be answered satisfactorily in some cases. In others, the questions remain unresolved. Mention should be made that the determination of lithium levels in blood has only limited usefulness as a warning of impending toxicity; levels associated with toxicity can vary widely. While some individuals will not show toxicity at lithium blood levels of 2.0 mEq/liter or higher, others will show it at more modest doses below 1.0 mEq/liter. It is likely that the intracellular concentration of the ion determines the toxic reaction. Elizur *et al.* (1972) undertook a preliminary investigation to explore the movement of lithium between plasma and the red blood cells (RBC). Their data suggest that RBC lithium concentration, and more specifically the RBC-to-plasma lithium ratio, may turn out to be a more sensitive indicator of incipient toxicity than the determination of plasma lithium levels alone. That lithium plasma levels are not necessarily an indicator for safe use or impending toxicity is also supported by the findings of lithium intolerance, neurotoxicity, and EEG changes that did not correspond to plasma lithium concentration (Shopsin *et al.*, 1970, 1971). Thus, monitoring serum-plasma lithium is no substitute for responsible clinical following. If there is even the slightest possibility of poisoning or neurotoxicity, a conservative approach with cessation (temporary) of medication is in order.

7.5. Complications of Lithium Treatment

The possible value of lithium as a prophylactic treatment for manic-depressive disorder necessitates the careful evaluation of any side effect or complication developing during lithium ingestion. Over the years numerous reports dealing with various endocrine and metabolic effects related to lithium carbonate maintenance have appeared in the literature; except for thyroid dysfunction, the diverse array of side effects has been met with little concern, apparently overshadowed by the greater interest paid to lithium's clinical efficacy in the affective illnesses.

The antithyroid and goitrogenic effects of lithium have been well documented (Baastrup, 1967; Schou *et al.*, 1968a; Sedvall *et al.*, 1968; Wiggers, 1968; Shopsin *et al.*, 1969b; Berens *et al.*, 1970; Shopsin, 1970). Alterations in carbohydrate metabolism (Van der Velde and Gordon, 1969;

Plenge *et al.*, 1969; Heninger and Mueller, 1970; Shopsin *et al.*, 1972) and steroid metabolism (Platman and Fieve, 1968; Goodwin *et al.*, 1968; Murphy *et al.*, 1969; Shopsin and Gershon, 1971*b*) related to lithium therapy have also been recorded, as have pitressin-resistant diabetes-insipidus-like syndromes (Angrist *et al.*, 1970). Several investigators have reported a reversible lithium-related leukocytosis during administration of this drug to both man and animal (Radomski *et al.*, 1950; Rissetto and Gazzano, 1952; Mayfield and Brown, 1966; O'Connell, 1970; Shopsin *et al.*, 1971*a*; Murphy *et al.*, 1971). The reported efficacy of lithium in countering the symptoms of premenstrual tension (Sletten and Gershon, 1966) and controlling postpuerperal mania (Gershon and Yuwiler, 1960) strengthens the assumption that lithium may affect diverse metabolic and hormonal systems. Finally, the effects of lithium on adenyl cyclase (cyclic AMP) activity in different animal tissues explored may be a relevant link underlying these various endocrine and metabolic perturbations (Berens *et al.*, 1970; Abdulla and Hamadah, 1970; Ramsden, 1970; Dousa and Hechter, 1970). These effects have been dealt with comprehensively elsewhere (Shopsin and Gershon, 1973).

7.6. Neurological Side Effects of Lithium Maintenance

7.6.1. Extrapyramidal Symptoms

Until recently, extrapyramidal symptoms have not been among the many side effects attendant upon the use of this ion. Essential tremor is common; the absence of response to antiparkinsonian drugs had contributed to the conclusion that the tremor is not related to the extrapyramidal system. Kirk *et al.* (1972) in Scandinavia have reported that propranolol, a β-adrenergic blocker, can be helpful in cases of lithium-induced tremor. More recently, however, Shopsin and Gershon (1975) have reported findings of cogwheel rigidity (CWR) in 22 out of 27 outpatients receiving lithium carbonate for periods of 6 months to 5 years as prophylaxis for manic-depressive recurrences. This symptom is apparently not dependent upon the age, sex, lithium dosage, blood levels, or the bipolar/unipolar nature of illness, but on duration of treatment. The more severe CWR appears to occur in those individuals on lithium for longer periods. The CWR was more pronounced, more coarse, and more objectively visible and often perceived as pathology by the patient during the examination when taking lithium in periods in excess of 3–4 years. Intravenous benztropine, an antiparkinsonian agent, did not result in the disappearance of these symptoms of CWR. CWR is one of the two recognized varieties of parkinsonian rigidity; this latter is the most common example of muscular hypertonia due to an extrapyramidal lesion (Bannister, 1973).

The findings of extrapyramidal symptoms under conditions of lithium maintenance have since been confirmed by others (Branchey *et al.*, 1976).

The extrapyramidal symptoms recorded above occur in individuals who are not clinically lithium toxic and whose blood levels have been maintained within an "acceptable" well-tolerated range. Parkinsonism has been recorded in acutely psychotic individuals made neurotoxic with lithium, however. For example, Van der Velde (1971) reports 3 cases, all in elderly patients, of toxic (lithium) reactions. In one of the patients profuse diaphoresis, lethargy, and quivering facial muscles occurred, followed by deep coma, severe parkinsonian tremors, hyperreflexia, and cogwheel phenomena. The extrapyramidal syndrome was later supplanted by episodes of fine, fast tremors and generalized fasciculations. Within 12 days from onset the patient made a complete recovery. Parkinsonian syndromes have been observed by others under similar conditions of acute lithium toxicity (Peters, 1949; Duc and Maurel, 1953; and Sivadon and Chanoit, 1955).

7.6.2. Neurotoxicity with Lithium

Testifying to its apparent specificity in mania, a double-blind controlled evaluation of lithium and chlorpromazine (Johnson *et al.*, 1968) indicated that 85% of schizoaffective patients treated with lithium carbonate showed an overall worsening of their clinical status. A significant feature of this group was the appearance of symptoms of organicity such as disorientation, confusion, and reduced comprehension. Along with this change there was an increase in the severity of the basic psychopathology; the thought disturbance often became more pronounced with psychomotor excitation, delusional thought, and hallucinations. The occurrence of these apparent toxic effects was at blood levels between 1.16 and 1.97 mEq/liter, levels not usually associated with toxic phenomena in manic individuals. In this latter investigation, we allowed for the possibility of experimental design as accounting for toxicity and poor response in schizophrenic subjects. A follow-up study was carried out, where lithium or chlorpromazine was issued to schizophrenic patients under conditions where lithium medication was carefully monitored in efforts to avoid toxicity (Shopsin *et al.*, 1970). Despite this built-in precaution, we were able to substantiate our previous findings of neurotoxic symptoms in six of the 11 schizophrenic subjects given lithium. The mean blood lithium level for these 6 patients was ±0.750 mEq/liter, and no patient showed levels exceeding 1.28 mEq/liter. In addition, we have observed neurotoxic changes on modest lithium dosage and blood levels in a cyclic manic-depressive in interphase, and a patient manifesting an acute depressive episode.

Previous reports of a possible psychotogenic activity of lithium have appeared in the literature. Schou (1959) stated that lithium treatment in mania was, on occasion, accompanied by an aggravation of symptomatology, although this was a rare occurrence. He also stated that in a few instances lithium treatment gave rise to visual and tactile hallucinations (Bleuler, 1958; Hastrup, 1958). Mayfield and Brown (1966) described a manic patient whose behavioral state worsened with lithium treatment, and lithium-induced mental confusion had been cited in the early literature by Greenfield *et al.* (1950), Glessinger (1954), as well as Sivadon and Chanoit (1955). Such toxic phenomena are not always related to blood lithium levels and may in fact reflect intolerance or abnormal sensitivity to lithium (Schou, 1959). In addition to our cases (Shopsin *et al.*, 1970), other reports of lithium-related toxic confusional states have more recently appeared in the literature. Lehmann and Ban (1969) mention the appearance of confusional states in four manic-depressives during the course of lithium treatment, and six cases of confusion have been reported in lithium-medicated patients with affective disorder by Baldessarini and Stephens (1970). Reports of lithium-induced delirium have continued to appear sporadically (Greenfield *et al.*, 1950; Glessinger, 1954), and in a recent study by Spring *et al.* (1970), three patients reportedly showed a delirium-like picture during lithium ingestion.

In a review of eight cases of neurotoxicity, Shopsin *et al.* (1970) deal comprehensively with various neurotoxic changes appearing during treatment with lithium carbonate. These cases underscored the apparent disease-specific therapeutic effect of lithium. Blood lithium levels were quite modest in all instances. The data suggest a central sensitivity to the drug with decreased threshold tolerance. The most consistent laboratory abnormalities consisted of EEG changes which included alterations in the α-activity, diffuse slowing, accentuation of previous focal abnormalities, and/or the appearance of previously absent focal changes. The occurrence of neurotoxicity corresponds, therefore, to the presence and severity of EEG changes rather than lithium blood levels.

Serum levels of lithium, therefore, can be misleading. There are now at least 11 papers reporting on at least 30 patients who have developed severe toxic reactions with serum levels lower than 2.0 mEq/liter (Mayfield and Brown, 1966; Baldessarini and Stephens, 1970; Spring *et al.*, 1970; Shopsin *et al.*, 1970; Van der Velde, 1971; Agulnick *et al.*, 1972; Herrero, 1973; Rifkin *et al.*, 1973; Cohen and Cohen, 1974; Thornton and Pray, 1975). In the 24 cases where lithium dose is reported, the mean dose was 1545 mg/day. Of the 30 patients, 21 were diagnosed manic-depressive and in the remaining 9 the diagnosis of schizophrenia was either suspected or actually made. In the report by Agulnick *et al.* (1972), for example, 3 cases of acute brain syndrome were reported in patients whose symptoms of disorientation, etc., appeared with serum lithium levels of 1.15–1.5 mEq/liter. All of these patients' lithium levels had been slow to rise upon institution of therapy, and all were receiving doses of 2.0 g or more of lithium daily. Agulnick *et al.* propose that the low serum lithium levels reflected an avidity of tissue compartments for the lithium ion against the concentration gradient, which is even steeper than that known to exist in most manic patients (Trautner *et al.*, 1955; Greenspan *et al.*, 1968). These support the notion that toxic levels may exist therefore in tissue, even though normal levels appear in serum.

Red blood cell lithium levels, or the RBC-to-plasma lithium ratio may be a more sensitive indicator of incipient toxicity than the determination of plasma lithium levels alone (Elizur *et al.*, 1972).

Of the 11 papers reviewed with regard to toxicity unrelated to serum lithium levels, 10 of the 30 patients so recorded were reported to be receiving concurrently either an antipsychotic or a tricyclic antidepressant in addition to lithium; at least 7 of these 10 received antipsychotic drugs, among them haloperidol, perphenazine, and chlorpromazine. The most frequent symptoms included disorientation and confusion.

In view of the clinician's inability to rely completely on serum lithium levels, the EEG may be useful in following suspected lithium poisoning. Several reports (Mayfield and Brown, 1966; Shopsin *et al.*, 1970; Johnson *et al.*, 1970) have demonstrated a high correlation between the presence and severity of EEG changes and neurotoxicity in patients who exhibited lethargy, ataxia, tremor, slurring of speech, confusion, and other symptoms of lithium toxicity with blood levels of lithium well under 2.0 mEq/liter.

In one of their depressed patients (Shopsin *et al.*, 1970) local EEG abnormalities accompanied a bout of aphasia, and in another paroxysmal EEG activity, together with seizure-like motor movements, suggested a convulsive disorder of a psychomotor type, although the motor movements were not similar to those seen in focal or generalized seizures. Schou *et al.* (1967) have reported a very similar case characterized by attacks of hyperextension of arms and legs, sometimes combined with gasping grunts, and wide-eyed gazing. The attacks lasted from seconds to half a minute and appeared spontaneously or after stimulation. Passouant *et al.* (1953) cited the appearance of paroxysmal EEG activity in lithium-treated patients resembling changes seen in temporal-lobe epilepsy. In another of our patients, there was evidence of focal EEG abnormalities, including spiking with the appearance of a toxic confusional state. In all of our cases, lithium dosage and blood levels were not excessive. Transitory neurological asymmetries simulating organic involvement (e.g., cerebral hemorrhage) have been reported during treatment with lithium (Schou, 1968). The occurrence of seizures has also been observed on several previous occasions during treatment with lithium or withdrawal from lithium medication (Roberts, 1950; Glessinger, 1954; Schou, 1957, 1968; Schou *et al.*, 1967; Wharton, 1969). A grand mal seizure (Baldessarini and Stephens, 1970) has been reported in a 42-year-old white male receiving 600 mg of lithium carbonate daily with serum lithium concentrations between 0.6 and 0.7 mEq/liter. The patient had no previous history of neurological diseases at the time, and the medication was continued without sequelae for more than 1 year.

Lithium bromide was widely used in the treatment of epilepsy (Squire, 1916) and listed in the *British Pharmaceutical Codex* of 1950 as a form of medication in this disease. Gershon and Yuwiler (1960) have reported decreased seizures and behavioral improvement between seizures in epileptics treated with lithium carbonate. It is interesting and paradoxical, therefore, that treatment with lithium salts can also lead to epileptiform seizures and status epilepticus (Noack and Trautner, 1951a,b; Teulie et al., 1955).

There is a conspicuous lack of experimental work on the effect of lithium on the CNS. Evidence is presented here to suggest that this property of lithium may be the result of a direct action on the brain.

Lithium-induced EEG changes had been reported by several authors in the early to mid-1950s (Reyss-Brion and Grambert, 1951; Duc and Maurel, 1953; Daumezon et al., 1955). That lithium produces EEG changes in man suggestive of a direct neurotoxic effect was first mentioned by Corcoran et al. (1949). The EEG changes showed a severe generalized high-voltage slow dysrhythmia. Schou et al. (1954, 1955) described similar changes in lithium-treated patients with no signs or only slight signs of clinical intoxication (slow-wave discharges and increased voltage). The lithium-induced EEG changes appeared 1–2 weeks following initiation of treatment with moderate lithium doses, and disappeared about 1 week after lithium was discontinued. Transient EEG changes in patients without clinical signs of intoxication have been reported by others (Passouant et al., 1953; Andreani et al., 1958; Schou, 1962; Mayfield and Brown, 1966; Itil et al., 1968; Fieve, 1970). Lithium-induced EEG changes were studied in greater detail by Andreani et al. (1958), who stated that lithium causes increased synchronization of the cerebral potentials with a normalization of previously desynchronized ones. However, there was no correlation made between EEG and serum levels or behavior. Mayfield and Brown (1966) reported EEG changes with chronic lithium administration, suggesting a correlation with serum lithium levels and clinical psychiatric change. In a detailed study by Johnson et al. (1970), chronic lithium administration produced marked EEG, behavioral, and toxic manifestations. The changes ranged from minimal changes in α amplitude and increased β activity, to severe generalized disturbances with dominant bilateral slow-wave changes. Paroxysmal activity and accentuation of focal abnormalities were seen. The presence of abnormal baseline EEG tracings correlated highly with moderate to marked EEG changes and neurotoxicity on chronic lithium therapy. Similar to the case reports presented by Shopsin et al. (1970), there was a marked correlation between clinical neurotoxic changes and EEG abnormalities. A direct relationship to serum lithium levels was not apparent.

In a previous study from our unit relating lithium and EEG abnormalities (Johnson et al., 1970), the most significant changes in EEG during chronic lithium administration were noted in individuals showing baseline abnormalities. Underlining the possible relevance of premorbid conditions as responsible for such changes, some studies (Rochford et al., 1970) indicate that neurologic abnormalities are found in almost 40% of young adult psychiatric patients and are significantly higher than controls (5%). The incidence of neurologic impairment does not differ significantly from one diagnostic group to another, with the exception of those patients with affective disorders. Interestingly, no neurologic abnormality was found among subjects in this latter diagnostic category. It may be anticipated from such findings that neurotoxicity following lithium administration to acutely ill patients would be highest in other than primary affective disorders; that is, in subjects that are not diagnosed manic-depressive, manic phase. This is supported by our findings in a number of studies reviewed here. Indications are that such patients, by whatever mechanism, exhibit a decreased threshold tolerance or sensitivity for the lithium ion which exposes them to CNS toxicity at moderate or even low levels of serum lithium.

7.7. "Irreversible" Lithium Toxicity

In our prepared lithium toxicity checklist, a number of neuromuscular, CNS, and miscellaneous symptoms of lithium toxicity have been cited. General muscle weakness, ataxia, tremor, muscle hyperirritability, hyperactive deep tendon reflexes, and choreoathetotic movements have all been seen in reversible lithium-toxic patients. In addition cutaneous anesthesia, incontinence, slurred speech, blurred vision, dizziness, vertigo, and epileptiform seizures are among the described CNS side effects. Severe lethargy has been reported. Schou *et al.* (1967), in discussing 8 cases of lithium poisoning, describe a clinical picture dominated by severe and protracted impairment of consciousness, preceded by a prodrome of sluggishness, coarse tremor, muscle twitching, dysarthria, loss of appetite, vomiting, and/or diarrhea. In several cases there were transient neurological signs such as facial paralysis, conjugate lateral deviation of the eyes, lateral rotation of the head, and one-sided extensor plantar reflex, stiffness of the neck, and vertical nystagmus.

Glessinger (1954) reported the appearance of CNS signs in 4 psychotic patients receiving lithium which he considered "beyond any doubt" due to encephalopathies. His patients manifested weakness, lethargy, drowsiness, slurred speech, nystagmus, and slight ataxia. Glessinger went to great lengths to point out that some of the manifestations of lithium poisoning reflect CNS involvement and not general poisoning. This author describes one case, which ended fatally, of a 45-year-old male patient who insidiously developed ataxia, followed by several epileptiform fits. The patient became confused and anoretic with a fatal outcome 2 weeks later. Postmortem examination showed both macroscopic and microscopic changes, indicating "encephalitis." In the cases of lithium-induced encephalopathy and/or death reported by Stern (1949), Corcoran *et al.* (1949), Hanlon *et al.* (1949), Roberts (1950), Duc and Maurel (1953), and Trautner *et al.* (1955), necroscopy offered no indication of structural brain damage, but microscopic examination of histological specimens were not carried out.

Although most of the symptoms of lithium toxicity appear reversible, some cases have been reported (Von Hartitzsch *et al.*, 1972; Cohen and Cohen, 1974) *of irreversible brain damage after lithium toxicity. In only one instance was lithium given alone.* Von Hartitzsch *et al.* (1972) reported two such patients. The first patient was also on 100–200 mg of chlorpromazine and had an acute syndrome consisting of lethargy and ataxia, progressing to stupor and coma, grand-mal seizures, generalized hyperreflexia, and extensor plantar reflexes. Her serum level was 5 mEq/liter maximum on an outpatient prescribed dose of 1600 mg lithium daily. She received peritoneal dialysis and regained consciousness, yet was ataxic with frequent choreoathetoid movements one year later. The second patient recorded by Von Hartitzsch was not receiving any other psychotropic agent than lithium carbonate, 1600 mg daily, with a maximum serum level of 2.3 mEq/liter. She developed an acute syndrome of disorientation, ataxia, coarse tremor, a grand-mal seizure, progressing to stupor and twitching of the face and limbs, hyperreflexia, and bilateral extensor plantar responses. She received hemodialysis and recovered, but six months later she remained ataxic and had choreiform movements involving head, tongue, and limbs, and a compound rhythmic tremor affecting particularly the right hand.

Cohen and Cohen (1974) report four cases of "irreversible" brain damage following combined haloperidol and lithium treatment. The irreversible outcomes were in two cases dementia, with masklike fascies, occasional opsoclonus, generalized weakness and hypotonia, and general devastation of ability to function. The first of these had snout, palmomental, and bilateral grasp reflexes. In two other cases the outcomes were buccofacial dyskinesia, choreoathetotic movements, resting tremor, and cogwheel movements. All these cases began with an identical acute syndrome: weakness, lethargy, fever, tremulousness, and increasing confusion; severe extrapyramidal pictures and cerebellar signs developed; and all showed the same physiological and chemical reactions of leukocytosis and elevated levels of serum enzymes, BUN, and FBG that returned to normal within 10 days after cessation of lithium carbonate/haloperidol therapy. One of the patients was diaphoretic. Nearly every feature of the acute syndrome displayed by their patients has been reported with either lithium or haloperidol given alone.

Because of the unfortunate negative effect this report has generated, and the possibility that untold numbers of patients may be deprived of a safe and effective treatment approach, there is a compelling need to critically evaluate the JAMA report. It is not the documentation of findings by neurologists (Cohen and Cohen) that is at issue but their spurious interpretation of data. There is little question that any polypharmacy should be approached cautiously, but equal care must be taken not to do harm to patients by withholding medications. The authors dogmatically and without firm foundation imply a specific toxic synergism between lithium and haloperidol. Let us more carefully examine the available data.

The report of Von Hartitzsch *et al.* on lithium toxicity mentioned above contradicts this notion. The two patients they report had permanent symptoms similar to the JAMA report of cases. However, neither was on haloperidol; one was on chlorpromazine and the other lithium alone. Thus haloperidol seems not to be necessary for lithium toxicity to produce permanent brain damage.

The presence of the "frontal release signs" of a snout in some of the JAMA cases should have provided a direct indication to the doctors responsible that an unusual reaction was taking place. These signs, when present in adults, are generally signs of supranuclear pyramidal tract involvement, diffuse brain disease, and cerebral degenerations (De Johng, 1967).

A major issue in the cases cited by Cohen and Cohen is the problem of baseline psychopathology and/or organicity in these four cases. Specifically, a review of the clinical material, sparse as it is, would most seriously question the diagnoses of mania in any given patient. At least two of the patients appear to have had some baseline organicity. Inasmuch as lithium appears to exert therapeutic specificity based on diagnostic accuracy, the importance of these latter issues may be critical.

The question of an encephalitis as responsible for these symptoms has really not been fully ruled out. In this regard, the fact that all patients ran fevers and showed elevated serum enzymes is telling. Also, in two cases in which irreversible, widespread "devastating" damage persisted, the descriptions of these patients are almost identical to those of patients showing postencephalopathic syndromes of viral origin. Then, too, the fact that four patients, in the same hospital setting and within a relatively short period of time, all developed similar encephalopathies would suggest that some weighty consideration be given to a viral origin.

ACKNOWLEDGMENTS

This work was supported by USPHS Grant MH-17436.

8. REFERENCES

ABDULLA, Y. H., and HAMADAH, K., 1970, 3,5-Cyclic adenosine monophosphate in depression and mania, *Lancet* **1**:378.

AGULNICK, P. L., DIMASCIO, A., and MOORE, P., 1972, Acute brain syndrome associated with lithium therapy, *Am. J. Psychiatry* **129**:621–623.

ALLAN, R. N., and WHITE, H. C., 1972, Side effects of parenteral long-acting phenothiazines, *Br. Med. J.* **1**:221.

ALLGEN, L. G., 1969, Laboratory experience of lithium toxicity in man, *Acta Psychiatr. Scand. Suppl.* **207**:98.

AMDISEN, A., 1967, Serum lithium determination for clinical use, *Scand. J. Clin. Lab. Invest.* **20**:104.

AMDISEN, A., 1975, Monitoring of lithium treatment through determination of lithium concentration, *Dan. Med. Bull.* **22**:277–291.

AMDISEN, A., and SKJOLDBORG, H., 1969, Haemodialysis for lithium poisoning, *Lancet* **2:**213.

ANDREANI, G., CASELLI, A., and MARTELLI, G., 1958, Clinical and electrographic findings in the treatment of mania with lithium salts, *G. Psichiatr. Neuropatol.* **83:**273–328.

ANGRIST, B. M., GERSHON, S., LEVITAN, S. J., and BLUMBERG, A. G., 1970, Lithium induced diabetes insipidus-like syndrome, *Compr. Psychiatry* **11:**141.

ANGST, J., 1966, Etiological and nosological considerations in endogenous depressive psychosis, in: *Monographien aus dem Gesamtgeliete der Neurologie und Psychiatrie*, p. 112, Springer-Verlag, Berlin.

ANGST, J., WEIS, P., GROF, P., BAASTRUP, P. C., and SCHOU, M., 1970, Lithium prophylaxis in recurrent affective disorders, *Br. J. Psychiatry* **116:**599.

ANNELL, A. L., 1969*a*, Manic-depressive illness in children and effect of treatment with lithium carbonate, *Acta Paedopsychiatr.* **36:**292–361.

ANNELL, A. L., 1969*b*, Lithium in the treatment of children and adolescents, *Acta Psychiatr. Scand.* **207** (Suppl.):19–30.

ARONOFF, M. S., and EPSTEIN, R. S., 1969, Lithium failure in mania: A clinical study, read at the annual meeting of the American Psychiatric Assn., Bal Harbor, Florida.

BAASTRUP, P. C., 1967, Report to symposium, Lithium and Goitre, Risskov, Denmark.

BAASTRUP, P. C., 1968, Supplementary information about lithium treatment of manic-depressive disorders, *Acta Psychiatr. Scand.* **203:**149.

BAASTRUP, P. C., POULSEN, J. C., SCHOU, M., THOMSEN, K., and AMDISEN, A., 1970, Prophylactic lithium: Double-blind discontinuation in manic-depressive and recurrent-depressive disorders, *Lancet* **2:**326.

BALDESSARINI, R. J., and STEPHENS, J. J., 1970, Lithium carbonate for affective disorders, *Arch. Gen. Psychiatry* **22:**72–77.

BAN, T. A., 1969, The butyrophenones, in: *Psychopharmacology*, Williams and Wilkins, Baltimore.

BANNISTER, R., 1973, *Brains Clinical Neurology*, 4th ed. Oxford Medical Publications, Baltimore.

BARON, M., GERSHON, E. S., RUDY, V., *et al.*, 1975, Lithium carbonate response in depression. Prediction by unipolar/bipolar illness, averaged evoked response, catechol-*O*-methyl transferase and family history, *Arch. Gen. Psychiatry* **32**(9):1107–1111.

BECK, A. T., 1967, *Depression: Clinical, Experimental and Theoretical Aspects*, Harper and Row, New York.

BERENS, S. A., BERNSTEIN, R. S., ROBBINS, J., and WOLFF, J., 1970, Antithyroid effects of lithium, *J. Clin. Invest.* **49:**1356.

BLEULER, M., 1970, Personal communication to Schou, in *Neurotoxicity with Lithium: Differential Drug Responsiveness*, by Shopsin, B., Johnson, G., and Gershon, S., *Int. Pharmacopsychiat.* **5:**170–182.

BLINDER, M. G., 1968, Some observations on the use of lithium carbonate, *Int. J. Neurol.* **4**(1):26.

BRANCHEY, M., CHARLES, J., and SIMPSON, G. M., 1976, Extrapyramidal side effects in lithium maintenance therapy, *Am. J. Psychiatry* **133:**4, 444–445.

BUHL, J., and HANSEN, O. E., 1968, Lithiumforgiftning. Meddelelse om 3 tilfaelde, *Ugeskrift Laeg.* **130:**1525.

BUNNEY, W. E., JR., GOODWIN, F. K., DAVIS, M. J., *et al.*, 1968, A behavioral–biochemical study of lithium treatment, *Am. J. Psychiatry* **125:**499–511.

CADE, J. F. J., 1949, Lithium salts in the treatment of psychotic excitement, *Med. J. Aust.* **2:**349–352.

CAMPBELL, M., FISH, B., DAVID, R., SHAPIRO, T., COLLINS, P., and KOH, C., 1972, Response to triiodothyronine and dextro-amphetamine: A study of preschool schizophrenic children, *J. Autism Child. Schizophr.* **2:**343–358.

CARMEN, J. S., POST, R. M., TEPLITZ, T. A., *et al.*, 1974, Divalent cations in predicting antidepressant response to lithium, *Lancet* **2:**1454.

COATS, D. A., TRAUTNER, E. M., and GERSHON, S., 1957, The treatment of lithium poisoning, *Aust. Ann. Med.* **6:**11.

COHEN, W. J., and COHEN, N. H., 1974, Lithium carbonate, haloperidol and irreversible brain damage, *J. Am. Med. Assoc.* **230**(9):1283–1287.

COOPER, T. B., BERGNER, P. E. E., SIMPSON, G. M., 1973, The 24-hour serum lithium level as a prognosticator of dosage requirements, *Am. J. Psychiatry* **13:**601–603.

CORCORAN, A. C., TAYLOR, R. D., and PAGE, I. H., 1949, Lithium poisoning from the use of salt substitutes, *J. Am. Med. Assoc.* **139:**685–688.

DALEN, P., 1973, Lithium therapy in Huntington's chorea and tardive dyskinesia, *Lancet* **1:**107–108.

DAUMEZON, G., BUIBERT, M., and CHANOIT, P., 1955, Un cas d'intoxication grave par le lithium, *Ann. Med. Psychol.* **113:** 673–679.

DE JOHNG, R. N., *The Neurologic Examination,* 1967, Harper and Row, New York.

DELAY, J., and DENIKER, P., 1968, Drug induced extrapyramidal syndromes, Chapt. 10 in: *Handbook of Clinical Neurology,* Vol. 6 (P. J. Vinken and G. W. Bruyn, eds.), pp. 248–266, American Elsevier, New York.

DILLON, J. B., 1972, Parenteral long-acting phenothiazines, *Br. Med. J.* **1:**807.

DOERR, P., and STAMM, D., 1968, Flammenphotometrische Lithiumbestimmung im Serum. *Klin. Chem.* **6:**178.

DOUSA, T., and HECHTER, O., 1970, The effect of NaCl and LiCl on vasopressin-sensitive adenyl cyclase, *Life Sci.* **9:**765.

DUC, N., and MAUREL, H., 1953, Le traitement des états d'agitation psychomatrice par le lithium, *Concourt Med.* **75:**1817.

DYSON, W., and MENDELS, J., 1968, Lithium and depression, *Curr. Ther. Res.* **10:**601–608.

ELIZUR, A., SHOPSIN, B., GERSHON, S., and EHLENBERGER, A., 1972, Intra–extracellular lithium ratios and clinical course in affective states, *Clin. Pharmacol. Ther.* **13:**947–952.

FEIGHNER, J. P., ROBINS, E., GUZE, S. B., WOODRUFF, R. A., JR., WINOKUR, G., and MUNOZ, R., 1972, Diagnostic criteria for use in psychiatric research, *Arch. Gen. Psychiatry* **26:**57–63.

FIEVE, R., 1970, Lithium studies and manic-depressive illness, 16th Ann. Meet. of Amer. Psychopathol. Assoc. (APPA), New York.

FIEVE, R., PLATMAN, S. R., and PLUTCHIK, R. R., 1968, The use of lithium in affective disorders. I. Acute endogenous depression, *Am. J. Psychiatry* **125:**487–498.

FRIES, H., 1969, Experience with lithium carbonate treatment at a psychiatric department in the period 1964–1967, *Acta Psychiatr. Scand. Suppl.* **207:**41.

FROMMER, E., 1968, Depressive illness in childhood, in: *Recent Developments in Affective Disorders: A Symposium* (A. Coppen and A. Walk, eds.), pp. 117–136, British Journal Psychiatry Special Publication No. 2.

GEISLER, A., and SCHOU, M., 1969, Lithium ved tvangsneuroser. *Nord. Psykiatr. Tidsskr.* **23:**493.

GERLACK, J., THORSEN, K., and MUNKVAD, I., 1975, Effect of lithium on neuroleptic-induced tardive dyskinesia compared with placebo in a double blind crossover trial, *Pharmakopsychiatrie* **8:**51–56.

GERSHON, S., and SHOPSIN, B., 1973, Toxicology of the lithium ion, in: *Lithium: Its Role in Psychiatric Research and Treatment* (S. Gershon and B. Shopsin, eds.), pp. 107–146, Plenum Press, New York.

GERSHON, S., and YUWILER, A., 1960, Lithium ion: A specific psychopharmacological approach to the treatment of mania, *J. Neuropsychiatry* **1:**229.

GLESSINGER, B., 1954, Evaluation of lithium in treatment of psychotic excitement, *Med. J. Aust.* **41:**277.

GOODMAN, I. K., and EBERT, M. H., 1973, Lithium in mania: Clinical trials and controlled studies, in: *Lithium: Its Role in Psychiatric Research and Treatment* (S. Gershon and B. Shopsin, eds.), pp. 237–252, Plenum Press, New York.

GOODWIN, F. K., and POST, R. M., 1974, Brain serotonin, affective illness, and antidepressant drugs. Cerebrospinal fluid studies with probenecid, in: *Serotonin—New Vistas* (E. Costa, G. L. Gessa, and M. Sandler, eds.), pp. 341–355, Raven Press, New York.

GOODWIN, F. K., MURPHY, D. L., and BUNNEY, W. E., JR., 1968, Lithium in mania and depression: A double-blind behavioral and biochemical study. Presented at American Psychiatric Assoc. Annual Meeting, Boston, Massachusetts.

GOODWIN, F. K., MURPHY, D. L., and BUNNEY, W. E., JR., 1969, Lithium carbonate treatment in depression and mania, *Arch. Gen. Psychiatry* **21:**486–496.

GOODWIN, F. K., MURPHY, D. L., DUNNER, D. L., *et al.*, 1972, Lithium response in unipolar versus bipolar depression, *Am. J. Psychiatry* **129:**44–47.

GRAM, L. F., and RAFAELSEN, O. J., 1972, Lithium in psychotic children. A controlled clinical trial, *Acta Psychiatr. Scand.* **48:**253–260.

GREENFIELD, I., ZUGER, M., BLEAK, R. M., and BAKAL, S. F., 1950, Lithium chloride intoxication, *N.Y. State J. Med.* **50:**459–460.

GREENHILL, L., and REIDER, R. O., 1973, Lithium carbonate in the treatment of hyperactive children, *Arch. Gen. Psychiatry* **28:**636–640.

GREENSPAN, K., GOODWIN, F. K., BUNNEY, W. E., *et al.*, 1968, Lithium ion retention: Patterns during acute mania and normothymia, *Arch. Gen. Psychiatry* **19:**664–673.

HAMILTON, M., and WHITE, J. M., 1959, Clinical syndromes in depressive states, *J. Ment. Sci.* **105:**985–998.

HANLON, L. W., ROMAINE, M., GILROY, F. J., and DEITRICK, J. E., 1949, Lithium chloride as a substitute for sodium chloride in the diet, *J. Am. Med. Assoc.* **139:**688.

HANSEN, J. L., 1968, The measurement of serum and urine lithium by atomic absorption spectrophotometry, *Am. J. Med. Technol.* **34:**625.

HARTIGAN, G. P., 1963, The use of lithium salts in affective disorders, *Br. J. Psychiatry* **109:**810–814.

HASTRUP, J., 1958, Personal communication to Schou, in Shopsin *et al.,* 1971a.

HAWKINS, G. B., and DORKEN, P., 1969, Lithium, *Lancet* **1:**839.

HENINGER, G. R., and MUELLER, P. S., 1970, Carbohydrate metabolism in mania: Before and after lithium carbonate treatment, *Arch. Gen. Psychiatry* **23:**310.

HERRERO, F. A., 1973, Lithium carbonate toxicity, *J. Am. Med. Assoc.* **226:**1109–1110.

HIMMELHOCH, J. M., DETRE, T., KUPFER, D. J., *et al.*, 1972, Treatment of previously intractable depressions with tranylcypromine and lithium, *J. Nerv. Ment. Dis.* **155:**216–220.

ISHIDA, M., ORIHASHI, Y., IGARASHI, A., *et al.*, 1972, Therapeutic experience with lithium carbonate enteric coated tablets in patients with manic-depressive psychosis, *Iryo* **26:**229–237.

ITIL, T., GERSHON, S., and SLETTEN, I., 1968, Lithium effect on human EEG, Principle Investigative Meeting, VA-NIMH Study of Affective Disorders, St. Louis.

JOHNSON, G., GERSHON, S., and HEKIMIAN, L. F., 1968, Controlled evaluation of lithium and chlorpromazine in the treatment of manic states: An interim report, *Compr. Psychiatry* **9:**563–573.

JOHNSON, G., MACCARIO, M., GERSHON, S., and KOREIN, J., 1970, The effects of lithium on electroencephalogram, behavior and serum electrolytes, *J. Nerv. Ment. Dis.* **151**(4):273–289.

JOHNSON, G., GERSHON, S., BURDOCK, A. F., and HEKIMIAN, L., 1971, Comparative effects of lithium and chlorpromazine in the treatment of acute manic states, *Br. J. Psychiatry* **119:**267.

KILOH, L. G., and GARSIDE, R. F., 1963, The independence of neurotic depression and endogenous depression, *Br. J. Psychiatry* **109:**451–463.

KINGSTONE, E., 1960, The lithium treatment of hypomanic and manic states. *Compr. Psychiatry* **11:**317.

KIRK, L., BAASTRUP, P. C., and SCHOU, M., 1972, Propranolol and lithium induced tremor, *Lancet* **1:**839.

KLEIN, D. F., and DAVIS, J. M., 1969, *Diagnosis and Drug Treatment of Psychiatric Disorders*, Williams and Wilkins, Baltimore.

KLERMAN, G. L., 1973, Unipolar and bipolar depressions—theoretical and empirical issues in establishing the validity of nosological concepts in the classification of affective disorders. Presented at the Symposium on Classification and Prediction of Outcome of Depression, Erbach am Rhein.

KLINE, N. S., WREN, J. C., COOPER, T. B., VARGA, E., and CANAL, O., 1974, Evaluation of lithium therapy in chronic and periodic alcoholism. *Am. J. Med. Sci.* **268**(1):15–22.

LEHMAN, H. E., 1968, Clinical perspective on antidepressant therapy, *Am. J. Psychiatry* **124**:12–21.

LEHMANN, H. D., and BAN, T. A., 1969, Informal ECDEU report from the Douglas Hospital ECDEU Meeting, Washington.

LINGJAERDO, O., EDLUND, A. H., GORMSEN, C. A., *et al.*, 1974, The effect of lithium carbonate in combination with tricyclic anti-depressants in endogenous depression, *Acta Psychiatr. Scand.* **50**:233–242.

LYTTKENS, L., SÖDERBERG, A., WETTERBERG, L., 1976, Relationship between environment and lithium concentration as an index in psychiatric disease, *Ups. J. Med. Sci.* **81**(2):123–128.

MAGGS, R., 1963, Treatment of manic illness with lithium carbonate, *Br. J. Psychiatry* **109**:56–65.

MANYAM, N. V. B., and BRAVO-FERNANDEZ, E., 1973, Lithium carbonate in Huntington's chorea, *Lancet* **1**:1010.

MARHOLD, J., *et al.*, 1974, *Act. Nerv. Super.* **16**:199, cited in Ayd, F. J., 1975, Lithium-haloperidol for mania: Is it safe or hazardous? *Int. Drug Ther. Newslett.* **10**:29–36.

MATTSSON, B., 1973, Huntington's chorea and lithium therapy, *Lancet* **1**:718–719.

MAYFIELD, D., and BROWN, R. G., 1966, The clinical laboratory and electroencephalographic effects of lithium, *J. Psychiatr. Res.* **4**:207.

McKNELLY, W. V., JR., TUPIN, J., and DUNN, M., 1970, Lithium in hazardous circumstances with one case of lithium toxicity, *Compr. Psychiatry* **11**:279.

MELIA, P. I., 1970, Prophylactic lithium, a double-blind trial in recurrent affective disorders, *Br. J. Psychiatry* **116**:621.

MENDELS, J., and COCHRANE, C., 1970, Syndromes of depression and the response to ECT, cited in J. Mendels, *Concepts of Depression*, John Wiley & Sons, New York.

MENDELS, J., SECUNDA, S. K., and DYSON, W. L., 1972, A controlled study of the antidepressant effects of lithium, *Arch. Gen. Psychiatry* **26**:154–157.

MELTZER, H. Y., 1973, Rigidity, hyperpyrexia and coma following fluphenazine enanthate, *Psychopharmacologia* (Berlin) **29**:337–346.

MURPHY, D. L., GOODWIN, F. K., and BUNNEY, W. E., JR., 1969, Aldosterone and sodium response to lithium administration in man, *Lancet* **2**:458.

MURPHY, D. L., GOODWIN, F. K., and BUNNEY, W. E., JR., 1971, Leukocytosis during lithium treatment, *Am. J. Psychiatry* **127**:1559.

MYSCHETZKY, A., and LASSEN, N. A., 1963, Urea-induced osmotic diuresis and alkalization of urine in the acute barbiturate intoxication, *J. Am. Med. Assoc.* **185**:936–948.

NOACK, C. H., and TRAUTNER, E. M., 1951a, Lithium treatment of manic psychosis, *Med. J. Aust.* **2**:219.

NOACK, C. H., and TRAUTNER, E. M., 1951b, The lithium treatment of maniacal psychosis, *Med. J. Aust.* **38**:219–222.

NULLER, Y. L., and RABINOVICH, N. M., 1971, An assessment of lithium carbonate, haloperidol and 1B-503 in the treatment of manic conditions, *S. S. Kursakova (Muskva)* **71**:277–283.

O'CONNELL, R. A., 1970, Leukocytosis during lithium carbonate treatment, *Int. Pharmacopsychiatry* **4**:30.

PASSOUANT, P., DUC, N., and MAUREL, H., 1953, L'electro-encephalographie au cours du traitement par le carbonate de lithium, *Montpell. Med.* **A96**:38.

PERRIS, C., 1966, A study of bipolar (manic-depressive) and unipolar recurrent depressive psychoses, *Acta Psychiatr. Scand.* **42:**1–189.

PETERS, H. A., 1949, Lithium intoxication producing choreoathetoses with recovery, *Wis. Med. J.* **48:**1075.

PLATMAN, S., 1970, A comparison of lithium carbonate and chlorpromazine in mania, *Am. J. Psychiatry* **127:**351–353.

PLATMAN, S. R., and FIEVE, R. R., 1968, Lithium carbonate and plasma cortisol response in the affective disorders, *Arch. Gen. Psychiatry* **18:**591.

PLENGE, P., MELLERUP, E. T., and RAFAELSEN, O. J., 1969, Effects of lithium on carbohydrate metabolism, *Lancet* **1:**1012.

PRANGE, A. J., WILSON, I. C., MORRIS, C. F., and HALL, C. D., 1973, Preliminary experience with trytophan and lithium in treatment of tardive dyskinesia. *Psychopharmacol. Bull.* **9**(1):36–37.

PRIEN, R. F., CAFFEY, E. M., JR., and KLETT, C. J., 1971a, A comparison of lithium carbonate and chlorpromazine in the treatment of mania, *Coop. Stud. Psychiatry* **86.**

PRIEN, R. F., CAFFEY, E. M., and KLETT, C. J., 1971b, A comparison of lithium carbonate and chlorpromazine in the treatment of excited schizoaffectives. Cooperative Studies in Psychiatry, Report No. 89, VA-NIMH Collaborative Study Group, Perry Point, Maryland.

PRIEN, R. F., CAFFEY, E. M., and KLETT, C. J., 1972, Comparison of lithium carbonate and chlorpromazine in the treatment of mania, *Arch. Gen. Psychiatry* **26:**146.

QUITKIN, F., RIFKIN, A., and KLEIN, D. F., 1973, Lithium in other psychiatric disorders, in: *Lithium: Its Role in Psychiatric Research and Treatment* (S. Gershon and B. Shopsin, eds.), pp. 295–315, Plenum Press, New York.

RADOMSKI, J. L., FUYAT, H. N., NELSON, A. A., and SMITH, P. K., 1950, The toxic effects, excretion and distribution of lithium chloride, *J. Pharmacol.* **100:**429.

RAMSDEN, E. N., 1970, Cyclic AMP in depression and mania, *Lancet* **2:**108.

REDA, F. A., ESCOBAN, J. J., and SCANLAN, J. M., 1975, Lithium carbonate in the treatment of tardive dyskinesia. *Am. J. Psychiatry* **132:**560–652.

RIFKIN, A., QUITKIN, F., CARRILLO, C., BLUMBERG, A., and KLEIN, D. F., 1972, Lithium in emotionally unstable character disorder, *Arch. Gen. Psychiatry* **27:**519.

RIFKIN, A., QUITKIN, F., and KLEIN, D. F., 1973, Organic brain syndrome during lithium carbonate treatment, *Compr. Psychiatry* **14:**251–254.

REYSS-BRION, R., and GRAMBERT, J., 1951, Essai de traitement des etats d'excitation psychotique par le citrate de lithium, *J. Med., Lyon* **32:**985–989.

RISSETTO, G., and GAZZANO, G., 1952, Variazioni del sangue periferico nella intossicazione sperimentale da sali di litio, *Riv. Patol. Clin. Sper.* **7:**202.

ROBERTS, E. L., 1950, A case of chronic mania treated with lithium citrate and terminating fatally, *Med. J. Aust.* **37:**261–262.

ROBINS, E., and GUZE, S. B., 1972, Classification of affective disorders: The primary-secondary, the endogenous–reactive and the neurotic–psychotic concepts, in: *Recent Advances in the Psychobiology of the Depressive Illness* (T. A. Williams, M. M. Katz, J. A. Shields, eds.), U.S. Government Printing Office, Washington, D.C.

ROCHFORD, J. M., DETRE, T., TUCKER, G. J., and HARROW, M., 1970, Neuropsychological impairments in functional psychiatric disease, *Arch. Gen. Psychiatry* **22:**114–119.

ROSENTHAL, S. H., and KLERMAN, G. L., 1966, Content and consistency in the endogenous depressive pattern, *Br. J. Psychiatry* **112:**471–484.

SCHAAF, M., and PAYNE, C. A., 1966, Dystonic reactions to prochlorperazine in hypoparathyroidism, *N. Engl. J. Med.* **275:**991–995.

SCHLAGENHAUF, G. K., TUPIN, J. P., and WHITE, R. B., 1966, The use of lithium carbonate in the treatment of manic psychoses, *Am. J. Psychiatry* **123**(2):201.

SCHOU, M., 1957, Biology and pharmacology of the lithium ion, *Pharmacol. Rev.* **9:**17–58.

SCHOU, M., 1959, Lithium in psychiatric therapy (stock taking after 10 years), *Psychopharmacologia (Berlin)* **1:**65.

SCHOU, M., 1963, Electrocardiographic changes during treatment with lithium and with drugs of the imipramine-type, *Acta Psychiatr. Scand.* **38**:331–336.

SCHOU, M., 1968, Lithium in psychiatry, a review. Psychopharmacology, a review of progress 1957 through 1967. *Publ. Hlth. Serv., Wash.* **1836**:712.

SCHOU, M., 1973, Preparation, dosage and control, in: *Lithium: Its Role in Psychiatric Research and Treatment* (S. Gershon and B. Shopsin, eds.), pp. 189–200, Plenum Press, New York.

SCHOU, M., JUEL-NIELSON, N., STROMGREN, E., and VOLDBY, H., 1954, The treatment of manic psychoses by the administration of lithium salts, *J. Neurol. Psychiatry (London)* **17**:250–260.

SCHOU, M., JUEL-NIELSON, N., STROMGREN, E., and VOLDBY, H., 1955, Behandling af maniske psykoser med lithium, *Ugeskr. Laeg.* **117**:93–101.

SCHOU, M., AMDISON, A., and TRAP-JENSEN, J., 1967, Svaer lithium-forgiftning. Meddelelse om 8 tilfaelde. *Nord. Med.* **77**:831–837.

SCHOU, M., AMDISEN, A., ESKAJAER-JENSEN, S., and OLSEN, T., 1968a, Occurrence of goitre during lithium treatment, *Br. Med. J.* :710.

SCHOU, M., AMDISEN, A., and TRAP-JENSEN, J., 1968a, Lithium poisoning, *Am. J. Psychiatry* **125**:520.

SCHOU, M., BAASTRUP, P. C., GROF, P., WEIS, P., and ANGST, J., 1970a, Pharmacological and clinical problems of lithium prophylaxis, *Br. J. Psychiatry* **116**:615.

SCHOU, M., THOMSEN, K., and BAASTRUP, P. C., 1970b, Studies on the course of recurrent endogenous affective disorders. *Int. Pharmacopsychiatry* **5**:100.

SCHOU, M., AMDISEN, A., and BAASTRUP, P. C., 1975, The practical management of lithium treatment, *Br. J. Psychiatry Spec. No.* **9**:76–84.

SEDVALL, G., JOHNSON, B., PETTERSSON, U., and LEVIN, K., 1968, Effects of lithium salts on plasma protein bound iodine and uptake of I^{131} in thyroid gland of man and rat, *Life Sci.* **7**:1257.

SHEARD, M. H., 1971, Effect of lithium on human aggression, *Nature* **230**:113.

SHOPSIN, B., 1970, Effects of lithium on thyroid function: A review. *Dis. Nerv. Sys.* **31**:237.

SHOPSIN, B., and GERSHON, S., 1971a, Chemotherapy of manic-depressive disorder, in: *Brain Chemistry and Mental Disease* (B. T. Ho and W. M. McIsaac, eds.), pp. 319–377, Plenum Press, New York.

SHOPSIN, B., and GERSHON, S., 1971b, Plasma cortisol response to dexamethasone suppression in depressed and control patients, *Arch. Gen. Psychiatry* **24**:320.

SHOPSIN, B., and GERSHON, S., 1973, Pharmacology–toxicology of the lithium ion, in: *Lithium: Its Role in Psychiatric Research and Treatment* (S. Gershon and B. Shopsin, eds.), pp. 107–146, Plenum|Press, New York.

SHOPSIN, B., and GERSHON, S., 1975, Cogwheel rigidity related to lithium maintenance, *Am. J. Psychiatry* **132**:560–562.

SHOPSIN, B., HEKIMIAN, L. J., GERSHON, S., *et al.*, 1969a, A controlled evaluation of haloperidol, chlorpromazine and sodium amobarbital: Intramuscular short-term use in acute psychotic patients, *Curr. Ther. Res.* **11**:561–573.

SHOPSIN, B., BLUM, M., and GERSHON, S., 1969b, Lithium-induced thyroid disturbance: Case report and review, *Comp. Psychiatry* **10**:215.

SHOPSIN, B., JOHNSON, G., and GERSHON, S., 1970, Neurotoxicity with lithium: Differential drug responsiveness. *Int. Pharmacopsychiatry* **5**:170–182.

SHOPSIN, B., FRIEDMANN, R., and GERSHON, S., 1971a, Lithium and leukocytosis, *Clin. Pharmacol. Ther.* **12**:923.

SHOPSIN, B., KIM, S., and GERSHON, S., 1971b, A controlled study of lithium vs. chlorpromazine in acute schizophrenics. Presented at VA Conference, Texas, April, 1970; *Br. J. Psychiatry* **119**:435–440.

SHOPSIN, B., STERN, S., and GERSHON, S., 1972, Altered carbohydrate metabolism during treatment with lithium carbonate, *Arch. Gen. Psychiatry* **26**:566.

SHOPSIN, B., GERSHON, S., THOMPSON, H., and COLLINS, P., 1975, Psychoactive drugs in mania: A controlled comparison of lithium carbonate, chlorpromazine and haloperidol, *Arch. Gen. Psychiatry* **32:**34–42.

SHOPSIN, B., SATHANANTHAN, G., and GERSHON, S., 1976, in preparation.

SIMPSON, B. M., 1973, Letter to the editor, Tardive dyskinesia, *Br. J. Psychiatry,* **122:**618.

SIMPSON, G. M., and ANGUS, J. W. S., 1970, A rating scale for extrapyramidal side effects, *Acta Psychiatr. Scand. Suppl.* **212:**11–19.

SIMPSON, G. M., and ANGUS, J. W. S., 1975, A rating scale for tardive dyskinesia, in preparation.

SIMPSON, G. M., BRANCHEY, M. H., LEE, J. H., VOITASHEVSKY, A., and ZOUBOK, B., 1976, Lithium in tardive dyskinesia, *Pharmakopsychiatrie* **9:**76–80.

SIVADON, P., and CHANOIT, P., 1955, L'emploi du lithium dans l'agitation psychomatrice à-propos d'une expérience clinique, *Ann. Med. Psychol.* **113:**790.

SLETTEN, I. W., and GERSHON, S., 1966, The premenstrual syndrome: A discussion of its pathophysiology and treatment with the lithium ion, *Comp. Psychiatry* **7:**198.

SMALL, J. G., KELLAMS, J. J., MILSTEIN, V., and MOORE, J., 1975, A placebo-controlled study of lithium combined with neuroleptics in chronic schizophrenic patients, *Am. J. Psychiatry* **132:**1315–1317.

SPRING, G., SCHWEID, D., GRAY, G., *et al.,* 1970, A double-blind comparison of lithium and chlorpromazine in the treatment of manic states. *Am. J. Psychiatry* **126:**1306–1309.

SQUIRE, P. W., 1916, *Companion to the British Pharmacopeia 19th Ed.,* Churchill, London.

STERN, R. L., 1949, Severe lithium chloride poisoning with complete recovery, *J. Am. Med. Assoc.* **139:**710–711.

TAKAHASHI, R., SAKUMA, A., ITOH, K., KURIHARA, M., SAITO, M., and WATANABE, M., 1975, Comparison of efficacy of lithium carbonate and chlorpromazine in mania, *Arch. Gen. Psychiatry* **32:**1310–1318.

TEULIE, M., FOLLIN, P., and BEGOIN, G., 1955, Etude de l'action des sels de lithium dans les etats d'excitation psychomotrice, *Encephale* **44:**266–285.

THOMSEN, K., and SCHOU, M., 1968, Renal lithium excretion in man, *Am. J. Physiol.* **215:**823.

THORNTON, W. E., and PRAY, B. J., 1975, Lithium intoxication: A report of two cases, *Can. Psychiatr. Assoc. J.* **20:**281–282.

TRAUTNER, E. M., MORRIS, R., NOACK, C. H., *et al.,* 1955, The excretion and retention of ingested lithium and its effect on the ionic balance of man, *Med. J. Aust.* **42:**280–291.

TUPIN, J., 1970, The use of lithium for manic-depressive psychosis, *Hosp. Commun. Psychiatry* **21:**73.

VAN DER VELDE, C. D., 1970, Effectiveness of lithium carbonate in the treatment of manic-depressive illness, *Am. J. Psychiatry* **127:**345–351.

VAN DER VELDE, C. D., 1971, Toxicity of lithium carbonate in elderly patients, *Am. J. Psychiatry* **127:**1075–1077.

VAN DER VELDE, C. D., and GORDON, M. W., 1969, Manic-depressive illness, diabetes mellitus and lithium carbonate treatment, *Arch. Gen. Psychiatry* **21:**478.

VAN PRANG, H. M., ULEMAN, A. M., and SPITZ, J. C., 1965, The vital syndrome interview: A structured standard interview for the recognition and registration of the vital depressive symptom complex, *Psychiatr. Neurol. Neurochir.* **68:**329–346.

VERBOV, J. L., PHILLIPS, J. D., and FIFE, P. G., 1965, A case of lithium intoxication, *Postgrad. Med. J.* **41:**190.

VOJTECHOVSKY, M., 1968, Zkusenosti s lecbou solemi lithia, in: *Probelmy Psychiatrie V Prasci A Ve Vyskumu,* Praha, 1957, quoted by M. Schou, in Lithium in psychiatry—a review, *J. Psychiatr. Res.* **5:**67–95.

VON HARTITZSCH, B., NOENICH, N. A., LEIGH, R. H., *et al.,* 1972, Permanent neurologic sequelae despite hemodialysis for lithium intoxication, *Br. Med. J.* **4:**757–759.

WARICK, L. H., 1966, Lithium salts in treatment of manic states, *Dis. Nerv. Syst.* **27:**527.

WEINSTEIN, M. R., and GOLDFIELD, M. D., 1973, Pharmacology—Lithium teratology, Chapt. 8, in: *Lithium: Its Role in Psychiatric Research and Treatment* (S. Gershon and B. Shopsin, eds.), pp. 147–165, Plenum Press, New York.

WENDER, P., 1972, Personal communication to Quitkin, Rifkin and Klein; Chapter 12 in: *Lithium in Other Psychiatric Disorders* (S. Gershon and B. Shopsin, eds.), Plenum Press, New York.

WHARTON, R. N., 1969, Grand mal seizures with lithium treatment (letters to the editor), *Am. J. Psychiatry* :152.

WHITEHEAD, P. L., and CLARK, L. D., 1970, Effect of lithium carbonate, placebo and thioridazine on hyperactive children, *Am. J. Psychiatry* **127:**824–825.

WHARTON, R. N., and FIEVE, R. R., 1966, The use of lithium in the affective psychoses, *Am. J. Psychiatry* **123:**706.

WIGGERS, S., 1968, Lithiumpavirkning af glandula thyreoidea, *Ugeskr. Laeg.* **130:**1523.

WINOKUR, G., 1973, The types of affective disorders, *J. Nerv. Ment. Dis.* **156:**82–96.

WINOKUR, G., CLAYTON, P. J., and REICH, T., 1969, *Manic-Depressive Illness,* C. V. Mosby, St. Louis.

WREN, J. C., KLINE, N. S., COOPER, T. B., VARGA, E., and CANAL, O., 1974, Evaluation of lithium therapy in chronic alcoholism, *Clin. Med.* **81**(1):33–36.

ZALL, H., THERMAN, P. O. G., and MYERS, J. M., 1968, Lithium carbonate: A clinical study, *Am. J. Psychiatry* **125:**549–555.

8

LITHIUM PROPHYLAXIS AND EXPERIMENTAL RUBIDIUM THERAPY IN AFFECTIVE DISORDERS

R. R. Fieve and H. L. Meltzer

1. FACTORS IN ASSESSING PROPHYLAXIS

The prophylactic effect of lithium was first studied and reported on by Hartigan (1963), who found that maintenance doses of lithium carbonate could prevent future attacks of mania and depression in patients with a history of frequent attacks. Baastrup (1964) and Baastrup and Schou (1967) observed a similar effect. These latter researchers concluded that "lithium is the first drug for which a clear-cut prophylactic action against one of the major psychoses has been demonstrated."

Subsequently a large number of prophylactic trials have been reported. However, the methodological problems involved in such trials are complex. According to Grof *et al.* (1970), the methodology of prophylactic trials differs from that of conventional therapeutic trials in many respects, particularly because the time factor is of special importance. Therapeutic trials require weeks; prophylactic trials may require months or years. There are also ethical problems involved in the use of control groups, which may receive placebo though disposed toward suicide (Laurell and Ottoson, 1968). Furthermore, researchers differ as to what constitutes "prophylaxis." For some, the term implies actual prevention; for others, early treatment or stabilization of a

R. R. Fieve and H. L. Meltzer • Lithium Clinic and Metabolic Research Unit, Columbia Presbyterian Medical Center; Milhausen Depression Center Program, Atchley Pavilion; Foundation for Depression and Manic Depression, New York, New York.

recent remission. Evaluation of prophylaxis has also varied. For some researchers, hospitalization or the use of additional medication are valid indices of relapse. Others have evaluated outcome by these and more sensitive measures, such as mood rating scales and clinic attendance.

Prophylactic trials are also complicated by variations in diagnostic categories. Early European trials reported results in patients with "recurrent affective disorders," a term so loose as to be virtually unintelligible to other researchers (Fieve, 1973). Under this rubric were included manic-depressives, recurrent endogenous depressives, and patients with schizoaffective disorder. Since 1972 the bipolar–unipolar classification system (Leonhard, *et al.*, 1962; Perris, 1966; Angst, 1966; Winokur *et al.*, 1969) has been used in all prophylactic trials of import. This system defines as *bipolar I* manic-depressives who have been hospitalized (or required equivalent medical supervision at home) for mania. *Bipolar II* patients are those who also have a history of highs and lows, but who have been hospitalized (or the equivalent) for depression. Often in these patients the highs are so mild as to be barely detectable. *Unipolar* patients are those with recurrent depressions only, at least one serious enough to warrant hospitalization (or medical management at home).

The question of diagnostic categories is of great importance because, as subsequent prophylactic trials and genetic research are making more and more apparent, the different subgroups may have different responses to lithium treatment. Winokur (1972) has postulated on the basis of clinical response that the unipolar category can be further divided into two subgroups: *unipolar I*, patients with no family history of mania or hypomania, and *unipolar II*, patients with a positive family history for mania. Dunner and Fieve (1974) and Dunner *et al.* (1976c) detected an additional subgroup within the bipolar category, "rapid cyclers." These patients have a history of four or more episodes per year, and a consistently poor lithium response. Other factors, such as severity of attacks, previous history of lithium treatment (Fieve and Mendlewicz, 1972), and family history of mania (Dunner *et al.*, 1970) may also influence the outcome of trials, and therefore must be taken into account.

2. METHODOLOGY OF PROPHYLACTIC TRIALS

Prophylactic trials with lithium are of three types (Coppen *et al.*, 1973a):

1. Before-and-after trials, in which the morbidity of a group of patients over a given period of time before starting lithium is compared with the morbidity in the same group of patients who have been kept on lithium for a comparable period of time.

2. Discontinuation trials, where a sample from a group of patients who

have been kept on lithium have placebo-lithium tablets substituted for lithium. The morbidity of the two groups is then compared.

3. Prospective trials, in which the patient is randomized to either lithium or placebo for a given period of time and then the morbidity of the two groups is measured. This is called the "start design" by Schou and Thomsen (1975).

In addition, trials are either "open" or "double-blind," i.e., lithium is given with the knowledge of patients and observers (nonblind) or else both researchers and patients are "blind" to whether lithium or placebo was given. Early trials, such as that of Baastrup and Schou (1967), were criticized for being both open and longitudinal. The before-and-after design assumes that the recurrences of affective episodes will occur consistently in the history of a patient, an assumption not universally accepted (Blackwell and Shepherd, 1968). Furthermore, in open trials the possibility exists that observer bias can influence the results. Consequently, most recent studies have been double-blind prospective trials, with an increasingly careful discrimination between affective subtypes.

3. EARLY TRIALS

The first systematic prophylactic trial was that of Baastrup and Schou (1967), in which a group of 88 female patients with "recurrent affective disorders" were given lithium for up to five years, and the morbidity compared before and after the administration of lithium salts. Baastrup and Schou found a marked reduction of morbidity, from an average of 13 weeks per year with an affective episode before treatment; during treatment patients averaged less than two weeks per year with an episode. Lithium was found to be equally effective in preventing episodes of mania and depression. In the United States the first prophylactic study was a single-blind trial reported by Fieve et al., (1968), who found evidence of lithium prophylaxis in mania and depression in 36 patients given lithium, imipramine, or placebo. These results were confirmed in a similar trial by Angst et al. (1970). This and other studies reported a marked reduction in morbidity during lithium treatment compared to pretreatment morbidity in both unipolar (recurrent depressive) and bipolar (manic-depressive) patients.

One-group open studies of lithium prophylaxis now number close to 100. The majority include large patient groups followed for long periods of time and are of value primarily insofar as they corroborate the findings of later double-blind trials that lithium has a clear-cut prophylactic effect in bipolar and unipolar illness. However, despite the fact that trials such as that of Baastrup and Schou (1967) were criticized for poor experimental design [selection of patients with a high frequency of pretreatment attacks, statistical errors in evaluating results, observer bias (Blackwell and Shepherd, 1968)], such trials have shed light on certain other aspects of lithium prophylaxis.

Some trials included observations on lithium maintenance in schizoaffective patients, a group later often excluded. Angst *et al*. (1970) found lithium's action was less pronounced in this subtype than in unipolar and bipolar illness. This study analyzed lithium's effect on the duration of episodes and duration of cycles (episode plus period of normal functioning) in bipolar and schizoaffective disorder and found that episodes were shorter in bipolar patients on lithium and unchanged in unipolar and schizoaffective patients on lithium. In contrast, duration of cycles (and intervals) was markedly longer. In bipolar and unipolar patients the cycles were prolonged 61% ($P <$ 0.001) and 76% ($P < 0.001$), respectively. In schizoaffectives, the prolongation was only 30% ($P < 0.01$). However, these figures underestimated prophylactic effect because cycles not concluded at the end of the trial were counted as if a relapse had occurred at that time.

Nonblind trials were defended on the basis that observer bias and psychological effects of treatment would not affect significantly the patient response. Schou *et al*. (1970) compared rate of relapse in patients after double-blind and non-double-blind discontinuation of treatment and found no difference in rate of relapse. If patient and physician attitudes exerted prophylactic action, there should have been a lower rate of relapse in placebo patients than in patients given no treatment. These researchers concluded that patient and physician attitude, i.e., positive expectation, does not significantly influence outcome.

The one-group studies selected patients with a high frequency of attacks before treatment (one or more episodes per year for 2–3 years) on the assumption that these patients would be likely to continue the high frequency of attacks in the absence of prophylactic treatment. Laurell and Ottoson (1968) and Angst *et al*. (1970) found that groups of patients selected for having high episode frequency in one period were just as likely to continue high episode frequency in a comparable following period. However, Saran (1970), in a group of 32 patients with manic-depressive psychosis or atypical psychosis not given prophylactic treatment, showed a 75% decrease in episodes in comparable periods. Schou (1974) notes that extensive studies have shown that recurrent affective disorders, including bipolar, unipolar, and schizoaffective types, tend to show an increase in frequency of episodes with the passage of time. Therefore, although selection procedure in the early, open studies would tend to lower the frequency of relapses from the prelithium to the lithium period, the spontaneous course of the disease would tend to raise it.

4. DOUBLE-BLIND TRIALS

These trials differ widely in design, presentation of data, indices of efficiency, and evaluation of results (Table 1). Double-blind trials are either "discontinuation," when patients already on lithium are randomized to either lithium or placebo, or "prospective" (the "start design"), when patients not previously treated with lithium are randomly allocated to either placebo or lithium salts. To date (January 1976) eight major double-blind two-group studies of lithium prophylaxis of mania and depression in bipolar and unipolar patients have been reported.

The first double-blind lithium–placebo study was a discontinuation trial by Baastrup *et al.* (1970). Fifty manic-depressive patients and 34 patients with recurrent endogenous depressions who had been on open lithium treatment for at least a year took part in double-blind discontinuance studies to compare lithium carbonate and placebo. Within each diagnostic group matched pairs were randomly allocated to lithium or placebo. Relapses occurring first in the lithium partners constituted placebo preferences, and those occurring first in the placebo partners, lithium preferences. A relapse was recorded as the occurrence of a mania or depression severe enough to necessitate either admission to the hospital or supervision at home with supplementary drugs. Serum lithium levels were monitored. Each patient was evaluated by clinicians who were blind. The trials terminated in significant preference for lithium in both manic-depressive and unipolar depressive disorders. This happened when 9 patients in each group had relapsed on placebo, and none on lithium (55% of the manic-depressive group; 53% of the recurrent depressive group). During the whole trial, which lasted 5 months, 21 placebo patients and none of the lithium patients relapsed. Before the trials, patients had been on lithium for up to 7 years. Even after this long period, the authors noted, there was still risk of relapse on withdrawal of the drug.

This study was important as the first clear-cut evidence of prophylaxis in any recurrent affective illness. However, it was criticized on the grounds that the sample was highly selective, since it consisted of females treated successfully with lithium for at least one year. Possibly prophylactic response would have been less marked in a group of patients chosen at random and beginning lithium for the first time.

In England, two trials by Coppen and associates confirmed the results of Baastrup *et al.* (1970). In the first, a double-blind trial designed to last two years, 65 patients hospitalized for mania or depression were selected (Coppen *et al.*, 1971). Twenty-six patients were bipolar and 39 unipolar. At discharge they were randomly assigned to lithium or placebo. All patients had at least two affective episodes in the two years before the study. Treatment outcome was evaluated by means of global assessments by a psychiatrist and psychiatric social worker at the end of the trial. Although evaluations were blind, the treating physician was not blind. Criteria for treatment outcome were more sensitive than those used by Baastrup *et al.* They consisted of a self-rating inventory, need for other medication, and ECT, inpatient periods, outpatient periods, episodes, and plasma lithium levels. Morbidity was thus measured in terms of (1) duration of episode and (2) severity of episode.

TABLE 1

Double-Blind Trials of Lithium Prophylaxis in Unipolar and Bipolar Illness

Investigator	Design	Mos. in study	Indices	Treatment	Failures	Depressive failures	Manic failures	Mean number months in study	Frequency of depressive ep per pt year	Severity			Dropouts
										Global scale—mean	Number of hospitalizations	Average duration of depression in days	
Unipolar													
Baastrup et al., 1970	Discon	5	Hosp/ add med	Li = 17	0 (0%)[a]	0 (0%)[a]	0						
				Pl = 17	9 (53%)	9 (53%)	0						
Coppen et al., 1971	Before–after	14	No improv over pretrt	Li = 11	1 (9%)[a]	Not indicated							
				Pl = 15	12 (80%)								
Cundall et al., 1972	Discon crossover	6	Hosp/ add med	Li = 4	3 (75%)	3 (75%)	0						
				Pl = 4	2 (50%)	2 (50%)	0						
Prien et al., 1973 VA-NIMH I	Random assign[a]	24	Hosp/ add med	Li = 27	13 (48%)[a]	12 (44%)[a]	3 (11%)						
				Pl = 26	24 (92%)	24 (92%)	2 (8%)						
				Im = 25	12 (48%)	12 (44%)	1 (4%)						
Coppen et al., 1975		24			Lithium statistically superior to Ludamil								
Fieve et al., 1975	Random assign[a]	48	Rating scale	Li = 14	8 (57%)	8 (57%)	0	20.52[a]	0.59[a]	1.87[a]	2	86.25	2
Fieve et al., 1976				Pl = 14	9 (64%)	9 (64%)	0	9.00	1.60	2.17	4	75.00	3

Bipolar	Design		Method	Group				Mean number manic episode/pt yr	Mean number depres episode/pt yr	Severity				Mean number months in study	Dropouts
										Frequency depressive ep per pt year	Global scale—mean	Number of hospitalizations	Average duration of depression in days		
Baastrup et al., 1970	Discon	5	Hosp/add med	Li = 28	0^a	6 (27%)	0^a								
				Pl = 22	12 (55%)	7 (32%)	7 (32%)								
Coppen et al., 1971	Before–after	14	No improv over pretrt	Li = 17	3 (18%)^a	Not indicated									
				Pl = 21	21 (100%)										
Fieve and Mendlewicz, 1972	Random assign^a	28	Add med/glob scale	Li = 25	11 (44%)^a	7 (28%)	5 (20%)^a	0.109^a	0.239^a						
				Pl = 27	25 (93%)	13 (48%)	15 (55%)	0.865	0.703						
Stallone et al., 1973															
Hullin et al., 1972	Discon	6	Readmis Hospital	Li = 18	1 (6%)^a	Not indicated									
				Pl = 18	6 (33%)										
Cundall et al., 1972	Discon crossover	6	Hosp/add med	Li = 12	4 (33%)^a	3 (25%)	1 (8%)^a								
				Pl = 12	10 (83%)	5 (42%)	9 (75%)								
Prien et al., 1973 VA-NIMH I	Random assign^a	24	Hosp/add med	Li = 101	43 (43%)^a	16 (16%)	32 (32%)^a								
				Pl = 104	84 (80%)	27 (26%)	71 (68%)								
Prien et al., 1973 VA-NIMH II	Random assign^a		Hosp/add med	Li = 18	5 (28%)^a	4 (22%)	2 (11%)								
				Pl = 13	10 (77%)	8 (62%)	5 (38%)								
				Im = 13	10 (77%) (Li vs. Imip. $= P < .02$)	4 (31%)	7 (54%)								
Dunner et al., 1976 BP-II	Random assign^a	16	Add med/glob scale	Li = 16	10 (62%)	9 (57%)	1 (6%)^a								
				Pl = 24	18 (75%)	12 (50%)	6 (25%)								
Fieve et al., 1976	Random assign^a	48	Rating scale	Li = 17^b	10 (59%)	5 (29%)	6 (25%)			0.194^a	2.30	3^a	58	40.12^a	2
				Pl = 18^b	17 (94%)	10 (44%)	—			0.853	2.44	9	48	18.2	19
				Li = 7^c	4 (57%)	4 (57%)	—			0.212^a	2.55	1	57^a	30.29	1
				Pl = 11^c	8 (73%)	7 (63%)	—			0.367	2.60	2	194	21.18	7

a Some patients previously on lithium.
b Bipolar I.
c Bipolar II.
d Statistically significant at 0.05 or better.

At the end of the study, global scales indicated that lithium was superior to placebo in both bipolar and unipolar patients. Ninety-five percent of placebo patients relapsed severely enough to require additional drugs or ECT. Fifty percent of patients on lithium did so. Neither age nor sex nor number of previous episodes was significantly related to subsequent morbidity in either lithium or placebo groups.

Given these results, the investigators considered that the prophylactic action of lithium had been demonstrated and no longer felt justified including a control group on placebo. Consequently, Coppen *et al.* (1973*a*) reported the results of both the double-blind and an additional open trial which had 34 patients. The same criteria for patient selection and evaluation were used. These investigators concluded that "lithium, when given in a prospective double-blind trial or in an open trial, gave remarkably similar results. Lithium is not a panacea, but this careful evaluation shows that the morbidity of affective disorders is reduced to about 20% of that experienced by conventionally treated patients." It was found that lithium was as effective in patients with unipolar illness as those with bipolar illness, and in bipolar patients lithium greatly reduced both manic and depressive attacks.

The first bipolar prophylactic study in America was reported by Fieve and Mendlewicz (1972) and later, an extension of this study was done by Stallone *et al.* (1973). Fifty-two bipolar patients were assigned to lithium or placebo during normal interval and followed for periods of up to 28 months. All had a history of at least two episodes in the two years preceding the study. Outcome was evaluated on the basis of a rating scale for mania and depression. A patient was considered relapsed if he required additional medication. Both raters and treating physicians were blind. At the end of the study, 93% of patients on placebo had had at least one episode, compared to 44% of patients on lithium. These authors reported that while there was clear prophylaxis of mania, the findings with respect to depression also showed prophylaxis but were less definite since a high rate of placebo patients experienced manic episodes and dropped out of the study.

Two interesting results were noted in this study. One was the finding that patients who had first- or second-degree relatives with a history of mania had more severe manic episodes and also responded better to lithium therapy than patients with no family history of mania. This is also reported by Mendlewicz *et al.* (1972*a,b*). It suggests that patients with a family history of mania may constitute a special subgroup of bipolar illness. The second finding of interest was that rapid cyclers (patients with a recent history of four or more episodes per year) had a much poorer response to lithium than did patients with histories of fewer episodes (Dunner and Fieve, 1974; Dunner *et al.*, 1976*c*).

An additional study of lithium prophylaxis in the U.S. consisted of two trials jointly sponsored by the Veterans Administration (VA) and the National Institute of Mental Health (NIMH). These studies, labeled study I and study II, were conducted concurrently at 18 public, private, and VA hospitals. In study I (Prien *et al.*, 1973*a*), 205 patients hospitalized with a diagnosis of manic-depressive illness, manic type, were treated upon discharge with either lithium or placebo for a two-year period. All patients were bipolar, since each entered the study following a manic episode. Patients were evaluated primarily in terms of occurrence of affective episodes, defined as manic or depressive attacks severe enough to require hospitalization or extensive treatment with supplementary medication. Patients were also evaluated with a large number of scales under double-blind conditions. The treating physician was not blind. As in the previous studies, lithium was found significantly more effective than placebo in preventing affective episodes: 42% of patients on lithium had affective episodes, compared to 80% on placebo. Approximately 75% of episodes were severe enough to require hospitalization. The other 25% were treated on an outpatient basis with supplementary drugs.

In study II (Prien *et al.*, 1973*b*), 122 patients hospitalized for acute depression were randomly assigned upon discharge to lithium, imipramine, or placebo. Procedures were identical to those employed in study I. The sample consisted of 44 bipolar and 78 unipolar patients who had had at least two affective episodes in the two years prior to the study. With bipolar patients, lithium was significantly more effective than imipramine and placebo. Only 20% of the patients on lithium had episodes, compared to 77% on imipramine and 77% on placebo. The difference between lithium and imipramine was attributable to both manic and depressive episodes. Unipolar patients responded equally well to lithium and imipramine; both treatments were more effective than placebo. Episodes occurred in 48% of the lithium patients, 48% of the imipramine patients, and 92% of the placebo patients.

One drawback of the VA–NIMH study is that it was not completely blind; decisions such as hospitalization were made by a nonblind physician. Therefore, the possibility of bias cannot be ruled out. However, scales completed by blind raters agreed with evaluations by treating psychiatrists and showed no systematic bias in their decisions (Prien, 1973*a*).

Hullin *et al.* (1972) subsequently reported positive results in a double-blind study of 69 patients with recurrent affective disorders given lithium. These patients were studied for an average period of 40 months (range 18–75 months). The sample included bipolar and unipolar patients as well as schizoaffective patients. They were selected on the basis of a previous history of an average of at least one admission to a hospital per year in the five years before treatment. The criteria for treatment evaluation were number of readmissions to the hospital and time spent in hospital. The mean number of admissions to hospital for episodes of depression and/or mania during lithium treatment was 0.55 compared with 3.36 during a similar period before lithium. Time spent in the hospital dropped from a group average of 26.9 weeks to 3.5 weeks. Forty-eight patients had no hospital admission while receiving lithium. Only two patients had higher readmission rates and longer time in the hospital than during the equivalent period before treatment. Fifteen of the 21 relapses occurred in the manic phase of manic-depressive psychosis, and there was biochemical evidence of low or zero lithium levels in 10 of these 15 cases. In a double-blind trial in 36 patients who had not required hospital admission for at least two years on prophylactic lithium, 6 out of the 18 patients on placebo relapsed within 6 months, compared to only one of the 18 patients continuing to receive lithium.

Two smaller studies of lithium prophylaxis are worth mentioning for completeness. Melia (1970), in a double-blind discontinuation trial of 18 bipolar and unipolar patients, found that the mean period of remission in the lithium group (433 days) was nearly twice as long as that of the placebo group (244 days). Cundall et al. (1972), in a lithium–placebo trial of a small (32) sample of bipolar patients, reported significant superiority of lithium over placebo.

The foregoing trials offer substantial evidence that lithium provides significant prophylaxis in the manic phase of bipolar illness. Its effect in bipolar depression, although less dramatic, is nonetheless marked (Baastrup et al., 1970; Melia, 1970; Coppen et al., 1971; Cundall et al., 1972). Fieve et al. (1968), in a single-blind longitudinal study of 43 outpatients, found that lithium produced a mild decrease in depth of depression scores among patients who had been on the drug for more than 7 months, as compared to patients who had been receiving lithium less than 7 months. These findings suggest that maintenance lithium may have a cumulative mild antidepressant effect, which, although it does not change the frequency of attacks, lessens the intensity of repeated depressions.

Although most prophylactic studies have involved far more bipolar cases than unipolar, in the general population unipolar disorders are thought to be far more prevalent than the bipolar type (Schou, 1974). Furthermore, in bipolar illness, depressive attacks are far more likely to occur than attacks of mania. Recent attention has focused increasingly on (1) lithium's putative prophylactic effect in the depressed phase of bipolar and unipolar illness, and (2) lithium's efficiency in comparison to that of other drugs, such as imipramine and tricyclic antidepressants.

5. PROPHYLAXIS IN DEPRESSION

Prien et al. (1973b) suggested that long-term imipramine treatment reduces depression episode frequency equivalent to prophylaxis achieved with lithium carbonate in unipolar patients. However, outcome in this trial was evaluated only in terms of need for hospitalization or additional medication. Fieve et al. (1976) compared the prophylactic efficacy of lithium to placebo in 28 unipolar patients, using as indices: frequency of episodes, depth of global depression scores, and rate of clinic attendance. The patients were followed up from 3 months to 4 years. A statistically significant decrease occurred in all three indices among the lithium group. These researchers suggested, therefore, that lithium carbonate and periodic use of tricyclic antidepressants might have several advantages over long-term tricyclic medication alone. Dunner *et al.* (1976), in a study of 40 bipolar II patients found a reduction in frequency of hypomanic episodes but no reduction in frequency of depressive attacks, although there was a suggestion that depressive attacks that occurred during lithium treatment might be attenuated. However, this study lasted a mean of only 16 months.

The most comprehensive trial of lithium prophylaxis in depression to date is a study of three depression subtypes (Fieve *et al.*, 1976). Thirty-five bipolar I patients, 18 bipolar II patients, and 28 unipolar patients were followed for 4 years. Four indices of prophylaxis were used:

1. Mean number of months in study
2. Frequency of episodes
3. Severity of depression as determined by:
    A. Global ratings
    B. Number of hospitalizations
    C. Duration of episodes
4. Dropout rates

It was found that lithium was highly effective as a prophylactic in bipolar I depression and was superior to placebo in bipolar II and unipolar depression. These researchers suggested that depression prophylaxis, in contrast to that of mania, requires an extended period of time to demonstrate [compare 4 years to the mean of 16 months in the study by Dunner *et al.* (1975), where no significant prophylaxis of depression was noted]. In addition, Fieve *et al.* (1976) noted, "it is possible that tricyclics combined with maintenance lithium may be superior to lithium or tricyclics alone in the overall group of unipolar depression that do better with lithium alone or with antidepressants alone."

Studies of Klerman *et al.* (1974) and Mindham *et al.* (1973) have shown that prophylactic tricyclic antidepressants can reduce affective morbidity in heterogeneous samples of depressed patients. Unfortunately, the precise effects on clearly defined bipolar and unipolar depressions were not studied by these groups. Trials with tricyclic antidepressants alone, monoamine oxidase (MAO) inhibitors alone, or either drug in combination with lithium for prophylaxis in clearly defined depression subtypes seem to be indicated.

6. CONSIDERATIONS IN PROPHYLAXIS: SUMMARY

Numerous prophylactic trials have confirmed the prophylactic action of lithium in the bipolar manic phase, and there is now strong evidence that lithium has prophylactic action in bipolar and unipolar depression as well.

Present genetic findings underscore the need to relate the response to lithium therapy to subtypes of depressive illness and genetic history. In severely ill patients who have had multiple attacks over the years, with many courses of electroshock therapy, one can now control the illness virtually without the use of shock treatments. It is likely that lithium will replace electroshock as a preferred and more specific method of preventing affective illness over extended periods of time. It appears that lithium in conjunction with other drugs (imipramine, amitryptilene, other tricyclic antidepressants, and chlorpromazine) can be used with good results in the majority of cases. Consequently, long-term lithium therapy with periodic conjoint medication is rapidly becoming the preferred mode of treatment in all subtypes of affective disorder.

Successful long-term management of lithium patients depends on acceptance of the concept of drug prophylaxis. Both physician and patient must understand that the drug is to be taken continuously, under close supervision with proper laboratory facilities, even though the patient may have been well for months and even years. This must be insisted upon because of the low toxic-to-therapeutic ratio with this ion. Furthermore, patient and physician should be aware of the stabilizing action of lithium on endogenous mood changes of less than psychotic intensity during the intervals between psychotic episodes, and on the gradual onset of lithium's full effect, particularly in the case of recurrent depression. Schou (1968) and Fieve (1970) have noted that lithium does not appear to interfere with normal intellectual activity, impair normal consciousness, or restrict the emotional range. However, some individuals, particularly creative cyclothymics who feel they do their best work in hypomanic periods, find the loss of the hypomanic phase may make life under lithium protection comparatively colorless. They may prefer to reject prophylaxis and take their chances without lithium carbonate. In contrast to this group of mildly ill, creative individuals, Polatin and Fieve (1971) have also described a limited number of highly creative, severely ill bipolar I manic-depressive patients who eagerly accepted lithium and did extremely well on the drug. These patients claimed an overall increase in productivity and creativity, in contrast to the prelithium period, when gross psychotic episodes disrupted their output. Finally, some patients are loath to accept lithium carbonate therapy as a lifetime need, since the idea of permanent dependence on a drug, periodic blood tests, and the stigma of incurable illness are unacceptable to them. Once stabilized on lithium some of these mildly cyclothymic patients feel so well that the possibility of another low becomes inconceivable and is denied by them.

When considering lithium therapy, both patient and physician must be aware that even after full stabilization has been achieved occasional periods will occur in which for a few weeks or days the patient becomes unstable and feels as if a psychotic episode were about to begin (Schou, 1974). Although no episode develops, to the inexperienced psychiatrist such prodromal symptoms may appear to indicate the administration—unnecessarily—of antidepressant therapy.

Because of the unpredictable nature of recurrent affective illness, a number of researchers have been led to develop statistical tools for estimating mathematical regularities in the parameters of its longitudinal course, both with and without lithium treatment.

7. THE LIFE TABLE

Most longitudinal studies of mental disorders call for the data to be collected at a limited number of time points following a subject's entry into the study (e.g., every 6 months after release from hospital, or every week after the start of treatment), and for the subsequent statistical analyses to be performed at each time point separately. A critique of such a "one-point-at-a-time" analytic strategy, and some potentially more informative methods, have been presented by May and his colleagues for the case of quantitive data (May, 1972*a,b*, 1973). The life table is a more informative method than those typically used in psychiatric research for the case of serially collected qualitative data.

The life table is a statistical technique for estimating such clinically important parameters of longitudinal course as the probability that a patient will experience the outcome under study within any specified time interval, and the mean and median length of time until the outcome occurs. The life table is the method of choice for estimating these parameters because it bases its estimates on data from *all* patients who were followed, whether for a short time (e.g., weeks) or a long time (e.g., years), and thus provides more precise estimates than does the one-point-at-a-time approach.

The life table is by no means a new tool in medical research, and in fact it is the standard means for estimating short- and long-term mortality risks associated with cancer (Berkson and Gage, 1950) and other diseases (Lew and Seltzer, 1970). With only rare exceptions, however (Kramer, 1969; Klerman *et al.*, 1974), it has not been employed in psychiatric follow-up studies.

Fleiss *et al.* (1976) used the life table to describe the long-term course of manic-depressive illness and the effects of lithium carbonate on this course. Ninety-six patients were followed on lithium treatment, and 38 were followed on control (either placebo or no) treatment; 31 patients contributed data to both the lithium and the control groups. All patients were followed from the start of their first week of continuous normal functioning (time 0) until the occurrence of the first of three possible outcomes, at which point the elapsed time (from time 0) was calculated.

A patient was judged to have *failed* if he experienced symptoms which required either hospitalization or the addition of further treatment (either a different drug or an increased dose of the original drug) or if he reported symptoms which did not require treatment but which persisted, as documented in his records, for at least 4 weeks.

A patient was recorded as having *terminated* the study *well* if he remained continuously well up to March 1, 1974, or if he was maintained well and was either discharged to private care or switched from one treatment group to the other before March 1, 1974.

Table 2 represents the first six rows of the life table for the 96 bipolar patients maintained on lithium. Figure 1 presents, separately for the bipolar patients followed on lithium and for those followed on control regimens (placebo or no treatment), a pair of curves describing the probabilities of remaining continuously well. One was derived by assuming that all dropouts were well at the time of dropping out, the other by assuming they were all ill at that time. The six values of P derived in Table 2 may be checked against the corresponding values in the second curve in Figure 1.

Fleiss *et al.* (1976) found that the control patient followed the longest failed during the 42nd study interval (i.e., between weeks 164 and 168). Table 3 illustrates the calculation of the summary chi-square statistic comparing the entire lithium course over the first 168 weeks of follow-up (assuming that all lithium dropouts failed at time of dropout) with the entire control course (assuming that all control dropouts were well at time of dropout). Only intervals during which failures actually occurred in either sample need to be recorded. Figure 2 shows the fit of predicted values (observed control course vs. course predicted by mathematical model) to be excellent.

The calculation of the quantities in a life table is itself relatively easy, but the determination of standard errors and the statistical comparison of results from different samples are more complicated than the usual analyses of longitudinal data. What is gained by applying the life table method to follow-up data is increased precision, the ability to estimate important parameters of

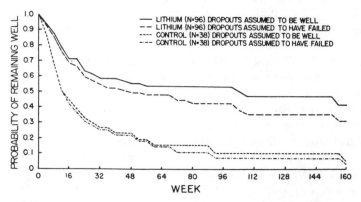

FIG. 1. Lithium carbonate vs. control course under two assumptions about dropouts.

TABLE 2

Portion of Life Table for Bipolar I Patients Already Maintained Well with Lithium Carbonate for Four Weeks

W to $W + 4$	a Number starting interval well (N_w)	b Number last observed well during interval (L_w)	c Adjusted number studied in interval ($N_w = [(a) - (b)/2]$)	d Number falling in interval (F_w)[a]	e Interval-specific probability of failure ($q_w = (d)/(c)$)	f Interval-specific probability of remaining well ($p_w = 1 - (e)$)	g Cumulative probability of remaining well ($P_{w+4} = \text{product}(f)$)
0–4	96	0	96	7	0.07	0.93	0.93
4–8	89	1	88.5	7	0.08	0.92	0.86
8–12	81	0	81	9	0.11	0.89	0.76
12–16	72	0	72	7	0.10	0.90	0.69
16–20	65	3	63.5	2	0.03	0.97	0.66
20–24	60	4	58	6	0.10	0.90	0.60

[a] Including dropouts.

TABLE 3

Calculation of Summary Chi-Square Statistics for Difference between Lithium Carbonate[a] and Control[b] Samples

Interval (weeks)	Lithium carbonate $N'^{(1)}$	Lithium carbonate $p^{(1)}$	Control $N'^{(2)}$	Control $p^{(2)}$	a $\dfrac{N'^{(1)} \times N'^{(2)}}{N'^{(1)} + N'^{(2)}}$	b $p^{(1)} - p^{(2)}$	c $(= a \times b)$	d $\bar{p}$	e $\bar{p}(1 - \bar{p})$	f $\dfrac{N'^{(1)} \times N'^{(2)}}{N'^{(1)} + N'^{(2)}} - 1$	g $(= e \times f)$
0–4	96	.93	37.5	0.87	26.97	0.06	1.62	0.91	0.08	27.17	2.17
4–8	88.5	.92	31.5	0.78	23.23	0.14	3.25	0.88	0.11	23.43	2.58
8–12	81	.89	24	0.75	18.51	0.14	2.59	0.86	0.12	18.69	2.24
12–16	72	.90	17.5	0.89	14.08	0.01	0.14	0.90	0.09	14.24	1.28
16–20	63.5	.97	15	0.87	12.13	0.10	1.21	0.95	0.05	12.29	0.61
20–24	58	.90	13	0.85	10.62	0.05	0.53	0.89	0.10	10.77	1.08
24–28	49.5	.96	11	0.91	9.00	0.05	0.45	0.95	0.05	9.15	0.46
28–32	47	.96	9.5	0.89	7.90	0.07	0.55	0.95	0.05	8.05	0.40
32–36	44.5	.96	8	1.00	6.78	−0.04	−0.27	0.97	0.03	6.91	0.21
36–40	42	1.00	7.5	0.87	6.36	0.13	0.83	0.98	0.02	6.49	0.13
40–44	41	.98	6	1.00	5.23	−0.02	−0.10	0.98	0.02	5.35	0.11
44–48	37.5	.97	6	1.00	5.17	−0.03	−0.16	0.97	0.03	5.29	0.16
48–52	34.5	1.00	6	0.83	5.11	0.17	0.87	0.97	0.03	5.24	0.16
52–56	33.5	.97	5	1.00	4.35	−0.03	−0.13	0.97	0.03	4.47	0.13
56–60	31.5	1.00	5	0.80	4.32	0.20	0.86	0.97	0.03	4.44	0.13
68–72	26	.93	3.5	1.00	3.08	−0.07	−0.22	0.94	0.06	3.19	0.19
76–80	22.5	.96	3	1.00	2.65	−0.04	−0.11	0.96	0.04	2.76	0.11
88–92	21	1.00	3	0.67	2.63	0.33	0.87	0.96	0.04	2.74	0.17
100–104	19	.89	2	1.00	1.81	−0.11	−0.20	0.90	0.09	1.90	0.17
104–108	16	.94	2	1.00	1.78	−0.06	−0.11	0.95	0.05	1.88	0.09
152–156	8.5	.88	2	1.00	1.62	−0.12	−0.19	0.90	0.09	1.79	0.16
156–160	7	1.00	2	0.50	1.56	0.50	0.78	0.89	0.10	1.75	0.18
164–168	6	.83	1	0.00	0.86	0.83	0.71	0.71	0.21	1.00	0.21
Sum							13.77				13.07

[a] Assuming all dropouts failed.
[b] Assuming all dropouts were well.

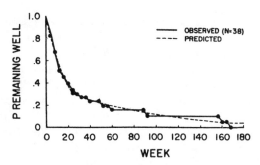

FIG. 2. Observed control course vs. course predicted by fitted mathematical model.

longitudinal course, and the opportunity to discover mathematical regularities which would otherwise remain hidden. These advantages are so great
that the life table should become as standard a tool in follow-up studies as,
say, the paired-sample test is in before-and-after studies. With these and
similar research tools it is hoped that in the future lithium may be given
prophylactically with optimal response to the millions of people now suffering from various forms of affective illness.

One of the most promising recent developments has been the discovery
that certain behavioral and biochemical effects of a related element, rubidium, appear to complement those of lithium and may elucidate what has
been hitherto unclear, i.e., lithium's mechanism of action, and, indirectly, the
etiology of affective disorder itself.

8. RUBIDIUM IN PSYCHIATRY

In 1860 Kirchoff and Bunsen discovered cesium, one of the group I
alkali metals, in a sample of mineral water. Bunsen subsequently obtained
larger quantities of rubidium and cesium by evaporating 40,000 liters of
mineral spring water and then studied the chemical properties of their salts.

The first report on the physiological effects of the new ion appeared in
1868, when Grandeau, comparing the effects of sodium, potassium, and
rubidium chlorides injected intravenously into dogs and rabbits, suggested
(Grandeau, 1864) that there might be some advantage to the use of rubidium
in medicine. His suggestion was based on the belief that undesirable side
effects of potassium iodide and potassium bromide (empiric treatments for
syphilis and epilepsy dating from 1835 and 1851, respectively) were due to
the potassium ion. However, the first application of rubidium salts to therapy
was in a different area. In 1887–1888 Botkin, working for a doctoral thesis in
the laboratory of Ivan Pavlov, administered rubidium chloride to 10 seriously
ill cardiac patients (Botkin, 1888). He reported that all of his patients
experienced a subjective sense of well-being, although no improvement in

the cardiac condition occurred. The maximum dose given was 300 mEq over a period of 25 days. The RbCl administration had been preceded by other cardiac medications, including cardiac glycosides.

Rubidium was also used extensively as a replacement cation for potassium in bromide therapy of epilepsy. Laufenauer (1889), who employed dosages of 200 mEq over a 15-day period, found no advantage or disadvantage with RbBr. A similar trial by Rottenbiller in 1889 again showed no untoward effects in 5 patients receiving up to 200 mEq (Rottenbiller, 1889).

Similarly, rubidium iodide was administered to syphilitics in place of KI. Leistikov (1893) employed a dosage schedule of 4 to 28 mEq/day for periods of up to 3 weeks. The RbI was as effective as KI in producing remission of symptoms. Side effects with RbI were all typical of KI therapy.

Other trials followed, none with any evidence of deleterious effects. From the reported literature it is certain that at least 60 patients received rubidium salts. The number is probably much higher since rubidium salts were sold in pharmacies throughout central Europe. Eventually more specific treatments were developed, and the use of the expensive rubidium salts was discontinued.

The initial experiments with rubidium salts were directed toward questions of its toxicity (Grandeau, 1864; Richet, 1882) and the extent of its physiological similarity to potassium (Ringer, 1882; Richet, 1882; Brunton and Cash, 1884; Harnack and Dietrich, 1885; Botkin, 1885). Richet's toxicity studies were particularly extensive, covering the effect of alkali salts on snails, crayfish, reptiles, amphibians, fish, birds, guinea pigs, and dogs. He observed that the dose size required to produce toxicity decreased when the site of injection facilitated rapid uptake by the blood stream.

Ringer (1882) suggested that rubidium and potassium had similar effects on the contractility of isolated frog heart. Brunton and Cash (1884) soon confirmed that the two ions caused an increase in strength and duration of muscle contraction. One year later the *in vivo* similarity of potassium and rubidium on dog heart was documented (Botkin, 1885).

Behavioral effects of rubidium salts were foreshadowed by Richet's toxicity studies (Richet, 1882) in which he concluded that, although acute intravenous injection of Li, K, or Rb produced a rapid cardiotoxic death, the much larger chronic subcutaneous injections required to produce death were preceded by presumed CNS effects such as "general weakening of the organism, staggering, hebetude, chill, weakening of motility and sensibility."

Mitchell *et al.* (1921) made specific mention of behavioral effects observed during the course of a study of the intracellular accumulation of RbCl by rats *in vivo*. They found that irritability, later followed by tetanic spasms and death, occurred when rats were fed a synthetic diet containing about 7 mEq Rb/kg/day. Twenty-two years later susceptibility by rats to audiogenic seizures were noted under similar conditions (Follis, 1943). Other incidental reports of irritability and convulsivity in rats soon followed (Pyke, 1956; Glendening *et al.*, 1956; Lambie *et al.*, 1959; Glasser and Ellis, 1961).

Hyperirritability was also reported by Sasser *et al.* (1969) as a consequence of feeding chicks with a Rb-containing diet.

The foregoing observations record behavioral effects that occurred incidental to other studies; the impetus to search for specific behavioral effects of rubidium arose after it was postulated (Meltzer *et al.*, 1969) that its biological actions were complementary to those of the known antimanic agent, lithium. Subsequently the effects on shock-elicited aggression (Stolk *et al.*, 1971; Eichelman *et al.*, 1973), amine-mediated excitement (Carroll and Sharp, 1971; Sanghvi and Gershon, 1973), and spontaneous motor activity (Yamauchi and Nakamura, 1972; Johnson, 1972) provided further support for the rationale of a clinical trial of rubidium in depression.

9. RECENT STUDIES

The major problem raised by chronic dosage of rubidium derives from its long biological half-life (50–70 days in humans), which makes it necessary to know the long-term effects. As a first approach to this problem rubidium chloride was added to the drinking water of rats, who were bred for three generations (Meltzer and Lieberman, 1971). Rubidium was present during conception, gestation, birth, weaning, and later development. Compared with controls, there were no effects on litter size, weight at weaning, or subsequent mortality. However, there was a slight tendency for mothers to attack their young. Plasma Rb levels ranged from 0.59 to 0.64 mEq/liter. A survey of the available literature supported the conclusion that the lack of toxicity in these experiments, compared to numerous previous reports of toxicity, was determined by the molar ingestion ratio of rubidium to potassium, which limited excessive tissue accumulation of rubidium.

We then conducted a subacute toxicity study in six beagle dogs, adding RbCl to foods to minimize gastric irritation and vomiting. The "low" dose level of 2 mEq/kg was administered to one male and one female dog. Additional levels of 4 and 8 mEq/kg were given to two other pairs of dogs. The 4 mEq/kg level could not be maintained beyond 24 days because of anorexia associated with other toxic effects of rubidium. The 8 mEq/kg level was administered for 5 days; subsequently it had to be reduced to 4 mEq/kg due to a period of anorexia.

Dogs receiving 2 mEq/kg tolerated the diet with some emesis, diarrhea, and very slight weight loss for 6 weeks. All four other dogs showed significant weight loss and died 26–35 days after initiating rubidium ingestion. For several days prior to death they had chronic convulsions. Three of these dogs also became very aggressive during the period in which convulsions were noted.

Except for some evidence of gastrointestinal irritation, no lesions were observed in any of the six dogs at necropsy. Electrocardiographic changes seen in the 4 and 8 mEq/kg groups included arrythmia and preventricular systoles. Plasma rubidium concentrations of 1.0 and 1.1 mEq/liter were attained in the two dogs receiving the 2 mEq/kg dose, and ranged from 1.6 to 2.4 in the others. For the two dogs with no serious toxicity, replacement of K by Rb (defined as Rb/Rb + K) in liver and muscle ranged from 22 to 33%, while for the four dogs on higher dose levels, replacement ranged from 43 to 53%.

We next studied the effect of lithium on rubidium toxicity in rats. In the first experiment, a group of four rats was given toxic doses of RbCl in the drinking water, and another group of four was given the same dose of Rb plus half as much LiCl. This group survived without evident toxicity until they were killed 3 months later; in contrast, rats in the group given only RbCl all died within 6 weeks. Analyses of tissues of two rats from each group showed that replacement in muscle and liver ranged from 26 to 32% in the surviving rats, while in those rats that died the replacement ranged from 44 to 51%. These results for dogs and rats, together with calculated replacement levels from the data of two other studies, one with rabbits (Bradbury, 1970) and an earlier study with rats (Relman et al., 1957), support the conclusion that serious toxicity is associated with a replacement of intracellular potassium by rubidium of 40–50%, while replacement levels of 30% or less are tolerated without evidence of toxicity.

The reduction of rubidium toxicity by lithium was explored further by giving rats free choice of rubidium or lithium drinking water. After a few days of seemingly random choice, they exhibited a large preference for rubidium in two such experiments with a total of 12 rats; the cumulative ingestion ratio of Rb/Li averaged 8. In these couples, as in those with a fixed ratio, Rb/Li intake alone was sufficient to produce severe toxicity. However, even at the low lithium intake level chosen, toxicity was absent or marginal (some loss of hair) with 11 rats. One rat died after 7 weeks.

10. ENDOGENOUS RUBIDIUM

Rubidium is ubiquitous in nature. Its content in the earth's crust is about one hundredth that of sodium and potassium. It occurs in particularly high concentration in some potassium-containing minerals, notably amazonite from Colorado and lepidolite from Massachusetts and southwest Africa, and also in carnallite salt deposits. In sea water its concentration ranges from 1.5 to 5 μEq/liter—about 1/2000 the concentration of potassium. The rubidium concentration in some mineral springs is ten times higher than its average sea-water concentration (Perelman, 1965).

Rubidium, like potassium, is concentrated intracellularly by most living tissue. It is found in all foods, and in particularly high concentration in soybeans and tomatoes (Glendening et al., 1956), sugar beets (LeFebvre and

Grandeau, 1862; Lippmann, 1888), coffee (Bertrand and Bertrand, 1954), and French wines (Bertrand and Bertrand, 1948). The average 70-kg man is estimated to contain 4.2 mEq of Rb (Yamagata, 1962)—about 1/800 of the potassium content. The possible use of Rb as a metabolic tracer of K would appear to be inconsistent with the known variability in total daily rubidium excretion (Burch *et al.*, 1955; Martin and Walker, 1958; Yamagata *et al.*, 1966). We have studied the excretion of naturally occurring (endogenous) Rb in hospitalized patients under careful metabolic controls (Meltzer *et al.*, 1973), and confirmed that the day-to-day variability cannot be reduced by controlling the daily Na and K ingestion. However, we did find that the daily excretion ratio, Rb/K, was relatively constant. Figure 3 shows data for a single patient over a 30-day period. Table 4 shows lists of ratios and standard deviations for 17 patients, demonstrating that Rb/K ratios range from 0.028 to 0.048 mEq of Rb per 100 mEq of K excreted daily in this group of unipolar and bipolar depressed patients. These ratios are consistent with those Rb/K ratios that we have calculated from two published studies of psychiatric normals. One, carried out in Utah (Wood, 1970), shows a mean ratio of 0.037 for 6 males and 0.036 for 6 females. The other, from France (Comar *et al.*, 1970), was an in-hospital longitudinal study of two females and one male, with mean ratios of 0.036, 0.034, and 0.036, respectively.

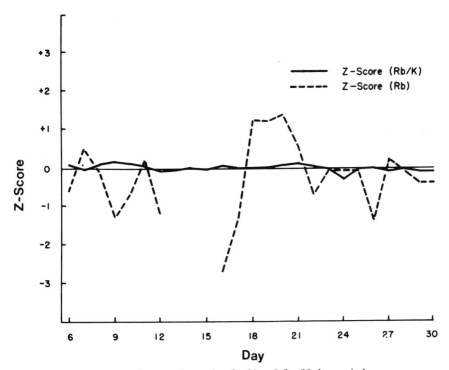

Fig. 3. Daily excretion ratio of subject 2 for 30-day period.

The conclusions implicit in this study were tested by experimentally manipulating the daily potassium ingestion level. These results demonstrate that endogenous Rb excretion is proportional to K excretion, and that at least from this point of view, Rb is a tracer of K metabolism. Endogenous Rb also accurately traces potassium distribution between plasma and cerebrospinal fluid (Dunner et al., 1974). Rb normally occurs in the CSF at about 70% of its concentration in plasma, and the same proportionate distribution occurs with potassium (Table 5).

We have also studied the distribution of endogenous Rb between blood plasma and erythrocytes. The analytical method (Lieberman and Meltzer, 1971) which is sufficiently sensitive to detect plasma levels yields data with considerable scatter; the mean plasma level was about 0.006 mEq/liter. Erythrocyte concentrations are about 30 times higher. Since the distribution ratio of K between erythrocytes and plasma seldom exceeds 25, it is evident that there is a relatively greater intracellular preference for endogenous Rb than for K, as has been found previously for rat tissues (Relman et al., 1957). Such selective accumulation is due either to selectivity of transport systems (Relman et al., 1957) or to intracellular binding (Menozzi et al., 1959). In either case, the selectivity mechanisms may also operate in the distal renal tubule cells, where Rb and K are exchanged for Na. Radioisotopes of Rb and K, simultaneously administered to dogs (Love et al., 1954), rabbits, and man

TABLE 4

Ratio of Naturally Occurring Rubidium to Potassium in Urine of
Hospitalized Patients

Subject No.	N^a	Mean (Rb/K) $\times$ 100	Standard deviation
1	22	0.028	0.0042
2	29	0.032	0.0036
3	23	0.031	0.0040
4	26	0.041	0.0101
5	33	0.028	0.0030
6	58	0.039	0.0049
7	15	0.042	0.0066
8	30	0.036	0.0042
9	22	0.037	0.0044
10	21	0.029	0.0028
11	23	0.048	0.0101
12	33	0.037	0.0045
13	21	0.037	0.0037
14	26	0.044	0.0039
15	27	0.039	0.0039
16	8	0.029	0.0023
17	62	0.038	0.0044

[a] N = number of days for which the mean ratio was computed.

TABLE 5

Endogenous Rubidium Concentration in CSF and Plasma[a]

Patient		CSF Rb	Plasma Rb	
Age	Sex	(mEq/liter)	(mEq/liter	Rb CSF/plasma
43	F	0.0020	0.0036	0.56
61	M	0.0029	0.0037	0.78
31	F	0.0016	0.0028	0.57
54	F	0.0023	0.0027	0.85
31	F	0.0034	0.0027	1.26
61	F	0.0015	0.0025	0.60
42	M	0.0014	0.0017	0.82
35	M	0.0028	0.0035	0.80
52	F	0.0016	0.0028	0.57
49	F	0.0017	0.0032	0.53
52	M	0.0005	0.0017	0.29
Mean ± SEM		0.0020 ± 0.0002	0.0028 ± 0.0002	0.69

[a] For the difference between CSF and plasma rubidium $t = 4.23$, $P < 0.01$, paired t test. The mean ratio Rb CSF/K Plasma for these patients was 1.01.

(Kilpatrick et al., 1956), distribute between urine and plasma such that the data can be summarized by the equation:

$$(Rb/K) \text{ urine} = S \times (Rb/K) \text{ plasma}$$

where the value of S, ranging from 0.6 to 0.8, indicates the selective preference of renal tubule cells for Rb with respect to K.

The long biological half-life of ingested Rb (50–70 days) (Iinuma et al., 1967; Fieve et al., 1973) implies an average daily excretion of about 1% of the total body load. An adult patient whose diet is sufficiently varied would be expected to excrete a quantity of Rb equal to the mean daily intake. It is important to recognize that the excretion of this "endogenous" Rb is not the same, molecule for molecule, as the Rb ingested each day. Only 2–3% of any newly ingested quantity is excreted during the next 24 hr (Fieve et al., 1971; Tyor and Eldridge, 1956), the remainder having been accumulated intracellularly. The bulk of the daily Rb excretion, therefore, arises from amounts previously stored in the body, principally in intracellular sites. These considerations are important for the interpretation of the metabolism of loading doses of Rb administered during the test for therapeutic potential.

11. CHRONIC ADMINISTRATION

Initially, before including chronic dosage of depressed patients, it was necessary to determine the rate of appearance of Rb in erythrocytes, plasma,

TABLE 6

Acute Administration to Four Subjects

Subject	Dose (mmol)	Peak plasma rubidium		Peak urine rubidium[a]		Ratio RBC/plasma rubidium		Half life (days)[a]
		(mmol/liter)	Time from dose (min)	(mmol/liter)	Time from dose (min)	At peak	24 hr	
H.L.M.	4.1	0.007	60			3[b]	c	55
	4.1	0.015	70	0.27	250			
M.H.	6.2	0.018	60			3.5	20	49
	6.2	0.024	90	0.17	450			
E.T.	8.2	0.041	45	0.09	200	2.5	19	21
A.B.	8.2	0.017	95	0.14	160	4.5	20	21

[a] Samples collected at 2 hr intervals.
[b] Approximate.
[c] Samples lost.
[d] Calculated from urinary excretion during the period 13–24 hr after rubidium administration.

TABLE 7

Increase in Intracellular Rubidium with Time

Time	RBC: Plasma Rb ratio
45 min	2.5
60 min	3.5
90 min	4.5
24 hr	20
3 days	30
10 days[a]	28–32[b]

[a] After ending a course of chronic dosage.
[b] Figures given are the range for all patients.

and urine after a small loading dose. Table 6 shows the results of acute administration to two normal volunteers and two hospitalized patients. The values for the 24-hr erythrocyte–plasma ratios are considerably removed from steady-state values (Table 7). The biological half-life, measured for the period 13–24 hr, was much longer for the normal subjects than for the two patients. This observation needs to be explored with larger numbers of volunteer subjects. The cautious nature of the first chronic trial is illustrated in Fig. 4, which is the longitudinal record of Rb administration. Total administered dose was raised to 45 mEq during the first 15 days, and then held constant for 3 weeks. The dose was then raised stepwise to a total of 268 mEq administered, and no more than 185 mEq retained. The estimation of

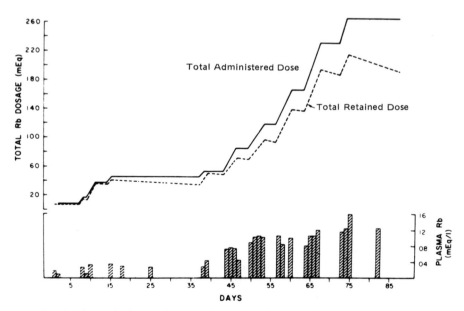

FIG. 4. Rb metabolism during chronic loading of rapid-cycling manic-depressive.

retained dose is based entirely on urinary excretion and is, therefore, overstated to a degree that varies in magnitude with excretion through extrarenal routes.

Another important calculation, bearing on safety, is the estimation of plasma Rb concentration resulting from any dose. To do this we assume that: the plasma Rb concentration is equal to total extracellular fluid concentration; the erythrocyte Rb concentration is always equal to the mean intracellular concentration of all body tissues; the retained dose is well represented by the difference between total administered dose and total urinary excretion (Meltzer, 1974). The first assumption is supported by ^{86}Rb data (Zipsen et al., 1953), from which it can be estimated that the half-time for equilibration of intravenously administered ^{86}Rb$_2$CO$_3$ between plasma and extracellular space is 3 min. The second assumption is verified by the successful application of the calculations outlined below. The third assumption, to the extent that it gives a falsely high value, results in calculated plasma levels that are erroneously high, in effect adding a safety factor to the dosage schedule.

After any given dose, Rb retained in the body will be distributed between intra- and extracellular space according to the equation:

$$\text{Rb retained} = ([\text{Rb}]_{\text{ECS}} \times V_{\text{ECS}}) = ([\text{Rb}]_{\text{ICS}} \times V_{\text{ICS}}) \tag{1}$$

where the expressions in brackets refer to concentrations. If the measurements are made after a steady state has been attained, the distribution of Rb between ICS and ECS will be constant:

$$[\text{Rb}]_{\text{ICS}}/[\text{Rb}]_{\text{ECS}} = D \tag{2}$$

Substituting in the previous equation and rearranging terms,

$$[\text{Rb}]_{\text{ECS}} = \text{Rb retained}/[V_{\text{ECS}} + (D \times V_{\text{ICS}})] \tag{3}$$

Several options are open at this point. First, V_{ECS} may be approximated as 20% of body weight, and V_{ICS} as 50% of body weight (Gamble, 1942). The value of D may be taken as 30, the mean value for the erythrocyte/plasma Rb ratio obtained at steady-state conditions. Then,

$$[\text{Rb}]_{\text{ECS}} = \text{Rb retained}/15.2 \times W_{\text{B}}$$

where W_{B} is the body weight in kilograms (Meltzer and Fieve, 1974).

Second, equation (3) may be used at non-steady-state conditions, if the distribution ratio, D, is measured at the time of sampling the blood. Third, equation (3) may be modified:

$$[\text{Rb}]_{\text{ECW}} = \text{Rb retained}/[V_{\text{ECW}} + (DW \times V_{\text{ICW}})] \tag{4}$$

where V_{ECW} and V_{ICW} represent volumes of extracellular water, and may be estimated by reference to published tables (Moore et al., 1963). DW then represents the distribution ratio between the water contained in intra- and extracellular space and may be approximated at 42 by multiplying the steady-state erythrocyte–plasma distribution by an appropriate correction factor for erythrocyte and plasma water.

Chronic administration of rubidium is known to displace exchangeable potassium (Relman *et al.*, 1957). We have estimated exchange of K for Rb by measuring erythrocyte Rb and K and also by measuring total body potassium by the method of whole-body counting of the naturally occurring radioactive ^{40}K. To date, replacement levels estimated by either method have not exceeded 12%. Figure 5 illustrates the course of potassium loss and regain for a single patient.

Displacement of intracellular K might possibly involve other metabolic disturbances. To examine this possibility we have obtained repeated SMA-12, SMA-6, CBC, and urinalyses for patients given Rb chronically. The data for four patients (Table 8) shows that chronic Rb administration is not accompanied by any consistent change (Fieve *et al.*, 1973).

Chronic administration of rubidium to patients maintained on metabolic balance has allowed us to study the biological half-life in detail. Two major points emerge. First, the daily excretion ratio of Rb to K is more constant than is total rubidium excretions (see above for endogenous Rb). Second, there are two components to the half-life. The early component, occurring during the day following a single dose, is characterized by excretion of 2–3% of the dose for most patients. The corresponding half-life is about 20–30 days. Thus, patient L.H. (Fig. 6) excreted 2.8% of the dose on the day following the initial dose, and 0.7–0.8% for the next 2 days. However, during 4 days of successive doses the excretion of the retained dose rose to 1.8–2.0%, only to fall again to 1.2% during the following dose-free days. Eventually, as the accumulated retained dose became significantly greater

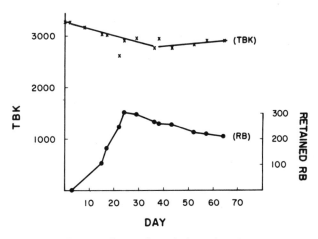

Fig. 5. K loss and regain in patient B.K.

TABLE 8
Plasma Enzymes During Chronic Rb Loading

Patient	Enzyme	Before	During	After
G.K.	Alkaline phosphatase	89	74	65
G.S.		88	80	88
L.H.		80	61	47
G.K.	Lactic acid dehydrogenase	129	132	165
G.S.		101	139	146
L.H.		182	163	156
G.K.	Serum glutamate oxaloacetic	27	20	19
G.S.	transaminase	29	15	19
L.H.		35	31	37

[a] Alkaline phosphatase.
[b] Lactic acid dehydroxyle.
[c] Serum glutamate oxaloacetic transaminase.

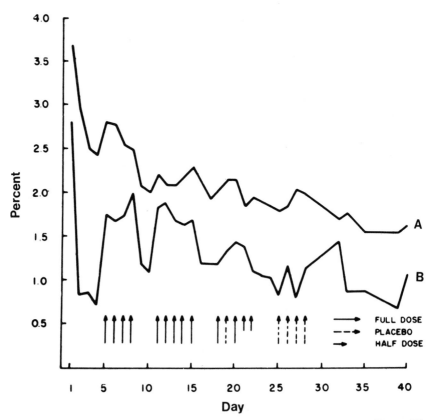

FIG. 6. Daily excretion as percent of remaining dose of Rb. (A) Percent E/K_{urine}; (B) percent E.

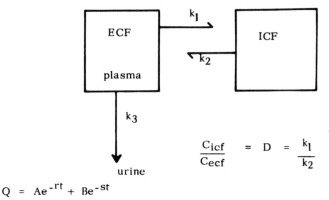

$$\frac{C_{icf}}{C_{ecf}} = D = \frac{k_1}{k_2}$$

$$Q = Ae^{-rt} + Be^{-st}$$

Fig. 7. Second component half-life as illustrated by two-compartment model. k_1, k_2, and k_3, rate constants; C, concentration; icf, intracellular fluid; ecf, extracellular fluid; Q, quantity (total); A and B, empirical constants

than any single daily dose, the excretion leveled off at about 1.2% of the retained dose, corresponding to the half-life of about 50 days.

The second component half-life is most likely accounted for by the two-compartment model shown in Fig. 7. Rb absorbed from the gut into the blood plasma is slowly incorporated intracellularly; attainment of a steady state may take 3 days. Thus during the first 12–24 hr a significant portion of the administered dose is available for urinary excretion.

At the end of this period of chronic dosage, there is a decline of retained rubidium which may be followed by a decrease in urinary Rb/K ratios and by a decrease in Rb concentration in CSF, erythrocytes, and plasma as well. The results (Dunner *et al.*, 1974) are illustrated for one patient in Fig. 8 and summarized in Table 9. Since the biological half-life of Rb, determined from decrements in either erythrocyte or plasma concentration, is similar to the half-life determined from the CSF, it appears likely that assessment of Rb in

TABLE 9

Biological Half-Life of Rubidium after Rubidium Loading[a]

Patient		Biological half-life (days)		
Age	Sex	CSF	Plasma	Erythrocytes
45	M	54.6	55.5	59.5
52	F	49.0	41.2	43.3
35	M	56.5	52.9	51.3
49	F	45.6	32.6	28.2
52	F	44.4	42.2	36.2
Mean ± SEM		50.0 ± 2.4	44.9 ± 4.2	42.7 ± 5.3

[a] 8 to 22 blood samples from each patient were analyzed over time periods ranging from 44 to 238 days. CSF data were computed for 2 LPs in each of 2 patients and 4 LPs in each of 3 patients.

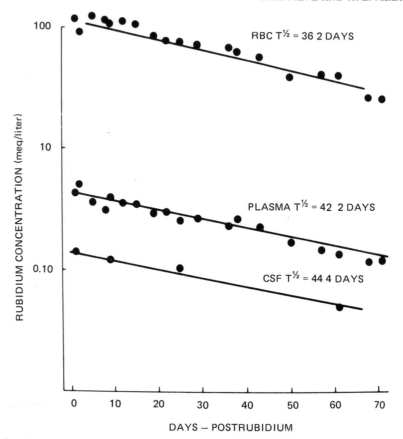

FIG. 8. Decline retained Rb and decrease urinary Rb/K ratios in patient B.S. (age 52).

the periphery reflects CNS Rb metabolism. This is an important consideration from the viewpoint of patient safety during clinical trials.

All of the metabolic studies support the conclusion that Rb metabolism
after chronic loading is not different from endogenous Rb metabolism, even
though body levels are increased 70-fold. This statement is true for distribution between intra- and extracellular space, distribution between CSF and
plasma (see below), and magnitude of biological half-life, whether measured
by percent excretion; decline in CSF, erythrocyte, or plasma level; or decline
in urinary Rb/K.

We have recently summarized our experience with chronic administration of Rb to 15 affectively ill patients (Fieve and Meltzer, 1974). Figures 9
through 13 illustrate mood and dosage data for 5 patients.

Patient B.K. is illustrated in Fig. 9 which shows that a total of about 325
mEq of rubidium were retained by 30 days and that the rubidium plasma
level reached a maximum of about 0.33 mEq/liter during the 20-day loading
period. If one follows the mood scores, it is apparent that there was no
substantial change in the slope of the curve. A mathematical analysis also

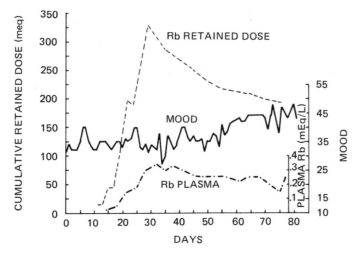

FIG. 9. Mood and dosage: patient B.K.

indicates that the slope of the dose–mood curve is not significantly different from zero.

Figure 10 illustrates in patient F.F. that 486 mEq of rubidium were retained by the 29th day and that the blood level achieved a maximum of 0.38 mEq/liter of rubidium over a 20-day period. Again, there was no appreciable statistically significant association between dose and mood score. This patient was a bipolar manic-depressive, whereas the patient in Fig. 9 was a unipolar patient.

Figure 11 for patient D.M. shows that 364 mEq of rubidium were retained in this bipolar II patient and that a maximum of 0.29 mEq/liter

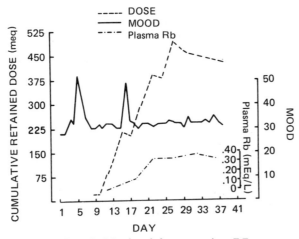

FIG. 10. Mood and dosage: patient F.F.

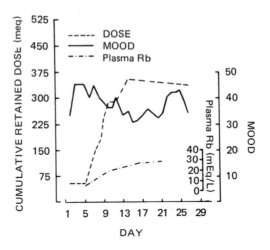

FIG. 11. Mood and dosage: patient D.M.

were reached in the blood. This was achieved over a short dose period of 13 days. If anything, there was correlation of decreasing mood with increasing rubidium dosage in this latter case.

Figure 12 for patient F.G. shows a unipolar patient who retained a total of 381 mEq of rubidium, achieving a maximum rubidium dose of 0.39 mEq/liter in plasma. There was a marked increase in the mood over the period of time that rubidium was administered, and there was a statistically significant correlation between the improvement in the mood score and the increasing dosage of rubidium.

Figure 13 for patient H.P. illustrates a total of 440 mEq retained in a bipolar II patient with an achievement of 0.40 mEq/liter of rubidium in

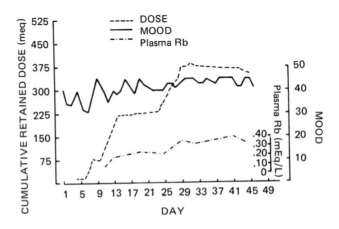

FIG. 12. Mood and dosage: patient F.G.

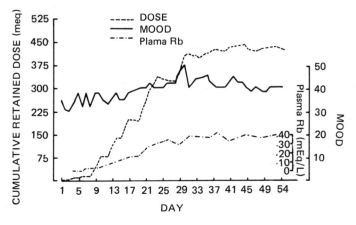

Fig. 13. Mood and dosage: patient H.P.

plasma. There is a marked increase in mood score in this patient as well and a statistically significant association between the improvement in mood score and the increasing dosage of rubidium. Table 10 lists the dosage and overall response, as evaluated by computer analysis of daily global mood scores.

Because safety considerations were always paramount, we began this series with low doses of Rb and have gradually increased the maximum retained dose. Table 10 is a retabulation of the mood response data with respect to maximum retained dose and maximum plasma level. Excluding

TABLE 10

Clinical Responses to Chronic Rubidium Administration

	Mood change			
	Decrease	No change	Slight change	Marked increase
A. By maximum retained dose				
140–200		4		
220–250		2		2
310–330		1	1	1
360–380	1	1	1	2
440–490	1	1		1
B. By peak plasma Rb				
0.12–0.17		4		1
0.28–0.30	2	1	1	2
0.33–0.39		4		2
0.40–0.43			1	1
Summary	2	9	2	6

the initial patient, a rapid cycler whose response was difficult to evaluate, 9 of
the 18 subjects showed no change in mood during chronic administration of
Rb, 2 showed a decline in mood, while there were marked improvements in
mood in 6 subjects and detectable increments in 2 others. Our data are,
therefore, equivocal: there is no firm basis for concluding that an antidepressant effect exists; on the other hand, we have not proved in this small sample
that Rb is totally without effect. Recently, however, there has been a
comparative study of rubidium and Tofranil in a group of 30 depressed
patients. The authors reported that rubidium was more specific than
Tofranil for treatment of retardation and other case symptoms of depression, and, in contrast to Tofranil, produced no side effects.

12. RUBIDIUM–LITHIUM INTERACTIONS

The ability of lithium to limit the intracellular displacement of K by Rb,
observed in rats (see above), is apparent also in studies of human Rb
metabolism in endogenous as well as chronically loaded subjects.

Lithium dosage has a turn-on, turn-off effect on the urinary Rb/K ratio
for naturally occurring Rb (Fig. 14). Ingestion of lithium promptly increases
the urinary Rb/K ratio above the stable pre-Li level. Cessation of Li dosage
leads within 1–2 days to a return to the baseline level (Table 11). The same
result was obtained when Li was given to patients who had received multiple
doses of Rb. In this case, however, the data are presented in a different
form. When Rb administration is discontinued, body Rb stores are slowly
depleted. The ratio of Rb to K in the urine therefore declines in direct
relation to the biological half-life of Rb. If the data are plotted semiloga-

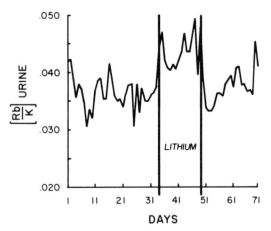

FIG. 14. Effect of lithium on urinary Rb/K.

TABLE 11
Effect of Lithium on Urinary Rb/K

Li dose	(Rb/K) × 100						x_1–x_2 significant at P less than:
	N	Mean (x_1)	SD	N	x_2	SD	
0.3–1.2	5	0.0309	0.0012	5	0.0370	0.0058	0.025
1.8	5	0.0360	0.0010	5	0.0432	0.0028	0.005
1.8	5	0.0359	0.0043	5	0.0400	0.0038	0.1
0.9	5	0.0343	0.0015	3	0.0410	0.0043	0.025
0.6	5	0.0316	0.0011	5	0.0341	0.0014	0.1
0.9		0.0316		2	0.0365	0.0007	0.005
1.2		0.0316		5	0.0387	0.0020	0.0005
0.6	5	1.82	0.14	7	1.97	0.24	0.025
0.9		1.82		7	2.16	0.09	0.005

rithmically, a straight line may be fitted to the data points. Extrapolation of the line indicates the expected Rb/K ratio at some future time. Figure 15 shows such a plot, whose data points, obtained when Li was administered, are well above the predicted line.

The urinary Rb/K ratio is increased by 15–20% and is due entirely to an increase in Rb excretion, without any significant change in K excretion. It has already been noted that the different ratios of plasma and urinary $^{42}K/^{86}Rb$ indicate a relative preference of renal tubule cells for Rb with respect to K. The average body intracellular preference for Rb over K is at least 20%. Thus the magnitude of the Li effect on urinary Rb/K strongly implies that Li

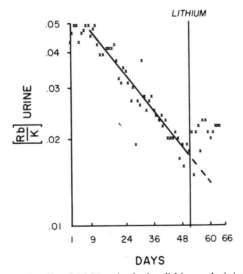

FIG. 15. Predicted Rb/K ratio during lithium administration.

has markedly reduced the difference between Rb and K. The same interpretation applies to the decreased Rb replacement of K in rats given Li. Similarly, the ratio of Rb/K in erythrocytes divided by the plasma Rb/K, which has been found to be about 1.15–1.2 after chronic Rb dosage, is reduced to 1.0–1.05 when Li is administered.

It would seem that the ability of Li to reduce selective Rb accumulation, already demonstrated inferentially for human renal tubule cells and directly for human erythrocytes and rat muscle and liver cells, is a widespread phenomenon. The possibility that the site of action may be at the cell membrane, where an ATPase "pump" is responsible for Na extrusion and Rb and K accumulation, is central to the hypothesis that will now be discussed.

13. A MEMBRANE TRANSPORT HYPOTHESIS

It is clear that both Li and Rb have behavioral and neurophysiological effects which may be designated as "opposite." Lithium interferes with the binding of both sodium and potassium to extracts of neuronal membranes; rubidium acts only on sodium binding (Meltzer et al., 1969). Lithium diverts catecholamine metabolism toward the deamination pathway (Colburn et al., 1967); rubidium enhances the O-methylation pathway (Stolk et al., 1970). Lithium increases, and rubidium decreases, the activity of ATPase (Tobin et al., 1974). Lithium decreases, and rubidium increases, the spontaneous motor activity of mice (Yamauchi and Nakamura, 1972). Lithium antagonizes, and rubidium potentiates, morphine-induced activation in mice (Carroll and Sharp, 1971). Lithium reduces (Sheard, 1970), and rubidium augments, shock-elicited aggression in rats (Stolk et al., 1971; Eichelman et al., 1973). Lithium reduces (Platman and Fieve, 1969), and rubidium increases (see below), the level of activation of the human electroencephalogram. Rb produces susceptibility to audiogenic seizures in normal rats (Alexander and Meltzer, 1975). Whether or not Rb is finally found to have antidepressant activity, the presently known contrasting activities of these simple ions remains to be explained. To date there is no satisfactory explanation for any of the known actions of lithium. It seems most reasonable to search for a common locus on which Li and Rb will have "opposite" actions.

We have hypothesized (Meltzer and Fieve, 1973) that the principal effect of these ions is on the shape of the neuronal action potential. Li allies the normal intracellular accumulation of Rb, perhaps by altering membrane selectivity (see above). Since Rb is qualitatively similar to K and passes through the same membrane channels, at least in erythrocytes (Solomon, 1952), there is a strong implication that the Li effect on Rb accumulation reflects a similar effect on K transport across membranes. The postulated Li–K interaction in the CNS may vary in extent at different intracellular sites since the distribution of Rb is different from that of K in various subcellular fractions of rat brain (Lieberman and Meltzer, 1971). While we might profitably investigate the effects of Li on synaptosomal mitochondria, or nuclear membranes of the neuron, the membrane of immediate interest would seem to be the axonal membrane, for it is here that the nerve action potential is generated. The action potential is accompanied by two changes in state of the membrane. There is first an increased inward rate of flow of Na, associated with the rising phase of the action potential, and then an increased outward rate of flow of K, associated with the somewhat slower falling phase. This is illustrated in the upper diagram of Fig. 16. If Rb is present intracellularly and moves through the same membrane channels as does K, as is known to be true for erythrocyte membranes (Solomon, 1952), then the slower movement of Rb will result in a delayed fall of the action potential (second diagram of Fig. 15). Prolonged action potentials have indeed been observed in the presence of Rb (Muller, 1963). If we now consider the case where Li is present intracellularly, and if we assume that Li acts on neuronal K as it does on Rb in other cells, then the increased rate of outward K movement will result in an abbreviated action potential (bottom diagram of Fig. 15).

We would hypothesize, then, that Li acts neurophysiologically and

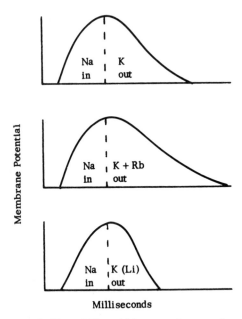

FIG. 16. Proposed effect of Rb and Li on membrane action potentials.

therapeutically by abbreviating the normal neuronal action potential in the CNS and that Rb acts neurophysiologically by extending the action potential.

If this is the principal mode of action of these ions, then what are we to make of the demonstrated (Eichelman *et al.*, 1973; Stolk *et al.*, 1970) effects of both Rb and Li on amine-transmitter metabolism? Regulation of synaptic levels of the amine transmitters is known to depend upon a number of factors, including synthesis, storage, and catabolism. All of these constitute, in effect, a chemostat which can provide a relatively constant supply of specialized molecules. This supply is drawn upon each time a neuronal impulse arrives in the synaptic region. It is reestablished in part by reuptake from the synaptic cleft of those molecules that have not been catabolized after release. Re-uptake and catabolism both serve to clear the synaptic cleft so that the arrival of a new impulse will lead to a discrete event. Thus the arriving neuronal impulse is an important factor in regulating transmitter levels and metabolic pathways.

We would, therefore, tentatively enlarge our hypothesis by suggesting that action potentials of greater or lesser duration produce greater or lesser release of transmitter into the synapses with the consequence that alteration in transmitter metabolism would be a secondary effect of the primary action of Rb or Li on the neuronal action potential. Finally, if all the preceding assumptions are accepted, it is reasonable to suggest that the information content of an action potential is altered by the presence of Rb or Li and that ultimately such informational changes ought to be reflected by changes in brain function, which in turn would result in alteration of behavioral states such as mania or depression. Thus, if Li and Rb restore normal function, they may do so by correcting a primary defect at the level of the axonal membrane.

14. REFERENCES

ALEXANDER, G. L., and MELTZER, H. L., 1975, Onset of audiogenic seizures in rodents after uptake of near-toxic doses of rubidium chloride, *J. Pharm. Exp. Ther.* **194**(3):480–487.

ANGST, J., 1966, Zur Atiologie und Nosologie endogener depressiver psychosen, *Monogr. Neurol. Psychiatr.* **112**:1.

ANGST, J., WEISS, P., GROF, P., BAASTRUP, P. C., and SCHOU, M., 1970, Lithium prophylaxis in recurrent affective disorders, *Br. J. Psychiatry* **116**:604–14.

BAASTRUP, P. C., 1964, The use of lithium in manic depressive psychosis. *Comp. Psychiatry* **5**:396–408.

BAASTRUP, P. C., and SCHOU, M., 1967, Lithium as a prophylactic agent: Its effects against recurrent depressions and manic-depressive psychosis, *Arch. Gen. Psychiatry* **16**:162–177.

BAASTRUP, P. C., POULSEN, J. C., SCHOU, M., THOMSEN, K., and AMDISEN, A., 1970, Prophylactic lithium: Double-blind discontinuation in manic depressive and recurrent depressive disorders, *Lancet* **2**:326–329.

BERKSON, J., GAGE, R. P., 1950, Calculations of survival rates for cancer, *Proc. Staff Meetings Mayo Clin.* **25**:270–286.

BERTRAND, G., and BERTRAND, D., 1948, The rubidium content of wines, *Ann. Agron.* **19**:887.

BERTRAND, G., and BERTRAND, D., 1954, The rubidium content of coffee, *C. R. Acad. Sci.* **238:**1684–1685.

BLACKWELL, B., and SHEPHERD, M., 1968, Prophylactic lithium: Another therapeutic myth? *Lancet* **1:**968–971.

BOTKIN, S., JR., 1885, Zurfrage über den Zusammenhaug der physiologische wirkung mit den chemischen Eigenschaften der alkali-metale der ersten gruppe nach mendeleyeff, Contralblatt fur die Medianische Wissenschaften **48:**849–852.

BOTKIN, S., 1888, The influence of the salts of rubidium and cesium upon the heart and circulation in connection with the laws of physiological action of alkali metals, St. Petersburg Military Academy doctoral dissertation. 41 pp.

BRADBURY, M. W. B., 1970, The effect of rubidium on the distribution and movement of potassium between blood, brain, and cerebrospinal fluid in the rabbit, *Brain Res.* **24:**311.

BRUNTON, T. L., and CASH, J. T., 1884, Contributions to our knowledge of the connection between chemical constitution, physiological action, and antagonism, *Phil. Trans. R. Soc. (London),* **1884:**174–224.

BURCH, G. E., THREEFOOT, S. A., and RAY, C. I., 1955, The rate of disappearance of rubidium-86 from the plasma: The biological decay rates of rubidium-86 and the applicability of rubidium-86, *J. Lab. Clin. Med.* **45:**371–395.

CAROLEI, A., SONSINI, U., CASACCHIA, M., AGNOL, A., and FAZIO, C., 1975, Azione farmziologia del cloruvo di rubidio: Effetto antidepressivo confronto con l'imipramino *La Clinica Terapeutica* **75:**469–478.

CARROLL, B. J., and SHARP, P. T., 1971, Rubidium and lithium: Opposite effects on amine-mediated excitement, *Science* **172:**1355.

COLBURN, R., GOODWIN, F., and BUNNEY, W. E., JR., 1967, Effect of lithium on the uptake of nonadrenaline by synaptosomes, *Nature* **215:**1395.

COMAR, D., LOC'H, C., RIVIERE, R., and KELLERSHOHN, C., 1970, The use of radio activation analysis and whole body counting in the study of Rb metabolism, *Strahlentherapie Sonderb.* **9:**245–252.

COPPEN, A., NOGUERA, R., BAILEY, J., BURNS, B. H., SWANI, M. S., HARE, E. H., GARDNER, R., and MAGGS, R., 1971, Prophylactic lithium in affective disorders: Controlled trial, *Lancet* **2:**275–279.

COPPEN, A., PEET, M., BAILEY, J., NOGUERA, R., BURNS, B. H., SWANI, M. S., MAGGS, R., and GARDNER, R., 1973*a*, Double-blind and open prospective studies of lithium prophylaxis in affective disorders. *Psychiatr. Neurol. Neurochir. (Amsterdam)* **76:**501–510.

COPPEN, A., PEET, M., and BAILEY, J., 1973*b*, The effect of long-term lithium treatment on the morbidity of affective disorders. Medical Research Council Neuropsychiatry Unit, Epsom, Surrey, England.

CUNDALL, R. L., BROOKS, P. N., and MURRAY, L. G., 1972, Controlled evaluation of lithium prophylaxis in affective disorders, *Psychol. Med.* **3:**308–311.

DUNNER, D. L., and FIEVE, R. R., 1974, Clinical factors in lithium carbonate prophylaxis failure, *Arch. Gen. Psychiatry* **30:**229–233.

DUNNER, D. L., GERSHON, E. S., and GOODWIN, F. K., 1970, Heritable factors in the severity of affective illness, *Sci. Proc. Am. Psychiatr. Assoc.* **123:**187.

DUNNER, D. L., MELTZER, H. L., and FIEVE, R. R., 1974, Cerebrospinal fluid rubidium metabolism in depression, *Psychopharm. (Berlin)* **37:**7–13.

DUNNER, D. L., STALLONE, F., FIEVE, R. R., 1976*a*, Lithium carbonate and affective disorders V. A Double-blind study of prophylaxis in affective illness, *Arch. Gen. Psychiatry* **33:**117–120.

DUNNER, D. L., PATRICK, V., and FIEVE, R. R., 1976*b*, Rapid-cycling manic-depressive patients. To be presented at Annual Meeting of American Psychiatric Association, Miami, Florida.

DUNNER, D. L., FLEISS, J. L., and FIEVE, R. R., 1976*c*, Lithium carbonate prophylaxis failure, *Br. J. Psychiatry* **129:**40–44.

EICHELMAN, B., THOA, N. B., and PEREZ-CRUET, J., 1973, Rubidium and cesium: Effects on aggression, adrenal enzymes and amine turnover, *J. Pharmacol. Biochem. Behav.* **1:**121–123.

FIEVE, R. R., 1970, Lithium in psychiatry, *Int. J. Psychiatry* **9:**375–412.

FIEVE, R. R., 1973, Overview of therapeutic and prophylactic trials of lithium in psychiatric patients, in: *Lithium: Its Role in Psychiatric Research and Treatment* (S. Gershon and B. Shopsin, eds.), New York, Plenum Press, New York.

FIEVE, R. R., and MENDLEWICZ, J., 1972, Lithium prophylaxis in bipolar manic-depressive illness (abstract), *Psychopharmacologia* **26**(Suppl.):93.

FIEVE, R. R., and MELTZER, H. L., 1974, Proceedings: Rubidium salts—toxic effects in humans and effects as an antidepressant drug, *Psychopharm. Bull.* **10:**38–50.

FIEVE, R. R., PLATMAN, S. R., and PLUTCHIK, R. R., 1968, The use of lithium in affective disorders, II: Prophylaxis of depression in chronic recurrent affective disorder, *Am. J. Psychiatry* **125:**492–498.

FIEVE, R. R., MELTZER, H. L., and TAYLOR, R. M., 1971, Rubidium chloride ingestion by volunteer subjects: Initial experience, *Psychopharmacologie* **20:**307–314.

FIEVE, R. R., MELTZER, H. L., DUNNER, D. L., LEVITT, M., MENDLEWICZ, J., and THOMAS, A., 1973, Rubidium: biochemical, behavioral, and metabolic studies in humans, *Am. J. Psychiatry* **130:**155.

FIEVE, R. R., KUMBARACHI, T., and DUNNER, D. L., 1976, Lithium prophylaxis of three depressive subtypes, *Am. J. Psychiatry* (in press).

FLEISS, J., DUNNER, D. L., STALLONE, F., and FIEVE, R. R., 1976, The life table: A method for analyzing longitudinal studies, *Arch. Gen. Psychiatry* **33:**107–112.

FOLLIS, R. H., 1943, Histological effects in rats resulting from adding rubidium or cesium to a diet deficient in potassium, *Am. J. Psychol.* **138:**246.

GAMBLE, J. L., 1942, *Chemical Anatomy, Physiology, and Pathology of Extracellular Fluid,* Harvard Univ. Press, Cambridge.

GLASSER, L., and ELLIS, J. T., 1961, The effects of rubidium on the adrenal cortex of normal and potassium deficient rats, *Am. J. Pathol.* **38:**103.

GLENDENING, B. L., SCHRENK, W. G., and PARRISH, D. B., 1956, Effects of rubidium in purified diets fed rats, *J. Nutr.* **60:**563.

GRANDEAU, L., 1864, Experiments on the physiological action of the salts of potassium, sodium and rubidium injected into veins, *J. Anat. Physiol.* **1:**378.

GROF, P., SCHOU, M., ANGST, J., BAASTRUP, P. C., and WEIS, P., 1970, Methodological problems of prophylactic trials in recurrent affective disorders, *Br. J. Psychiatry* **116:**599.

HARNACK, E., and DIETRICH, E., 1885, The effects of rubidium and cesium chlorides on the diagonally striped muscle of the frog. *Arch. Exp. Pathol. Pharm.* **19:**153.

HARTIGAN, G. P., 1963, The use of lithium salts in affective disorders, *Br. J. Psychiatry* **109:**810.

HULLIN, R. P., McDONALD, P., and ALLSOP, M. N. E., 1972, Prophylactic lithium in recurrent affective disorders, *Lancet* **1:**1044–1046.

IINUMA, T., WATARE, K., NAGAI, T., IWASHIMA, K., and YAMAGATA, N., 1967, Comparative studies of Cs^{132} and Rb^{86} turnover in man using a double tracer method, *J. Radiat. Res. (Tokyo)* **8:**100.

JOHNSON, F. N., 1972, Effects of alkali metal chlorides on activity in rats, *Nature* **238:**333.

KILPATRICK, R., MITTER, H., MUNRO, D. S., RENSCHLER, H., and WILSON, G. M., 1956, Comparison of the distribution of K^{42} and Rb^{86} in rabbit and man, *J. Physiol. (London)* **133:**194–200.

KLERMAN, G. L., DiMASCIO, A., WEISSMAN, M., PRUSOFF, B., and PARKER, E., 1974, Treatment of depression by drugs and psychotherapy, *Am. J. Psychiatry* **131:**186–191.

KRAMER, M., 1969, Applications of Mental Health Statistics. World Health Organization, Geneva.

LAMBIE, A. T., RELMAN, A. S., and SCHWARTZ, W. B., 1959, Electrolyte and acid–base balance during acute loading with rubidium chloride, *J. Clin. Invest.* **38:**1538–1543.

LAUFENAUER, K., 1889, On the therapeutic action of rubidium ammonium bromide. *C. R. Int. Med. Ment.* **109:**183–192.

LAURELL, B., and OTTOSON, I. O., 1968, Prophylactic lithium? *Lancet* **2**:1245.

LEFEBVRE, D., and GRANDEAU, L., 1862, Rubidium content in sugar beet, *Comptes Rendus* **55**:430.

LEISTIKOV, L., 1893, Rubidium iodide, *Monat. prak. Dermatol.* **17**:509.

LEONHARD, K., KORFF, I., and SCHULZ, H., 1962, Die Temperamente in den Familien der monopolaren und bipolaren phasischen Psychosen, *Psychiatr. Neurol.* **143**:416.

LEW, A., and SELTZER, F., 1970, Uses of the life table in public health, *Milbank Mem. Fund Q.* **48**:15–37.

LIEBERMAN, K. W., and MELTZER, H. L., 1971, Determination of rubidium in biological materials by atomic absorption spectrophotometry, *Anal. Lett.* **4**:547.

LIPPMAN, E. O., 1888, Uber einige seftenere Bestandtheile der Rübenosche, *Ber. Dtsch. Ges. (Berlin)* **21**:3492–3493.

LOVE, W. D., ROMNEY, R. B., and BURCH, G. E., 1954, A comparison of the distribution of potassium and exchangeable rubidium in the organs of dogs using rubidium-86, *Circ. Res.* **2**:112–122.

MARTIN, M. M., and WALKER, G., 1958, Rubidium-86 as a tracer of potassium in man, *Nature* **181**:705–706.

MAY, P. R. A., YALE, C., and DIXON, W. J., 1972a, Assessment of psychiatric outcome I: Cross section analysis, *J. Psychiatr. Res.* **9**:271–284.

MAY, P. R. A., POTEPAN, P., and YALE, C., 1972b, Assessment of psychiatric outcome II: Simple Simon analysis, *J. Psychiat. Res.* **9**:285–292.

MAY, P. R. A., YALE, C., and GARRETT, S., 1973, Assessment of psychiatric outcome III: Process analysis, *J. Psychiatr. Res.* **10**:31–42.

MELIA, P. I., 1970, Prophylactic lithium: A double-blind trial in recurrent affective disorders, *Br. J. Psychiatry* **116**:621–624.

MELIA, P. I., 1971, Lithium prophylaxis in recurrent affective disorders, *Br. J. Psychiatry* **118**:134.

MELTZER, H. L., 1974, Human and animal metabolism of rubidium, *Psychopharm. Bull.* **10**(1):43–50.

MELTZER, H. L., and FIEVE, R. R., 1973, Some metabolic interactions of rubidium and lithium: A membrane transport hypothesis for mechanism of action in the CNS. Ann. Mtg. of the Am. Psychiatr. Assoc., Honolulu.

MELTZER, H. L., and FIEVE, R. R., 1974, Chronic administration of rubidium to depressed patients. Prediction of its plasma level and displacement of total body potassium, *Excerpta Med. Int. Cong. Ser.* **359**:647–648.

MELTZER, H. L., and LIEBERMAN, K. W., 1971, Chronic ingestion of rubidium without toxicity. Implications for human therapy, *Experientia* **27**:672–674.

MELTZER, H. L., TAYLOR, R. M., PLATMAN, S. R., and FIEVE, R. R., 1969, Rubidium: A potential modifier of affect and behavior, *Nature* **223**:321–322.

MELTZER, H. L., LIEBERMAN, K. W., SHELLEY, E. M., STALLONE, F., and FIEVE, R. R., 1973, Metabolism of naturally occurring rubidium in the human: The constancy of urinary Rb/K, *Biochem. Med.* **7**:218–225.

MENDLEWICZ, J., FIEVE, R. R., RAINER, J. D., and FLEISS, J. L., 1972a, Manic depressive illness: A comparative study of patients with and without a family history, *Br. J. Psychiatry* **120**:523–530.

MENDLEWICZ, J., FIEVE, R. R., and STALLONE, F., 1972b, Genetic history as a predictor of lithium response in manic-depressive illness, *Lancet* **1**:599–600.

MENOZZI, P., NORMAN, D., POLLERI, A., LESTER, G., and HECTER, O., 1959, Specific intracellular binding of rubidium by rat diaphragm muscle, *Proc. Natl. Acad. Sci. U.S.A.* **45**:80–88.

MINDHAM, R. H., HOWLAND, C., SHEPHERD, M., 1973, An evaluation of continuation therapy with tricyclic antidepressants in depressive illness, *Psychol. Med.* **5**:5–17.

MITCHELL, P. H., WILSON, J. W., and STANTON, R. E., 1921, The relative absorption of potassium by animal cells. II. The cause of potassium retention as indicated by absorption of rubidium and cesium, *J. Gen. Physiol.* **4**:141–148.

MOORE, F. D., OLESON, K. H., McMURREY, J. D., PARKER, H. V., BALL, M. R., and BOYDEN, C. M., 1963, *The Body Cell Map and its Supporting Environment,* W. B. Saunders, Philadelphia.

MULLER, P. J., 1963, Potassium and rubidium exchange across the surface membrane of cardiac purkinje's fibers, *J. Physiol.* **177:**453–462.

PERELMAN, F. M., 1965, *Rubidium and Cesium,* Macmillan, New York.

PERRIS, C. (ed.), 1966, A study of bipolar (manic-depressive) and unipolar recurrent depressive psychoses, *Acta. Psychiatr. Scand. Suppl.* **194.**

PLATMAN, S. R., and FIEVE, R. R., 1969, The effect of lithium carbonate on the electroencephalogram of patients with affective disorders, *Br. J. Psychiatry* **115:**1185.

POLATIN, P., and FIEVE, R. R., 1971, Patient rejection of lithium carbonate prophylaxis, *J. Am. Med. Assoc.* **218:**864.

PRIEN, R. F., CAFFEY, E. M., and KLETT, C. J., 1973*a*, Prophylactic efficacy of lithium carbonate in manic-depressive illness, *Arch. Gen. Psychiatry* **28:**337–341.

PRIEN, R. F., KLETT, C. J., and CAFFEY, E. M., 1973*b*, Lithium carbonate and imipramine in prevention of affective episodes, *Arch. Gen. Psychiatry* **29:**420–425.

PYKE, R. E., 1956, Effects of certain nutrients and other factors on the physiological action of rubidium, University microfilms, doctoral dissertation, Kansas State College of Agriculture and Applied Science.

RELMAN, A. S., LAMBIE, A. T., BURROWS, B. A., ROY, A. E., CONNORS, H., and DELL, E. S., 1957, Cation accumulation by muscle tissue: The displacement of potassium by rubidium and cesium in the living animal, *J. Clin. Invest.* **36:**1249.

RICHET, C., 1882, Study of the comparative physiological action of alkali chlorides, *Arch. Physiol. Norm. Pathol.* 2, 10, 145, 366.

RINGER, S., 1882, An investigation concerning the action of rubidium and cesium salts compared with the action of potassium salts on the ventricles of the frog's heart, *J. Physiol. (London)* **4:**370.

ROTTENBILLER, J., 1889, The curative effects of rubidium bromide, *Gyogyoszat (Budapest)* **29:**505.

SANGHVI, I., and GERSHON, S., 1973, Rubidium and lithium: Evaluation as antidepressant and antimanic agents, *Res. Commun. Chem. Pathol. Pharmacol.* **6**(1):293–300.

SARAN, B. M., 1970, The course of recurrent depressive illness in selected patients from a defined population, *Int. Pharmacopsychiatry,* **5:**119–131.

SASSER, L. B., KEINHOLZ, E. E., and WARD, G. M., 1969, Interaction of rubidium and potassium in chick diets, *Poult. Sci.* **48:**114–118.

SCHOU, M., 1968, Lithium in psychiatric therapy and prophylaxis, *J. Psychiatr. Res.* **6:**67.

SCHOU, M., 1974, Lithium prophylaxis in recurrent affective disorders: Debate, development and documentation, in: *Factors in Depression,* (N. S. Kline, ed.), Raven Press, New York.

SCHOU, M., and THOMSEN, K., 1975, Lithium prophylaxis of recurrent endogenous affective disorders, in: *Lithium Research and Therapy* (F. N. Johnson, ed.), pp. 63–84, Academic Press, New York.

SCHOU, M., THOMSEN, K., and BAASTRUP, P. C., 1970, Studies on course of recurrent endogenous affective disorders, *Int. Pharmacopsychiatry* **5:**100–106.

SHEARD, M. H., 1970, Effects of lithium on footshock aggression in rats, *Nature* **228:**284.

SOLOMON, A. K., 1952, The permeability of the human erythrocyte to sodium and potassium, *J. Gen. Physiol.* **36:**57–110.

STALLONE, F., SHELLEY, E., MENDLEWICZ, J., and FIEVE, R. R., 1973, The use of lithium in affective disorders III: A double-blind study of prophylaxis in bipolar illness, *Am. J. Psychiatry* **130**(9):1006–1010.

STOLK, J. M., CONNER, R. L., and BARCHAS, J. D., 1971, Rubidium-induced increase in shock-elicited aggression in rats, *Psychopharmacologie* **22:**250.

STOLK, J. M., NOWACK, W. J., and BARCHAS, J. D., 1970, Brain norepinephrine enhanced turnover after rubidium treatment, *Science* **168:**501.

TOBIN, T., AKERA, T., and BRODY, T. M., 1974, Lithium, rubidium and $Na^+ + K^+$-ATPase: A molecular basis for their pharmacological actions, *Fed. Proc.* **33**(3):483 (abstract).

TYOR, M. P., and ELDRIDGE, J. S., 1956, A comparison of the metabolism of Rb-86 and K-42 following simultaneous injection into man, *Am. J. Med. Sci.* **232:**186–193.

WINOKUR, G., CLAYTON, P. J., and REICH, R., 1969, *Manic Depressive Illness*, C. V. Mosby, St. Louis.

WINOKUR, G., 1972, Depression spectrum disease: Description and family study, *Comp. Psychiatry* **13**(1):3.

WOOD, O. L., 1970, Determination of rubidium in human erythrocytes, plasma and urine by atomic absorption spectrophotometry, *Biochem. Med.* **3:**458.

YAMAGATA, N., 1962, Balance of K, Rb and Cs between Japanese people and diet and assessment of their biological halftimes, *J. Radiat. Res. (Tokyo)* **3:**9.

YAMAGATA, N., IWASHIMA, K., NAGAI, T., WATARI, K., and IINUMA, T., 1966, *In vivo* experiment on the metabolism of cesium in human blood with reference to rubidium and potassium, *J. Radiat. Res. (Tokyo)* **7:**29.

YAMAUCHI, Y., and NAKAMURA, M., 1972, Effects of alkali metals on spontaneous motor activities of mice, *Kurume Med. J.* **19**(3):175–178.

ZIPSER, A., PINTO, H. B., and FRIEDBERG, A. S., 1953, Distribution and turnover of administered rubidium (Rb-86) carbonate in blood and urine of man, *J. Appl. Physiol.* **5:**317–322.

INDEX